NUTRITION
FOR SPORT, EXERCISE AND PERFORMANCE

EDITED BY

Regina Belski • Adrienne Forsyth • Evangeline Mantzioris

NUTRITION
FOR SPORT, EXERCISE
AND PERFORMANCE

A practical guide for students, sports
enthusiasts and professionals

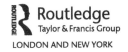

Routledge
Taylor & Francis Group

LONDON AND NEW YORK

CONTENTS

Part 3. Applied sports nutrition

LIST OF FIGURES, TABLES AND BOXES

TABLES

FIGURES

BOXES

CONTRIBUTORS

EDITORS

Regina Belski

Associate Professor Regina Belski is an Advanced Sports Dietitian, Advanced Accredited Practising Dietitian and founding course director of Dietetics at Swinburne University of Technology. Regina has worked as a sports dietitian for over a decade with athletes from Olympic level through to 'weekend warriors'. She is also a passionate researcher in sports nutrition, working on building the evidence base for the efficacy of sports dietitians, having recently led the team who developed and published the Nutrition for Sport Knowledge Questionnaire (NSKQ). Regina's contribution to nutrition education and teaching excellence has been further recognised by a National Citation for Outstanding Contribution to Student Learning from the Australian Government Office of Learning and Teaching.

Adrienne Forsyth

Dr Adrienne Forsyth is a senior lecturer in the School of Allied Health at La Trobe University, where she coordinates the Bachelor of Human Nutrition and leads sports nutrition teaching and research. Adrienne is an Advanced Sports Dietitian and Accredited Exercise Physiologist with research interests spanning sports and clinical nutrition, community health and education. She is an award-winning educator with a focus on creating engaging learning experiences to cultivate work-ready graduates.

Evangeline Mantzioris

Dr Evangeline Mantzioris is an Accredited Practising Dietitian and an Accredited Sports Dietitian. With over 25 years' practice in dietetics, she has experience in clinical dietetics, clinical teaching and private practice. She is now Program Director of the Nutrition and Food Science Degree at the University of South Australia, where she has taught many courses in nutrition, including sports nutrition. She is also on the editorial board of the journal *Nutrition and Dietetics*.

AUTHORS

Rebekah Alcock

Rebekah Alcock is an Accredited Practicing Dietitian and Accredited Sports Dietitian who is in her final year as a PhD student with the Australian Catholic University. Rebekah is also currently embedded at the Australian Institute of Sport as a PhD scholar. The topic of her doctorate is nutrition support for connective tissues in athletes, and she has a keen interest in nutrition support for rehabilitation from injury. Rebekah also currently works as the Melbourne Rebels Performance Dietitian.

Elizabeth Broad

Dr Liz Broad has been Senior Sports Dietitian, US Paralympics at the US Olympic Committee, since August 2013 and has worked at two Olympic Games and four Paralympic Games (London with Team Australia, and Sochi, Rio and PyeongChang with Team USA). Liz has been a sports dietitian for 25 years and is a Fellow of Sports Dietitians Australia, working with a wide range of sports in Australia, Scotland and the USA from development through to professional and elite Olympic and Paralympic athletes. Liz is also a Level 3 anthropometrist and has contributed to several book chapters and research articles, including being editor of *Sports Nutrition for Paralympic Athletes*.

Louise M. Burke, OAM

Professor Louise Burke, OAM, was the inaugural Head of Sports Nutrition at the Australian Institute of Sport, leading the team for almost three decades. She remains as Chief of Nutrition Strategy at the AIS and holds a Chair in Sports Nutrition at the Mary MacKillop Institute for Health Research at the Australian Catholic University. She has over 300 peer-reviewed papers and book chapters, as well as 20 books. Her primary research areas include nutritional periodisation—fat adaptation, fluid needs for optimal performance, carbohydrate metabolism and performance of exercise, and performance supplements. Louise is a director of the IOC Diploma in Sports Nutrition.

Anthea Clarke

Dr Anthea Clarke is a lecturer in the School of Allied Health at La Trobe University. Anthea is accredited as both a sports scientist and exercise scientist with Exercise and

Sports Science Australia. Anthea teaches in a variety of sport and exercise science subdisciplines, including sport and exercise physiology, sports analytics and performance analysis. Her research interests are in the areas of applied physiology and performance analysis in team sports, with a focus on the female athlete.

Matthew Cooke

Dr Matthew Cooke is a new senior lecturer at Swinburne University. Matthew has co-authored three book chapters and published over 35 papers and 60 abstracts in the area of exercise training and nutrition interventions in healthy, diseased and older populations. Matthew's current work focuses on nutrigenomics and the manipulation of energy balance in the understanding, prevention and treatment of lifestyle-related diseases.

Michelle Cort

Michelle Cort is an Advanced Sports Dietitian who currently works as the lead sports performance dietitian for Cricket Australia. Michelle's career has involved working within professional team sports and organisations as part of their high-performance units. She has worked with several Australian Football League (AFL), National Rugby League (NRL) and Super Rugby teams. Michelle also spent five years working at the AIS and attended the 2016 Olympics as part of the Australian sailing team support staff. Michelle has been a member of the AFL Anti-Doping Advisory Group and is a sessional lecturer in sports nutrition at various universities.

Gregory Cox

Dr Gregory Cox is an Associate Professor at Bond University having worked at the Australian Institute of Sport for 20 years. He has extensive experience in providing performance nutrition support to athletes in numerous sports and is the Nutrition Lead for Triathlon Australia. Greg has attended three Olympics and was Nutrition Lead for the Australian Olympic Team at Rio 2016. He has published numerous peer-reviewed journal articles, book chapters and lay publications. Greg is curious about athlete's nutrition habits and behaviours, their iron status, and dietary manipulations that enhance endurance exercise. He is a Fellow of Sports Dietitians Australia and continues to be competitive in endurance sports, having held both world and Australian titles in triathlon and surf lifesaving.

Ben Desbrow

Associate Professor Ben Desbrow is the program convenor of the Bachelor of Nutrition and Dietetics (Hon) program at Griffith University on the Gold Coast. Following a decade of work as a clinical dietitian, Ben was awarded the first Nestlé Fellowship in Sports Nutrition at the AIS. Ben is an Advanced Sports Dietitian and active researcher in the areas of applied sports and clinical nutrition.

Brooke Devlin

Dr Brooke Devlin is a postdoctoral researcher and the research dietitian within the Exercise and Nutrition Research Program in the Mary MacKillop Institute for Health Research at the Australian Catholic University. Brooke completed her PhD at La Trobe University in 2016. She is an Accredited Practising Dietitian, Accredited Sports Dietitian and an Accredited Exercise Scientist. Her current research interests include a range of exercise and nutrition interventions for optimal blood glucose control.

Stephanie K. Gaskell

Steph Gaskell is an Advanced Sports Dietitian and former national competitive ultra-endurance runner who has worked in gastrointestinal nutrition private practice for over a decade and is currently studying for her honours degree in the area of gastrointestinal sports nutrition. Steph works with recreational, high-level and elite-level athletes, including athletes who have represented Australia in the Olympics. She has been an invited speaker to national and international conferences in the area of gastrointestinal and sports nutrition, written two recipe books, developed portion plates and co-authored a chapter in *Clinical Sports Nutrition*, 5th edn.

Janelle Gifford

Dr Janelle Gifford is a senior lecturer in nutrition within the discipline of Exercise and Sport Science, Faculty of Health Sciences at the University of Sydney. She is an Advanced Accredited Practising Dietitian and Advanced Sports Dietitian. Her current research interests include sports nutrition in masters athletes and nutrition literacy.

Andrew Govus

Dr Andrew Govus is a lecturer in sport and exercise science in the School of Allied Health at La Trobe University. Andrew's research interests are exercise-induced iron deficiency, altitude training, training-load monitoring and applied statistics in sports science. In his spare time, Andrew enjoys distance running, watching football, reading and drinking craft beer.

Shona L. Halson

Dr Shona Halson is a senior physiologist at the AIS, where her role involves service provision, education and scientific research. She has a PhD in exercise physiology and has been involved in conducting research into the areas of recovery, fatigue, sleep and travel. She is an associate editor of the *International Journal of Sports Physiology and Performance*. Shona was selected as the Director of the Australian Olympic Committee Recovery Centre for the 2008 Beijing Olympic Games, the 2012 London Olympic Games and the 2016 Rio de Janeiro Olympic Games. She has published numerous peer-reviewed articles and has authored several book chapters on sleep, fatigue and recovery.

Patria Hume

Patria Hume is Professor of Human Performance at Auckland University of Technology, New Zealand. Patria has a PhD in sports injury biomechanics, and an MSc (Hons) and BSc in exercise physiology and sports psychology. Patria was the inaugural director of the Sports Performance Research Institute New Zealand (SPRINZ) from 2000 to 2012 and is director of the SPRINZ J.E. Lindsay Carter Kinanthropometry Clinic and Archive. Patria's research focuses on improving sport performance using sports biomechanics and sports anthropometry, and reducing sporting injuries by investigating injury mechanisms, injury prevention methods and using sports epidemiology analyses. She received the 2016 Geoffrey Dyson award from the International Society for Biomechanics in Sports, and the 2016 Auckland University of Technology Research Medal.

Christopher Irwin

Dr Christopher Irwin is a nutrition academic at Griffith University on the Gold Coast and teaches in the undergraduate nutrition and dietetics program in the areas of nutrition and food science as well as exercise and sports nutrition. He is actively involved in several areas of research, with particular focus on hydration practices and the role of fluid composition and food ingestion for rehydration after exercise. Chris is an Accredited Practising Dietitian and an associate member of Sports Dietitians Australia.

Stephen Keenan

Stephen Keenan is a postgraduate researcher at Swinburne University of Technology. He is an Accredited Practising Dietitian and Accredited Sports Dietitian and has provided dietetic services to elite Australian soccer players, working with professional male, female and youth teams.

Annie-Claude M. Lassemillante

Dr Annie Lassemillante is an Accredited Practising Dietitian and lecturer at Swinburne University of Technology. She brings together her passion for food, understanding of human physiology and her drive to help people achieve a healthier life through evidence-based strategies.

Michael Leveritt

Dr Michael Leveritt is a Senior Lecturer in Nutrition and Dietetics at the University of Queensland. His research and teaching activities focus on developing a better understanding of how nutrition can positively enhance athlete participation, wellbeing and performance in a variety of sport and exercise contexts. Michael is a passionate educator, practitioner and researcher with over 100 peer-reviewed research publications and his career to date has included positions with the Australian Institute of Sport and the Queensland Academy of Sport as well as academic positions in New Zealand and the United Kingdom.

Dana M. Lis

Dr Dana Lis has worked as a high-performance sports dietitian for over a decade and has had the honour of working with several of Canada's top athletes, sport scientists and many professional athletes internationally, expanding her focus from practical work in the field with athletes to receiving a doctorate from the University of Tasmania and postdoctoral research at the University of California, Davis. Her primary research areas include the effects of gluten-free diet's short-chain carbohydrates (FODMAPs) on athletes' gastrointestinal health and nutrition strategies to improve connective tissue health and performance in athletes. With one foot in research and the other in practice, Dana continues to strive to push the envelope of evidence-influenced sports nutrition.

Bronwen Lundy

Bronwen Lundy is an Accredited Practising Dietitian and Advanced Sports Dietitian. She is a senior sports dietitian at the AIS and the lead dietitian for Rowing Australia. Bronwen has an interest in relative energy deficiency in sport (RED-S) and tools for its identification.

Alan McCubbin

Alan McCubbin is an Accredited Sports Dietitian (Advanced) and lecturer in the Department of Nutrition, Dietetics and Food at Monash University. He has consulted to athletes across many sports over a period of 15 years, including athletes at both Summer and Winter Olympics, and the world's hottest, coldest and highest altitude ultramarathons. Alan is currently completing a PhD on sodium consumption, sweat losses and the implications for endurance athletes, and has competed at international level in sailing, and recreationally in endurance mountain biking.

Anthony Meade

Anthony Meade is an Accredited Sports Dietitian in Adelaide, South Australia. He has worked in the AFL with both Adelaide teams, the AIS cricket and track cycling programs and since 2006 has worked with A-League club Adelaide United FC. He continues to work in private practice and takes pride in mentoring budding sports dietitians and providing practical advice to athletes to achieve their goals.

Kane Middleton

Dr Kane Middleton is a lecturer in the School of Allied Health at La Trobe University. Kane is a sports scientist who specialises in sport, exercise and occupational biomechanics. His main research interests are the enhancement of human performance and reduction of injury risk in both sporting and occupational contexts. Dr Middleton has consulted for a number of professional organisations, including the International Cricket Council, Red Bull, Vicon Motion Systems Ltd and the Defence Science and Technology Group.

Michelle Minehan

Dr Michelle Minehan is an Advanced Sports Dietitian and Accredited Practising Dietitian. She has been a dietitian for over 20 years and worked at the AIS for several years where she worked with a wide range of elite athletes. Michelle is currently an academic at the University of Canberra where she teaches many nutrition units, including sports nutrition.

Lachlan Mitchell

Dr Lachlan Mitchell is an Accredited Practising Dietitian and exercise scientist who has worked with amateur and semi-professional athletes both in Australia and internationally. His current research at the University of Sydney focuses on dietary and training practices of bodybuilders, while he also teaches in the undergraduate and postgraduate exercise physiology degrees.

Helen O'Connor

Associate Professor Helen O'Connor is a sports dietitian with extensive clinical and research experience. She is an academic at the University of Sydney where she teaches nutrition to students studying exercise science. Helen is a Fellow, and was the inaugural president, of Sports Dietitians Australia.

Yasmine C. Probst

Dr Yasmine Probst is a senior lecturer with the School of Medicine at the University of Wollongong and Research Fellow at the Illawarra Health and Medical Research Institute. She holds dual masters qualifications in dietetics and health informatics, has been recognised as a fellow of the Australasian College of Health Informatics and is an Advanced Accredited Practising Dietitian with the Dietitians Association of Australia. Yasmine leads the virtual multidisciplinary Centre for Nutrition Informatics, has held consecutive NHMRC funding 2007 to 2016 and has served on NHMRC committees for food and nutrient policies. Her research focuses on nutrition informatics targeting food composition and its application to nutrition practice including development of new food composition data and analysis of national health survey data. Yasmine has published numerous book chapters and scientific journal articles and presented her work at a number of national and international conferences.

Georgia Romyn

Georgia Romyn is a PhD scholar in physiology and performance recovery at the AIS and the School of Human, Health and Social Sciences at Central Queensland

University. Her research focuses on the impact of sleep and daytime napping on athletic and cognitive performance, as well as best-practice travel strategies to reduce jet lag and travel fatigue in athletes. Georgia is accredited as both a sports scientist and exercise scientist with Exercise and Sports Science Australia.

Greg Shaw

Greg Shaw is a senior sports dietitian at the AIS who has worked in professional team sports for 15 years. This involvement has led him to investigate and develop nutrition strategies to shorten rehabilitation periods from major injuries.

Frankie Pui Lam Siu

Frankie Siu is a senior sports dietitian at the Hong Kong Sports Institute, where his duties include individual nutrition consultation (such as weight management, hydration strategies, recovery nutrition, training and competition nutrition strategies and the use of nutritional supplements), small group nutrition education for coaches and athletes, supervising the athletes' dining hall and applied nutrition research. Frankie also travels with different sports teams to provide on-field nutrition support to ensure every athlete fuels and hydrates optimally for training, competition and recovery.

Gary Slater

Associate Professor Gary Slater is an Advanced Sports Dietitian who has been working in elite sport since 1996. He currently divides his time between coordinating a masters degree in sports nutrition at the University of the Sunshine Coast and consultancy work within the elite sport environment. Gary has authored or co-authored 103 scholarly publications, including 70 peer-reviewed scientific papers and 14 textbook chapters.

Tim Stewart

Tim Stewart is a lecturer in clinical and sports nutrition in the School of Allied Health at La Trobe University. Tim is an experienced sports and clinical dietitian who has worked in the AFL along with elite individual endurance athletes. Tim enjoys competing in cross-country running and is building an interest in trail running.

Gina Trakman

Dr Gina Trakman is a sports dietitian, lecturer and nutrition researcher. She completed her PhD thesis on the nutrition knowledge of elite and non-elite Australian athletes. Her research interests include survey validation, sports nutrition, dietary additives and the gut microbiota.

Sam S.X. Wu

Dr Sam Wu is an exercise scientist and lecturer at Swinburne University of Technology. His work focuses on exercise performance and physiology, in particular pacing within endurance events. His interests also expand into improving health and discovering best practice for individuals with exercise. He applies his research to practice, having competed in various short to long distance triathlon events.

ABBREVIATIONS

AA	arachidonic acid
ABV	alcohol by volume
ADP	adenosine diphosphate
AFL	Australian Football League (AFL)
AI	acceptable intake
AIHW	Australian Institute of Health and Welfare
AIS	Australian Institute of Sport
ALA	alpha-linolenic acid
AMDR	acceptable macronutrient distribution range
AMP	adenosine monophosphate
ATP	adenosine triphosphate
ATP-PCr	alactacid
AUSNUT	Australian Nutrient (databases)
BHI	beverage hydration index
BIA	bioelectrical impedance analysis
BM	body mass
BMD	bone mineral density
BMI	body mass index
BW	body weight
CCK	cholecystokinin
CHO	carbohydrate
CoA	coenzyme A
Cr	Creatine
CT	computed tomography
CTE	chronic traumatic encephalopathy
CVD	cardiovascular disease
DASH	dietary approaches to stop hypertension
DHA	docosahexaenoic acid
DVT	deep-vein thrombosis
DXA	dual energy X-ray absorptiometry
EA	energy availability
EAH	exercise-associated hyponatraemia
EAR	estimated average requirements
EER	estimated energy requirements
EGCG	epigallocatechin

EPA	eicosapentaenoic acid
EPOC	excess post-exercise oxygen consumption
ER	endoplasmic reticulum
ESSA	Exercise and Sports Science Australia
ETC	electron transport chain
FFM	fat-free mass
FGID	functional gastrointestinal disorders
FITT	frequency, intensity, time, and type
FM	fat mass
FODMAP	fermentable oligosaccharides, disaccharides, monosaccharides and polyols
GFD	gluten-free diets
GI	glycaemic index
GL	glycaemic load
GORD	gastroesophageal reflux disorder
GTP	guanosine triphosphate
Hb	haemoglobin
HBV	high biological value
HCl	hydrochloric acid
HDL-C	high-density lipoprotein cholesterol-C
HDL	high-density lipoprotein
HMB	b-Hydroxy-b-methylbutyrate
HRR	heart rate reserve
IBS	irritable bowel syndrome
IDA	iron deficiency anaemia
IOC	International Olympic Committee
IPC	International Paralympic Committee
ISAK	International Society for the Advancement of Kinanthropometry
IU	international units
LA	linoleic acid
LCHF	low-carbohydrate, high-fat diet
LDL-C	low-density lipoprotein cholesterol-C
LDL	low-density lipoprotein
LEA	low-energy availability
LEAF-Q	Low Energy Availability in Females questionnaire
MCV	mean cell volume
MEOS	microsomal ethanol-oxidising system
MRI	magnetic resonance imaging

MUFA	monounsaturated fatty acids
NHMRC	National Health and Medical Research Council
NRL	National Rugby League
NRV	nutrient reference values
NSAID	non-steroidal anti-inflammatory drugs
NUTTAB	nutrient tables
OA	osteoarthritis
PAL	physical activity level
PCr	phosphocreatine
PEM	protein-energy malnutrition
Pi	inorganic phosphate
PUFA	polyunsaturated fatty acids
RDI	recommended dietary intake
RED-S	relative energy deficiency in sport
RER	respiratory exchange ratio
RM	repetition maximum
RMR	resting metabolic rate
RPE	rating of perceived exertion
SCFA	short-chain fatty acids
SCI	spinal cord injuries
SF	serum ferritin
SGLT-1	sodium-glucose linked transporter 1
SPRINZ	Sports Performance Research Institute New Zealand
TBI	traumatic brain injury
TBW	total body water
TFA	trans fatty acids
TIBC	total iron binding capacity
UL	upper level of intake
URTI	upper respiratory tract infection
USG	urine specific gravity
UTI	urinary tract infections
UV	ultraviolet
UVB	ultraviolet B
VFA	volatile fatty acids
WADA	World Anti-Doping Agency
WPI	whey protein isolate

INTRODUCTION

As academics in nutrition, dietetics and sports science teaching sports nutrition to undergraduate students, we have struggled to find a standalone textbook on sports nutrition that is pitched at the right level—containing enough evidence-based scientific information to support university-level students, written for an Australian and New Zealand context and designed in a straightforward manner that makes it easy to find, understand and apply information. We feel that with this textbook we have created a learning and teaching tool that will support a range of interests in sports nutrition, from recreational athletes to developing sports and nutrition professionals. It will also be a great reference text for athletes and those working with athletes.

This book has been developed in three parts.

Part 1: The science of nutrition and sport
The chapters contained in this section will help you to develop the underlying knowledge in physiology, nutrition and assessment required to understand and apply concepts in sports nutrition. Some of these chapters may serve as review or reference material for students who have completed previous study in nutrition and exercise physiology.

Part 2: Nutrition for exercise
These chapters will provide you with evidence-based recommendations on what to eat and when, and support you in developing plans for individual athletes and teams.

Part 3: Applied sports nutrition
In this section, you will become familiar with the nutrition requirements of athletes participating in a range of sports, and with the unique nutrition needs of athletes at different developmental stages and with other special needs.

The support website for the book provides additional resources, including further reading lists for each chapter, questions to test your understanding, study questions and case studies.

Before we jump ahead to the main content of the book, it is important to clarify a few important terms and concepts related to sports nutrition.

Elite sport versus recreational sport and exercise

The nutrition demands of athletes will vary depending on a range of factors, including age, sex, experience, training and the sport itself. The demands of athletes participating at an elite level may or may not differ from those of an athlete participating at a recreational level or exercising for fitness. Elite athletes often have the opportunity to train more, and will have higher energy and nutrition requirements due to their training load (although this is not always the case; for some elite athletes, stringent requirements related to body weight, body composition or image may lead them to consume diets lower in energy). In general, the elite athlete will be better adapted to perform in their chosen sport, and may be looking to nutrition to gain a slight edge on the competition. For recreational athletes and exercisers, nutrition may play an important role in increasing their ability to train and perform by reducing gastrointestinal discomfort and increasing energy levels before, during and after training. Throughout this textbook, you will be provided with examples of how modifying dietary intake before, during and after training or performance can improve the comfort, energy and performance of athletes at all levels, as well as promoting a healthy diet for long-term health benefits.

Sports nutrition and scope of practice

There is a range of roles nutrition professionals can play in sport. The work that you do and the information and recommendations that you provide should be guided by the scope of practice of your role and training.

Completion of a subject in sports nutrition does not make you a sports nutrition professional, but it does provide you with the foundational knowledge to undertake further study toward a career in sports nutrition, or to work in a role supporting other sports nutrition professionals.

If you are studying sports or exercise science, you should be guided by the scope of practice guidelines developed by Exercise and Sports Science Australia (ESSA). On completion of an accredited course in sports or exercise science, you will be able to perform basic nutritional assessments and provide nutrition advice in line with national nutrition guidelines such as the Australian Dietary Guidelines and the Australian Guide to Healthy Eating; depending on the level of qualification, you may be able to undertake sports nutrition-related research. Undertaking more advanced nutrition assessment, providing medical nutrition interventions or prescribing nutritional supplements are beyond the scope of practice of exercise professionals unless they have completed relevant additional training.

If you are studying human nutrition, you will be able to perform similar activities to those described above. You may undertake basic nutritional assessments and provide advice for general health and wellbeing in line with national nutrition guidelines. Individualised dietary advice and recommendations related to specific medical conditions should be provided only by dietitians who have completed an accredited course in dietetics.

Accredited sports dietitians are the only professionals who are accredited to practice in sports nutrition in Australia. These professionals complete an accredited undergraduate or postgraduate course in dietetics, gain experience in clinical dietetics, then apply to Sports Dietitians Australia to undertake additional training in sports nutrition. After completing this training, passing an exam, and acquiring substantial experience related to sports nutrition, a dietitian may gain accreditation as a sports dietitian. Accredited sports dietitians work in roles supporting elite sporting organisations, in private practice with individual athletes, or as consultants to sporting clubs. Sports dietitians may be supported by other dietitians, nutritionists and exercise or sports scientists in these roles.

Sifting through the evidence: How to source and interpret the literature

This textbook will be a great reference for sports nutrition information. However, there is a lot of great research taking place and the evidence and recommendations for sports nutrition are constantly evolving. It is likely that there will be times when you are confronted with new ideas about food and nutrition in sport. So, how can you tell if what you are reading about is new information based on scientific research, or the latest fad being promoted by a celebrity? Given the implications for performance and health, it is important that you are able to separate credible information from popular anecdotes.

These days, we receive information from a variety of sources—traditional books, journals and newspapers, as well as television, radio, and online and social media. When assessing the credibility of new evidence, start by looking at who has written and published the evidence. Is the author an expert in the field? What other work have they done, and are they associated with an education or research institution? Is the work published by a reputable journal or a government website, or is it reported in a popular magazine or blog? Popular media such as television, radio and social media can present some credible information, but it is best to identify their source, and access and assess the original source of information for credibility. Sometimes, book and magazine articles can be written by someone with great interest but no qualifications in nutrition, and may contain ideas that are attractive and promise great things, but are not based on scientific evidence. In addition to checking the qualifications of the author and the credibility of the publisher, also identify what evidence is used to support any nutrition claims. Are claims based on quality, up-to-date research? Be wary of claims made with no supporting scientific studies, or those with only very old studies (evidence in nutrition is constantly evolving!), as well as any claims made by someone with a financial interest. Food and supplement companies can sometimes produce and report on high-quality research, but it is in their own financial interest to tell you about findings that support their products, so make sure you also identify some independent evidence.

So, where can you go to obtain credible and unbiased information? The support website has suggestions for additional reading with links to books, journal articles and websites. The Sports Dietitians Australia website (www.sportsdietitians.com.au/) has a large range of easy-to-read sports nutrition factsheets written by sports dietitians based on the latest scientific evidence. For those wanting to read more original research, PubMed (www.ncbi.nlm.nih.gov/pubmed/) provides access to a huge range of research articles published in high-quality journals. Be sure to also read journal articles with a critical eye, checking that they have used appropriate methods and that their conclusions were justified based on the results.

We trust that you will find this textbook to be a source of reliable nutrition information that is easy to understand and apply in sports settings.

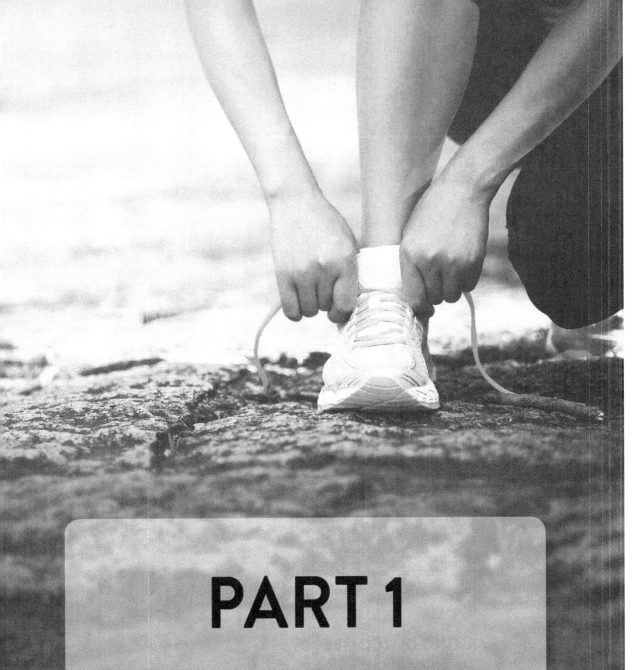

PART 1

THE SCIENCE OF NUTRITION AND SPORT

CHAPTER 1

Introduction to sport and exercise

Kane Middleton, Andrew Govus, Anthea Clarke and Adrienne Forsyth

You may be reading this book because you are an athlete, you work with athletes, or you would like to work with athletes in the future. To provide appropriate nutrition advice to athletes, it is important that you understand the practical and physiological impacts of physical activity, exercise and sport. This chapter will provide you with an overview of key concepts related to sport, exercise and performance, and outline the body's responses and adaptations to exercise.

LEARNING OUTCOMES

Upon completion of this chapter you will be able to:
- compare and contrast physical activity, exercise and sport
- describe different types of sport and exercise, and relate these to differing physiological processes and adaptations
- measure exercise performance and intensity
- describe the principles of exercise prescription
- describe muscle types and actions

- explain the body's physiological response and chronic adaptations to exercise
- outline how the body recovers from exercise.

PHYSICAL ACTIVITY, EXERCISE AND SPORT

Although often used interchangeably, there is a distinct conceptual difference between physical activity, exercise and sport. **Physical activity** is any movement that we perform that expends energy. The simplest categorisation of physical activity is based on proportioning activities in daily life—namely, sleep, work and leisure. The energy expenditure during sleep is obviously very small, whereas the energy expenditure during work would depend on the type of employment. A nurse who spends a lot of time walking around a hospital ward would expend much more energy than an office worker who spends the majority of the work day sitting down. In regard to leisure time physical activity, humans typically perform this incidentally (such as walking to the shops), in the household (such as gardening), or during exercise and sport.

Physical activity
Any bodily movement produced by skeletal muscles that results in energy expenditure.

Exercise
Physical activity that is planned, structured, repetitive and purposeful with the aim to improve or maintain one or more components of physical fitness.

Exercise is a subcategory of physical activity. Although it still includes body movements that result in energy expenditure, it is different to physical activity in that it is planned, structured and repetitive. The purpose of exercise is to improve or maintain components of physical fitness, including:

- aerobic and anaerobic capacity (described later in this chapter)
- muscular endurance, strength and power
- body composition (see Chapter 13)
- flexibility
- balance.

Aerobic capacity
The ability of the body to take in and distribute oxygen to the working muscles during exercise.

Accredited Exercise Scientist
A specialist in the assessment, design and delivery of exercise and physical activity programs (Exercise and Sports Science Australia 2018).

Examples of structured exercise include a running program to promote fat loss and/or increase **aerobic capacity**, a conditioning program to increase muscular strength or a stretching program to increase joint flexibility. If we take the example of a conditioning program, for it to be most effective it would be planned before beginning, ideally by an **Accredited Exercise Scientist**. The plan would incorporate purposeful exercise and progress the exerciser through mental stages of readiness to change (see Chapter 8 for the transtheoretical model of change). The program would be delivered in a structured, repetitive manner, taking into account the concepts of periodisation and progressive overload (this is discussed in more detail later in this chapter under **Chronic Adaptations to Exercise**).

It has been difficult to develop a universally approved definition of sport. Currently, the most accepted definition is that of the Global Association of International Sports Federations, which states that the following criteria must be met in order for a sport to become a member of the Association (Global Association of International Sports Federations 2012):

- The sport proposed should include an element of competition.
- The sport should not rely on any element of 'luck' specifically integrated into the sport.
- The sport should not be judged to pose an undue risk to the health and safety of its athletes or participants.
- The sport proposed should in no way be harmful to any living creature.
- The sport should not rely on equipment that is provided by a single supplier.

Sport
'A human activity capable of achieving a result requiring physical exertion and/or physical skill which, by its nature and organisation, is competitive and is generally accepted as being a sport' (Australian Sports Commission 2018).

In Australia, the Australian Sports Commission currently (at time of print) recognises 95 national sporting organisations. Their definition of **sport** focuses more on physical effort and skill that includes a competitive element.

TYPES OF SPORT

Due to the large variety of sports in existence, the Global Association of International Sports Federations has also developed categories of sports. These categories are based on the primary (not exclusive) type of activities that make up the sport. The list of categories and examples of sports in those categories can be found in Table 1.1. Note that many sports may belong to multiple categories.

Table 1.1. Categories of sport

Category	Examples of sports
Physical	Football, Basketball, Athletics
Mind	Chess, Draughts, eSports
Motorised	Formula One, Motorcycling
Coordination	Lawn Bowls, Billiards, Shooting
Animal-supported	Horse Racing, Equestrian, Polo

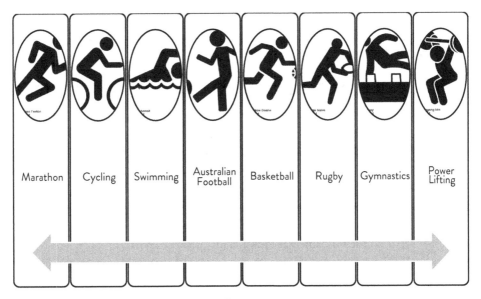

Figure 1.1. Endurance–power continuum of sport

Primarily physical sports are by far the most common and best known, and it could be strongly argued that nutrition is more important in these types of sports. Whether a sport is individual or team-based, the physical requirements of that sport will lie somewhere on an endurance–power continuum (Figure 1.1). Sports such as marathon running and triathlon are on the endurance end of the continuum, where repeated movement cycles are performed over a sustained period of time. In contrast, power lifting and track and field throws are on the power end of the continuum, where a single movement is performed at high intensity and often at high speed. To complicate this, sports often have different requirements for the disciplines within the sport or playing position within a team. In track and field, a 100-metre sprinter has a different physical requirement than a 10,000-metre runner. In American Football, a defensive tackle is usually the biggest and strongest player on the team, whereas running backs tend to be smaller but fast and agile.

Sporting activities are also sometimes categorised as **aerobic** or **anaerobic**. Endurance sports, which are performed at a somewhat lower intensity over a long period of time, are predominantly aerobic, meaning that the body is able to breathe in enough oxygen to support metabolic processes and fuel muscle activity. High-energy bursts of activity in

Aerobic

Exercise at an intensity that is low enough to allow the body's need for oxygen (to break down macronutrients) to be matched to the oxygen supply available.

Anaerobic

Exercise at an intensity where the body's demand for oxygen is greater than the oxygen supply available, therefore relying on anaerobic metabolism and the production of lactate.

power sports are usually performed at such a high intensity that athletes are unable to breathe in enough oxygen and rely on anaerobic metabolic processes to fuel the muscles.

LEVELS OF SPORTS PARTICIPATION AND COMPETITION

Levels of sports participation can be thought of as a pyramid (Figure 1.2) that generally represents the inverse relationship between competition level and participation rate. The foundation level of competitive sport most often occurs at a young age, when people are first introduced to a sport. In Australia and New Zealand, this would typically occur during physical education classes. Sporting organisations and recreation centres also contribute to the foundation level by offering introductory programs, such as the AFL Auskick (Australian football) or in2CRICKET (cricket) programs that focus on the fundamental motor skills of those sports.

Once someone advances from an introduction to a sport to regularly engaging with that sport, they enter the participation level. As a large number of people are introduced to a variety of sports at the foundation level, there is an inevitable decline in numbers reaching the participation level. The engagement at this level is generally recreational in nature, such as social sport; although competition is present, i.e. there is a winner and a loser, the main aim of participating is enjoying the activity itself rather than the final outcome.

The aim of competition changes from enjoyment to winning at the performance level. Whereas the skill level of people at the participation level is not overly important, performance athletes are often selected in teams or for competition based on, as the name suggests, their performance. They will often represent a club or team in these competitions, which are generally administered by official sporting organisations with standard rules and regulations. Representative sport will generally start in high

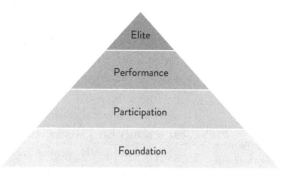

Figure 1.2. Levels of sports participation

school and continue through to adult competition. The critical development period from 18 to 23 years of age coincides with tertiary education for many high-achieving athletes. In Australia and New Zealand, the progress of these athletes is supported by national sporting organisations and state-based academies and institutes of sport. This stage is different around the world, with a contrasting system in the United States of America. The United States has established a college-based sports system, regulated by organisations such as the National Collegiate Athletic Association, and organised and funded by the colleges themselves.

The peak of sports participation is the elite level. This is very similar to the performance level but only includes the very best representatives of a sport, meaning that this level has the fewest athletes of all the levels of the sports participation pyramid. The delineation of elite athletes from other high-performing athletes is difficult, but elite athletes often compete at the national or international level. Although the Olympic Games is still the pinnacle of elite amateur sport around the world, the evolution of elite sport has coincided with growing professionalism due to the resources dedicated to preparation, training and competition. The large investments in professional sport make winning 'big business' and, given that the performance differential between athletes at the elite level is very small, nutritional interventions such as supplementation can have a large impact on performance and competition outcomes (see Chapter 12 for more information on this topic).

MONITORING EXERCISE

Cardiorespiratory exercise
Whole-body, dynamic exercise that taxes predominantly the cardiovascular and respiratory systems, such as running, cycling and swimming.

Resistance exercise
Exercise that predominantly involves the musculoskeletal system.

Skeletal muscle
Voluntary muscle attached to bones that move a part of the skeleton when stimulated with a nerve impulse.

Biomechanical
Pertaining to the mechanical nature of the body's biological processes, such as movements of the skeleton and muscles.

Exercise can be categorised into two main types: **cardiorespiratory exercise** (involving the **cardiovascular** and **respiratory system**) and **resistance exercise** (predominantly involving the **musculoskeletal system**). Whereas cardiorespiratory exercise involves predominantly whole-body, dynamic exercise involving a large **skeletal muscle** mass, resistance exercise aims to develop **physiological**, **neurological** and **biomechanical** properties of skeletal muscle. Cardiorespiratory exercise is predominantly aerobic, while resistance exercise is predominantly anaerobic.

The intensity of cardiorespiratory and resistance exercise can be expressed in either absolute or relative terms. **Absolute exercise intensity** refers to the total amount of energy expended (expressed in **kilojoules** or **kilocalories**) to produce mechanical work, in the form of skeletal muscle contraction. Note that in Australia we follow the internationally agreed

Kilojoules

A unit of energy equal to 1000 joules. A joule is a unit of energy equal to the amount of work done by a force of 1 Newton (the force required to accelerate 1 kilogram of mass at the rate of 1 metre per second squared in the direction of the applied force) to move an object 1 metre.

Kilocalories

A unit of energy equal to 1000 calories. A calorie is the energy required to increase the temperature of 1 gram of water by 1°C.

decimal system of measurement (metric system), which will be used in this textbook (1 calorie = 4.18 kilojoules). See Chapter 2 for a more detailed discussion of energy, work and power.

Absolute exercise intensity can be expressed in **metabolic equivalents** (METs), which describe exercise intensity as a multiple of the amount of energy required by the body at rest. One MET is approximately equivalent to an oxygen uptake of 3.5 mL.kg$^{-1} \cdot$min^{-1}, although the exact value will vary between individuals and should be measured directly (see Chapter 2 for more information about measurement of energy expenditure). For example, the oxygen consumption for a 70 kilogram male exercising at an absolute exercise intensity of five METs for 30 minutes would be calculated as:

$$Oxygen\ consumption\ (\dot{V}O_2) = 5 \times 3.5\ mL \cdot kg^{-1} \cdot min^{-1} = 17.5\ mL \cdot kg^{-1} \cdot min^{-1}\ O_2$$

$$Oxygen\ consumption\ (\dot{V}O_2) = 17.5\ mL \cdot kg^{-1} \cdot min^{-1} \times 70\ kg = 1225\ mL \cdot min^{-1}\ O_2$$

$$Oxygen\ consumption\ (\dot{V}O_2) = 1225\ mL \cdot min^{-1} \times 30\ min = 36750\ mL\ O_2$$

$$Oxygen\ consumption\ (\dot{V}O_2) = \frac{36750\ mL}{1000} = 36.75\ L\ O_2$$

From the estimated oxygen consumption we can calculate the energy expenditure during exercise, since each litre of oxygen yields ~5 kcal (see Chapter 2 for a detailed explanation). Therefore, the estimated energy expenditure for the example above is:

$$Energy\ expenditure\ (kcal) = 36.75\ L\ O_2 \times 5\ kcal = 183.75\ kcal$$

$$To\ convert\ kilocalories\ to\ kilojoules\ (kJ) = 183.75\ kcal \times 4.18\ kj/kcal = {\sim}768\ kj$$

Maximum aerobic power ($\dot{V}O_{2max}$)

The maximum amount of oxygen an individual can take up per minute during dynamic exercise using large muscle groups.

Oxygen reserve (%$\dot{V}O_2R$)

The difference between resting oxygen consumption and maximal oxygen consumption.

In comparison, **relative exercise intensity** refers to exercise that is expressed relative to an individual's maximal capacity for a given task or activity. The intensity of cardiorespiratory exercise is commonly expressed as a percentage of an individual's **maximum aerobic power** ($\dot{V}O_{2max}$), heart rate (HR$_{max}$) or rating of perceived exertion (RPE).

The most accurate method of monitoring the intensity of submaximal exercise is by expressing the exercise intensity as a percentage of the individual's maximal oxygen uptake ($\%\ \dot{V}O_{2max}$) or **oxygen reserve** ($\%\ \dot{V}O_2R$).

$$\text{Per cent maximal oxygen uptake } (\%\ \dot{V}O_{2max}) = \dot{V}O_{2max} \times \text{intensity } (\%)$$

$$\text{Per cent oxygen reserve } (\%\ \dot{V}O_2R) = [\dot{V}O_{2max} - \dot{V}O_{2rest}] \times \text{intensity } (\%) + \dot{V}O_{2rest}$$

A linear relationship exists between heart rate and oxygen uptake during incremental exercise (Figure 1.3), so an individual's heart rate, rather than their oxygen uptake, is more regularly used to monitor their exercise intensity, since heart rate monitoring is both cheaper and less invasive than measuring oxygen consumption.

Several different equations exist to estimate an individual's HR_{max} and the equation used should be appropriate for the population being measured. One common formula is that of Gellish et al. (2007):

$$\text{Maximum heart rate } (HR_{max}) = 207 - [0.70 \times \text{Age (years)}]$$

Per cent heart rate reserve (%HRR)
Heart rate reserve multiplied by the desired percentage of exercise intensity.

Another method of estimating exercise intensity using heart rate methods is by calculating the percentage of **heart rate reserve (%HRR)**. Heart rate reserve is often known as the Karvonen formula (Karvonen 1957). The HRR and %HRR are calculated using the equations below.

$$\text{Heart rate reserve } (HRR) = (HR_{max} - HR_{rest}) + HR_{rest}$$

$$\text{Per cent heart rate reserve } (\%HRR) = [(HR_{max} - HR_{rest}) \times \text{intensity } (\%)] + HR_{rest}$$

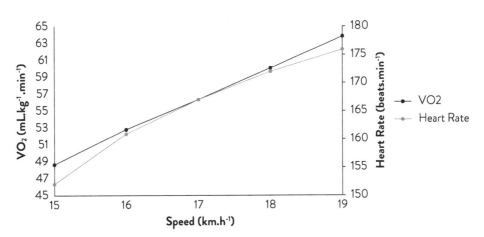

Figure 1.3. The relationship between oxygen uptake ($\dot{V}O_2$) and heart rate during treadmill running

The advantages and disadvantages of using heart rate-based methods to monitor the intensity of cardiorespiratory exercise are summarised in Table 1.2.

In addition to measuring oxygen consumption or heart rate, exercise intensity can be expressed as an individual's current level of effort or exertion, relative to their perceived maximal exertion. The most common method of measuring an individual's perceptual response to exercise is by using visual analogue scales such as Borg's 6–20 scale of perceived exertion (Borg 1982) (Table 1.3) or the Foster's Category Ratio (CR) 10 scale (Foster et al. 2001) (Table 1.4).

In comparison, resistance exercise may be expressed relative to the maximum amount of mass that a particular muscle group can lift successfully for one repetition, which is known as the one repetition maximum (1 RM), or by using perceptual methods such as the RPE. Exercise intensity for resistance training can then be expressed as a percentage of an individual's 1 RM. For example, an athlete with a 1 RM for the back-squat exercise of 120 kilograms wishes to develop their muscular strength, and so should lift ~85 per cent of their 1 RM in training. The mass they should lift in training can be calculated as follows:

$$85\% \ 1 \ RM = 0.85 \times 120 \ kg = 102 \ kg$$

Exercise intensity is stratified into categories related to the level of challenge experienced. This will vary from person to person depending on the individual's maximal physical capacity. The intensity of the stimulus applied during a training session (for example, the amount of weight lifted, or the speed of running) determines the

Table 1.2. Advantages and disadvantages of measuring exercise intensity using heart rate monitoring

Advantages	Disadvantages
Objective measurement	Need to know (or accurately estimate) maximum heart rate for effective exercise prescription
Easy to use in daily training	Average heart rate for a workout can be misleading if exercise intensity varies within a session
Heart rate and blood lactate response remain stable over time	Limited usefulness for very high-intensity intervals performed above the maximum heart rate
Useful to gauge perceptual methods of measuring exercise intensity such as RPE	The relationship between heart rate and workload is influenced by fatigue, heat, humidity and dehydration within a training session

Table 1.3. The Borg 6–20 scale of perceived exertion

Rating	Descriptor
6	No exertion at all
7	Extremely light
8	–
9	Very light
10	–
11	Light
12	–
13	Somewhat hard
14	–
15	Heavy
16	–
17	Very hard
18	–
19	Extremely hard
20	Maximal

physiological and mechanical loads placed upon the body during training and, consequently, the physiological adaptations that occur. Consistent with the Principle of Progressive Overload (discussed in more detail later in this chapter), the exercise intensity is one exercise prescription variable that can be manipulated to overload the body. Physiological and perceptual methods of monitoring exercise intensity are summarised in Table 1.5.

ACUTE RESPONSES TO CARDIORESPIRATORY EXERCISE

Acute exercise stresses several of the body's physiological systems, including the cardiovascular, respiratory and musculoskeletal systems. In response to cardiorespiratory exercise, the cardiovascular system increases oxygen delivery to the skeletal muscle

Table 1.4. The Foster Category Ratio scale

Rating	Descriptor
0	Rest
1	Very, very easy
2	Easy
3	Moderate
4	Somewhat hard
5	Hard
6	—
7	Very hard
8	—
9	—
10	Maximal

Table 1.5. Stratification of exercise intensity using various physiological and perceptual methods according to the American College of Sports Medicine (ACSM)

Intensity	HRR/$\dot{V}O_2R$ (%)	$\dot{V}O_{2max}$ (%)	HR_{max} (%)	RPE (6–20) (Borg 1982)
Very light	<30	37	<57	<9
Light	30–39	37–45	57–63	9–11
Moderate	40–59	46–63	64–76	12–13
Vigorous	60–89	64–90	77–95	14–17
Near maximal	≥90	≥91	>96	>17

Source: Adapted from American College of Sports Medicine 2010.

by increasing **cardiac output** as well as redistributing blood flow from non-essential organs. Furthermore, the skeletal muscle tissue extracts more oxygen from the blood to support the metabolic activities needed to fuel skeletal muscle activity.

During **steady-rate exercise** at low intensities, **pulmonary ventilation** increases by virtue of an increase in breathing frequency and tidal volume. In contrast, hyperventilation (over-breathing) occurs during **maximal exercise** intensities, in order to buffer

Cardiac output

The product of an individual's heart rate (the amount of times the heart contracts per minute) and stroke volume (the volume of blood ejected from the heart per minute).

Steady-state exercise

Exercise performed at an intensity whereby the body's physiological systems are maintained at a relatively constant value.

Pulmonary ventilation

The product of an individual's breathing frequency (the amount of breaths per minute) and tidal volume (the volume of gas inhaled per minute).

Maximal exercise

Exercise performed at an intensity equal to an individual's maximum capacity for the desired activity.

Submaximal exercise

Exercise performed at an intensity below an individual's maximum capacity for the desired activity.

Metabolism

Chemical processes that occur within a living organism to maintain life.

Metabolic acidosis

A decrease in blood pH below the body's normal pH of ~7.37–7.42.

Physiological conditions

The natural internal and/or external environmental conditions within which the body's physiological systems operate.

Buffer

A chemical system within the body that aims to counteract a change in the blood pH, defined by the blood [H+].

the acidic carbon dioxide that accumulates in the blood in response to anaerobic exercise. Common values for selected cardiorespiratory parameters at resting, **submaximal** and maximal exercise are presented in Table 1.6.

Buffers and maintaining acid–base balance

It is important to maintain acid–base balance during acute exercise to delay the onset of fatigue. **Metabolic acidosis** can impair energy substrate metabolism and result in a reduction in the desired power output. Under **physiological conditions**, lactic acid produced immediately dissociates into lactate ($C_3H_5O_3$-) and hydrogen ions (H^+) in solution. Hydrogen ions dissolved in a solution are acidic, and therefore decrease the blood pH. The pH scale, a measure of the relative acidity of a solution, ranges from 0 (extremely strong acid, such as hydrochloric acid) to 14 (extremely strong base, such as sodium hydroxide), with a pH of 7 indicating a neutral solution (such as water). Since many of the body's systems operate within an optimal pH range, the body counteracts increases in blood acidity by neutralising the rise in [H^+] using a combination of chemical (bicarbonate and phosphate), physiological (protein) and respiratory **buffers** to maintain blood pH within physiologic limits (pH = ~7.37–7.42).

The main method of controlling acid–base balance during acute exercise is by expiring (breathing out) excess CO_2 that accumulates within the blood. As the blood pH decreases (i.e. becomes more acidic), the respiratory frequency increases and raises the blood pH by expelling excess CO_2. In addition to the respiratory buffer, hydrogen carbonate ions (HCO_3^-) in the blood neutralise H^+, forming carbonic acid (H_2CO_3), which dissociates in the blood to water (H_2O) and CO_2 with the excess CO_2 expired. This process is summarised in the reversible chemical reaction below.

$$H^+ + HCO_3^- \leftrightarrow H_2CO_3 \leftrightarrow H_2O + CO_2$$

Blood pH is also maintained by the buffering effects of proteins in the blood and surrounding cells, which also act as

Table 1.6. Typical values for selected cardiorespiratory parameters during rest, submaximal and maximal exercise for a healthy adult male

Physiological Parameter	Rest	Submaximal Exercise	Maximal Exercise
Cardiac output	5 L/min	10–15 L/min	20–45 L/min
Stroke volume	50–80 mL/beat	110–130 mL/beat	110–130 mL/beat
Heart rate	50–70 beats/min	70–180 beats/min	180–220 beats/min
Skeletal muscle blood flow	15–20%	80–90%	80–90%
Systolic blood pressure	100–120 mmHg	120–180 mmHg	180–200 mmHg
Minute ventilation	5–6 L/min	35–150 L/min	150–200 L/min
Breath frequency	10–15 breaths/min	15–35 breaths/min	35–50 breaths/min
Tidal volume	0.5 L/min	0.5–3.0 L/min	3.0–5.0 L/min

Proton
A positively charged subatomic particle with a positive electric charge.

proton acceptors for H^+. Finally, phosphate ions (PO_4^-) act as proton acceptors in a similar way to HCO_3^-.

ACUTE RESPONSES TO MUSCULOSKELETAL EXERCISE

The musculoskeletal system also undergoes several different physiological responses during acute exercise to allow it to produce mechanical work. Such responses to acute exercise include an increase in **motor unit** and muscle fibre recruitment, muscle temperature and muscle enzyme activity.

Motor unit
A motor neuron (nerve cell) and the skeletal muscle fibres that it innervates (services).

Acute cardiorespiratory and/or resistance exercise requires repeated skeletal muscle action to complete the desired physical task. Skeletal muscle actions rely on the actions of smaller fibres (called myofilaments) consisting of myosin (a thick myofilament) and actin (a thin myofilament). Myosin and actin slide past each other during skeletal muscle actions; hence, the process underlying skeletal muscle action is known as the **sliding filament theory**.

When the external resistance is low, such as during low-intensity cardiorespiratory or resistance exercise, the body recruits predominantly slow-twitch (type I) skeletal muscle fibres, which are highly fatigue resistant but have low force-generation characteristics. In contrast, high external loads, such as those encountered during maximal strength training, activate fast-twitch (type II) skeletal muscle fibres, which are more

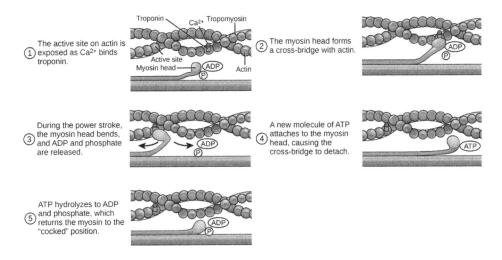

Figure 1.4. The sliding filament theory of skeletal muscle contraction

Source: Retrieved from www.oercommons.org/courseware/module/15136/overview.

susceptible to fatigue but are able to generate higher forces (see Table 1.7 for a comparison between the physiological characteristics of the different skeletal muscle fibre types). Collectively, slow- and fast-twitch skeletal muscle fibres produce the movements required during an acute exercise bout.

In addition, acute exercise may involve three different types of skeletal muscle actions; concentric, eccentric and isometric. Concentric muscle actions involve the shortening of skeletal muscle fibres and occur when the contractile force of the muscle is greater than the resistance force, whereas eccentric muscle actions involve the lengthening of skeletal muscle fibres and occur when the contractile force is less than the resistive force. The skeletal muscle length remains constant during an isometric muscle action, which occurs when the contractile and resistive forces are equal.

PRESCRIBING PHYSICAL ACTIVITY AND EXERCISE

Due to the strong association between physical activity and health outcomes such as chronic disease and obesity, the Australian Department of Health has developed age-specific guidelines for physical activity (Table 1.8). These guidelines are intended to help facilitate positive health outcomes for all Australians.

Whether you are undertaking exercise for general health, or to improve your competitive performance, when exercise sessions are repeated over multiple weeks and months chronic adaptations to exercise begin to occur. These chronic adaptations occur as a result of the specific loading and progression of exercise sessions and can be specific aerobic, anaerobic or strength adaptations, depending on the goals of the individual. One of the

Table 1.7. A comparison of the physiological, neurological and biomechanical properties of different skeletal muscle fibre types

Characteristic	Type I	Type IIa	Type IIx
Colour	Red	Red	White
Fibre size	Small	Medium	Large
Motor neuron size	Small	Large	Very large
Twitch velocity	Slow	Medium	Fast
Force production	Low	Medium	High
Phosphate resynthesis rate	Fast	Medium	Slow
Oxidative enzyme concentration	High	Medium	Low
Glycolytic enzyme concentration	Low	Medium	High
Major metabolic fuel source	Triacylglycerols	Phosphocreatine/ glycogen	Phosphocreatine/ glycogen
Mitochondrial density	High	High	Low
Capillary density	High	Medium	Low
Myoglobin content	High	Medium	Low

simplest and most common methods to monitor and progress your training program is by using the FITT (frequency, intensity, time, and type) Principle. An example of how you may target different exercise goals using the FITT Principle is provided in Table 1.9. By changing one or more of the elements within the FITT Principle, you can continue to overload the body to promote adaptations.

It is important to adjust training loads as an individual progresses through an exercise program to ensure adequate training stress is applied; this is termed **progressive overload**. Following an initial exercise stimulus, the body is transiently fatigued due to acute changes, and subsequently recovers and adapts to that initial stimulus. This results in the body having a new baseline level of performance,

Progressive overload
The continued incremental increase in training demand (duration or intensity) required to elicit an adaptive response.

Table 1.8. Australia's Physical Activity Guidelines

Age Range	Guideline
Birth–5 years	Infants (Birth–1 Year): 30 minutes of 'tummy time' per day Toddlers (1–2 Years): At least 180 minutes of activity including energetic play Pre-schoolers (3–5 Years): At least 180 minutes of activity with at least 60 minutes of energetic play
5–12 Years	At least 60 minutes of moderate-to-vigorous physical activity per day
13–17 Years	At least 60 minutes of moderate-to-vigorous physical activity per day
18–64 Years	150 to 300 minutes of moderate physical activity or 75 to 150 minutes of vigorous physical activity per week
Older Adults	At least 30 minutes of moderate physical activity per day

Source: Adapted from Department of Health 2017.

which therefore requires a greater exercise stimulus to promote the next adaptation. Figure 1.5 outlines the effect of subsequent exercise sessions on improving the performance level of the individual. If exercise is not followed by sufficient rest, it may result in the individual becoming over-trained. Conversely, if too much time follows between exercise bouts, the adaptations return to the initial baseline levels without

Table 1.9. Example application of the FITT principle for targeted physiological adaptation

	Cardiovascular Endurance	Muscular Endurance	Muscular Strength
Frequency (How often the exercise is performed)	3–5 times per week	3–5 times per week	3 times per week
Intensity (How hard the exercise is)	60–90% max heart rate	12+ repetitions, 2–4 sets	3–7 repetitions, 3–5 sets
Time (The duration of each individual exercise session)	>30 min	30–60 min	15–60 min
Type (The kind of activity completed)	Running Swimming Bicycling Walking	Free weights Circuit training Body-weight exercises	Free weights Resistance machines

Source: Adapted from ThePhysicalEducator.com.

Periodisation
The timing of exercise bouts to ensure sufficient exercise stimulus and recovery is provided to elicit the greatest response and adaptation.

further adaptation occurring. In this sense, the **periodisation** of training becomes important to ensure a sufficient balance between exercise stimulus and recovery.

CHRONIC ADAPTATIONS TO EXERCISE

Adaptations that occur as a response to exercise are specific to the training stimulus applied and include changes to the cardiovascular, metabolic, respiratory and muscular systems. Regular aerobic exercise, for example, enhances the ability of the body to use fat as fuel during exercise through increased transport of free fatty acids, fat **oxidation**

Oxidation
Part of a chemical reaction that results in the loss of electrons. During fat oxidation, triglycerides are broken down into three fatty acid chains and glycerol.

and mitochondrial biogenesis (increase in the number and mass of mitochondria), to name a few, and elicits the development of type I muscle fibres. All of these adaptations lead to an improved capacity to complete longer duration or higher intensity exercise while remaining within an aerobic state.

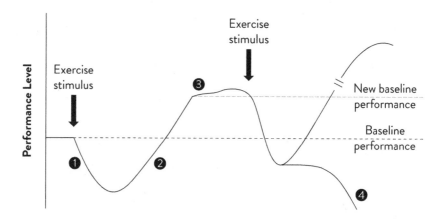

1. **Alarm phase:** Initial response to training where there is a fatigue response.
2. **Resistance phase:** Recovery and adaptation starts to occur and performance tracks back towards baseline.
3. **Supercompensation phase:** Adaptation results in a new level of performance capacity in response to the resistance phase.
4. **Overtraining phase:** If stimuli are too high with inadequate recovery between sessions, performance is further suppressed and overtraining syndrome can result.

Figure 1.5. The general adaptive syndrome and its application to periodisation

Source: Adapted from National Strength and Conditioning Association 2011.

Anabolic

An anabolic effect refers to the 'building up' and repair of tissues through increased protein synthesis and cell growth. It is the opposite of 'catabolism', which refers to the breakdown of molecules.

Wolff's Law

Bone in a healthy person will adapt to the loads under which it is placed. In this sense, an exercise stimulus results in bone remodelling that makes the bone stronger to resist that sort of loading.

Exercise and prolonged training also stimulate the release of a number of hormones, including testosterone and growth hormone, which promote an **anabolic** effect on the body. These hormones increase protein synthesis and cell growth, leading to an increase in lean muscle mass and decreased fat mass. This chronic adaptation of an individual's body composition, which increases the amount of active tissue in the body, also leads to an increased metabolic rate for the individual. Growth hormone also stimulates cartilage formation and skeletal growth, which encourages bone formation. The mechanical loading of exercise, such as during foot strike while running, also elicits the remodelling of bone to adapt to the load under which it is placed; this is known as **Wolff's Law**. As is the case with all chronic adaptations to training, when the exercise stimulus is removed these adaptations revert back to original baseline levels.

Along with the more commonly discussed changes to our cardiovascular, metabolic and muscular systems, exercise also affects our immune system. Following acute exercise, there is a reduction in white blood cell numbers and activity due to circulating hormones (catecholamines, growth hormone, cortisol, testosterone) and as a result of local inflammation. This acute-phase response can last from two to 72 hours post-exercise. The extent of these changes is influenced by the intensity and duration of exercise, with longer duration and higher intensity exercise eliciting a greater immunosuppressive response. The immune system can also be affected by travel and when in a team sport environment. Specific hygiene practices should be in place to reduce the duration and severity of illness, as well as to limit the spread of infection during periods of exercise. Over a period of time, there appears to be a J-shaped relationship between exercise and immune function (Figure 1.6). While sedentary behaviour or excessive/strenuous exercise can result in immune dysfunction and greater risk of illness, moderate amounts of exercise exert a protective effect on our immune system. Nutrition is also thought to play a role in maintaining immune function, through the adequate intake of specific micronutrients (for example, iron, zinc, vitamins A, E and B12) and sufficient carbohydrate availability during exercise bouts to help limit the rise in the stress hormone cortisol.

RECOVERING FROM EXERCISE

In order for the body to adapt to the exercise stimulus, sufficient recovery is required following each bout of exercise (short-term recovery) and training block (long-term recovery). It is during this recovery period that the body is able to replenish energy

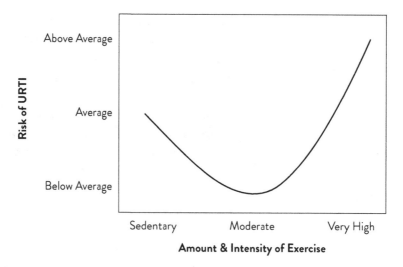

Figure 1.6. J-shaped relationship between exercise and risk of an upper respiratory tract infection (URTI)

Source: Adapted from Neiman 1994.

stores and repair damaged tissue to allow the body to develop and adapt in response to the stimulus. The simplest ways to recover from exercise are to have a rest day from training and to get good-quality sleep. Other common recovery methods include cold or contrast water immersion, compression garments, foam rolling and massage. Nutrition plays a big part in the recovery process through the sufficient intake and timing of key macro- and micronutrients. The nutritional recovery requirements are dependent on the demands of the activity and so will vary between endurance and power-based sports.

Amino acids
The building blocks of protein, composed of a central carbon to which is attached a hydrogen (H), an amino group (NH$_2$), a carboxylic acid group (COOH), and a side chain group.

As an example, endurance sports such as a marathon or game of Australian football will have key recovery strategies focusing on rehydration and the replenishment of carbohydrates, whereas power-based sports such as weightlifting have a greater focus on increasing protein-building amino acids to assist in muscle repair and growth following training. You can read more about these requirements in Chapters 15 and 16.

SUMMARY AND KEY MESSAGES

After reading this chapter, you should understand the importance of physical activity for human health. You will have an understanding of the types of sport played in Australia and New Zealand, and be familiar with physiological adaptations to sport and exercise. You will understand how exercise is measured and monitored, and be familiar with the principles of exercise prescription.

Key messages

- Physical activity is vital for our health and wellbeing, and our daily physical activity levels can be maximised through participation in intentional exercise and recreational or competitive sport.
- Exercise can be classed as endurance or power, aerobic or anaerobic, and cardiorespiratory or musculoskeletal.
- METs are used to describe the amount of work performed during exercise based on the amount of oxygen consumed relative to rest. The energy expended can be expressed using kilojoules or kilocalories.
- The intensity of exercise is often estimated using heart rate or perceived exertion.
- The body responds to cardiorespiratory exercise by increasing the blood flow to the muscle, increasing the volume of air inhaled, and increasing the amount of oxygen delivered from the blood to the working muscles.
- There are three types of muscle fibres, each with different properties that enable them to perform best in different types of activities.
- The body responds to musculoskeletal exercise by increasing the temperature and enzyme activity within the muscle, and by recruiting more muscle fibres.
- Exercise prescription involves the manipulation of frequency, intensity, time and type of exercise.
- Chronic adaptations that occur as a response to exercise are specific to the training stimulus applied and include changes to the cardiovascular, metabolic, respiratory and muscular systems.
- Rest is important to avoid overtraining, promote recovery and minimise risk of injury and illness.

REFERENCES

American College of Sports Medicine, 2010, *American College of Sports Medicine's Resource Manual for Guidelines for Exercise Testing and Prescription*, Philadelphia, PA: Lippincott Williams & Wilkins.

Australian Sports Commission, 2018, *ASC recognition*, ASC, retrieved from <www.ausport.gov.au/supporting/nso/asc_recognition>.

Borg, G.A., 1982, 'Psychophysical bases of perceived exertion', *Medicine & Science in Sports & Exercise*, vol. 14, no. 5, pp. 377–81.

Department of Health, 2017, *Australia's physical activity and sedentary behaviour guidelines*, retrieved from <www.health.gov.au/internet/main/publishing.nsf/content/health-pubhlth-strateg-phys-act-guidelines>.

Exercise and Sports Science Australia, 2018, *Accredited exercise scientist scope of practice*, retrieved from <www.essa.org.au/wp-content/uploads/2018/05/Accredited-Exercise-Scientist-Scope-of-Practice_2018.pdf>.

Foster, C., Florhaug, J.A., Franklin, J. et al., 2001, 'A new approach to monitoring exercise training', *Journal of Strength & Conditioning Research*, vol. 15, no. 1, pp. 109–15.

Gellish, R.L., Goslin, B.R., Olson, R.E. et al., 2007, 'Longitudinal modeling of the relationship between age and maximal heart rate', *Medicine & Science in Sports & Exercise*, vol. 39, no. 5, pp. 822–9.

Global Association of International Sports Federations, 2012, *Definition of sport*, retrieved from <https://web.archive.org/web/20121205004927/http://www.sportaccord.com/en/members/definition-of-sport>.

Karvonen, M.J., 1957, 'The effects of training on heart rate: A longitudinal study', *Annales Medicinae Experimentalis et Biologiae Fenniae*, vol. 35, no. 3, pp. 307–15.

Neiman, D., 1994, 'Exercise, upper respiratory tract infection, and the immune system', *Medicine & Science in Sports & Exercise*, vol. 26, no. 2, pp. 128–39.

National Strength and Conditioning Association, 2011, *NSCA's Guide to Program Design: Understand the general principles of periodization*, Champaign, IL: Human Kinetics.

CHAPTER

2

Energy for sport and exercise

Matthew Cooke and Sam S.X. Wu

Our bodies require a constant supply of energy to fuel our working organs, including the brain, heart, lungs and muscles. The major energy currency within the human body is an energy-rich molecule known as adenosine triphosphate, or ATP. In this chapter, we will explore how ATP is produced and the factors that impact how much we need. We will learn about methods used to estimate energy expenditure and how to calculate individual energy requirements. Finally, we will conclude the chapter with a focus on recovery from sport and exercise.

LEARNING OUTCOMES

Upon completion of this chapter, you will be able to:
- define and understand the association between 'energy', 'power' and 'work' and explain their relationship with exercise intensity and duration of exercise and sporting events
- compare and contrast the relative contributions of energy systems in relation to exercise intensity, duration and modality

- discuss methods used to assess energy expenditure and determine daily energy requirements of an individual
- explain the interplay between energy systems that allows physical exercise to occur, as well as those systems' contribution to recovery.

At rest, the demand for ATP is low; however, sport and exercise can increase this demand as much as a thousandfold, requiring a coordinated metabolic response by the energy systems to replenish ATP levels. The contribution of each energy system is determined by the interaction between the intensity and the duration of exercise, and is regulated by metabolic processes and the **central nervous system**.

THE RELATIONSHIP BETWEEN ENERGY, WORK AND POWER

Energy exists in many different forms. Although there are many specific types of energy, the two major forms are **kinetic energy** and **potential energy**. Kinetic energy is the energy in moving objects or mass, such as mechanical energy and electrical energy. Potential energy is any form of energy that has stored potential and can be put to future use such as nuclear energy and chemical energy (ATP). With exercise, energy is the capacity to do work and is calculated as follows:

Equation 1: Work done (Newton·metres [N·m] or Joules [J]) = Force (N) × Distance (m)

Work done, measured in **Newton metres** or **Joules** is calculated as force multiplied by distance. For example, the greater the force required to move an object, or the further the distance of the object to be moved, the greater the work done. Power, also known as work rate, is the amount of work done over time:

Equation 2: Power (Watts [W]) = Work done (J) ÷ Time (s)

Therefore, the faster the rate at which work is completed, the higher the power output. With sufficient training, athletes can develop physiological adaptations that allow them to perform a larger amount of work in a short period of time, thus generating higher power outputs (see Table 2.1). Power output is often used in sports such as cycling and rowing to quantify training loads or as a measure of exercise performance. It is not uncommon for professional riders in the Tour de France to produce more than 1600 watts in the final sprint and reach 75 km/h after two weeks of gruelling cycling over the French Alps and having just completed 200 kilometres immediately prior to the sprint!

Table 2.1. Adaptations from aerobic and anaerobic resistance training

Aerobic training	Anaerobic resistance training
Increases in:	Increases in:
• Aerobic power output	• Anaerobic power output
• Muscular endurance at prolonged submaximal intensities	• Muscular endurance at high power outputs
• Capillary density	• Strength production
• Mitochondrial density and size	• Muscle fibre size
• Proportion of Type I muscle fibres	• Proportion of Type II muscle fibres
• Aerobic enzymes	• Anaerobic substrates

ENERGY IN THE HUMAN BODY

Chemical energy is a form of potential energy that is stored in the bonds of atoms and molecules. Within the body, the major energy currency is the ATP molecule, which comprises three components: An adenine ring (as part of adenosine), ribose sugar and three phosphate groups (triphosphate) (Figure 2.1).

Carbohydrates, protein, fats and alcohol (discussed in more detail in Chapter 4) are sources of energy in the diet. Under normal circumstances, more than 95 per cent of this food energy is digested and absorbed from the gastrointestinal tract, providing the body with its chemical energy needs (see Chapter 3 for more detail on digestion and absorption).

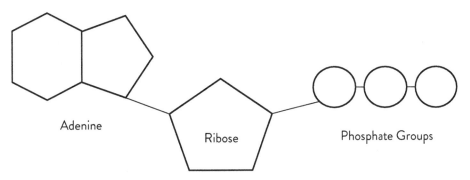

Adenine   Ribose   Phosphate Groups

Figure 2.1. An ATP molecule

Hydrolysis
The breakdown of a compound by chemical reaction with water.

Catabolic reactions
Biochemical reactions that result in the breakdown of large molecules and give off energy in the form of ATP.

Anabolic reactions
Small molecules join to form a larger molecule in the presence of energy (ATP).

In the presence of water, ATP can be broken down to form adenosine diphosphate (ADP). This process is known as **hydrolysis**. Living cells contain ten times more ATP than ADP. When ATP is hydrolysed to ADP, a large amount of energy is released. The release of this free energy from the high-energy bonds is used to drive energy-requiring reactions such as protein synthesis.

Reactions within a cell can be classed as either catabolic or anabolic. **Catabolic reactions** involve breaking molecules down into their smaller components; energy is released as a by-product of these reactions. **Anabolic reactions** involve combining simple molecules to form complex molecules, and energy in the form of ATP is required to support these reactions. Energy-yielding reactions (catabolic) within a cell are typically coupled to energy-requiring reactions (anabolic). The high-energy bonds of ATP thus play a central role in cell metabolism by serving as a usable storage form of free energy.

PRODUCTION OF ENERGY: THE ROLE OF METABOLIC PATHWAYS

Given the importance of energy, especially chemical energy in the form of ATP, it is not surprising that the human body has a number of important metabolic pathways to ensure its ATP levels remain relatively constant. A metabolic pathway is a linked series of **enzyme**-mediated biochemical reactions occurring within a cell.

Enzymes
Proteins that start or speed up a chemical reaction while undergoing no permanent change to their structure. Enzymes perform this function by lowering the minimum energy required (activation energy) to start a chemical reaction. Enzymes are involved in most biochemical reactions; without them, most organisms could not survive.

Cytoplasm
The semifluid substance contained within a cell.

The three main metabolic pathways for ATP resynthesis (Figure 2.2) are: (a) the phosphagen system (ATP-PCr, alactacid), (b) anaerobic glycolysis (lactic acid) and (c) oxidative phosphorylation (mitochondrial ATP production). Both the phosphagen system and glycolysis pathway occur in the **cytoplasm** (cytosol) of the cell. Oxidative phosphorylation occurs within the mitochondria. Mitochondria are known as the powerhouses of the cell. They are organelles that act like a digestive system to take in nutrients, break them down and create energy-rich molecules for the cell.

The phosphagen system

The phosphagen system is the quickest way to resynthesise ATP, and comprises three reactions (Table 2.2). Phosphocreatine (PCr) donates a phosphate to ADP to produce

Creatine supplementation
Supplementation with synthetic creatine can augment the level of creatine in the body and lead to enhanced performance of power activities.

ATP. Despite its ability to rapidly resynthesise ATP, the total capacity of this high-energy phosphate system to sustain maximal muscle contraction is about four seconds, assuming complete depletion of PCr and ATP. With this in mind, **creatine supplementation** has been investigated over the past few decades as a way to enhance exercise performance. Creatine supplementation can increase total creatine, specifically PCr levels stored in the muscle, and thus enhance the rephosphorylation of ADP to ATP. Numerous studies have shown the benefits of creatine supplementation on exercise performance, especially that involving short-burst, high-intensity power-type movements, such as power lifting (Cooper et al. 2012).

Table 2.2. Three reactions of the phosphagen system

Reactants	Products	Enzymes Used
ATP + Water (H_2O)	ADP + Pi + Energy	ATPase
PCr + ADP	ATP + Cr	Creatine kinase
ADP + ADP	ATP + AMP	Adenylate kinase

Note: ATP: Adenosine triphosphate; ADP: Adenosine diphosphate: AMP: Adenosine monophosphate; Pi: Inorganic phosphate; PCr: Phosphocreatine; Cr: Creatine

Glycolysis

A major source of cellular energy comes from the breakdown of carbohydrates, particularly glucose (see Chapter 4 for more detail about carbohydrates). The complete oxidative breakdown of glucose to carbon dioxide (CO_2) and water (H_2O) is written as follows:

$$C_6H_{12} + 6O_2 \rightarrow 6\ CO_2 + 6\ H_2O$$

Glycolysis
The breakdown of glucose to form two molecules of ATP.

Within cells, glucose is oxidised in a series of steps coupled to the synthesis of ATP. **Glycolysis** is common to virtually all cells and is the first step in the breakdown of glucose. It increases when oxygen is lacking (anaerobic) and the demand for ATP is high.

The terms 'aerobic' and 'anaerobic' are used to describe the different conditions by which oxidation of food molecules especially glucose, fatty acids and proteins occur (known as respiration). Aerobic respiration occurs when adequate oxygen is present, anaerobic respiration occurs when lack of oxygen is present and the demand for ATP is high. Check out Box 2.1 for more information.

Anaerobic glycolysis involves a series of ten steps (see Figure 2.2) that utilise glucose, either circulating in the blood or from the stored form of glycogen, to produce two ATP molecules, pyruvate and reduced coenzyme NADH. Glycolysis also produces **lactic acid**, predominately during exercise performed at high intensities (see Chapter 1 for more information about lactic acid and buffering). Although the production of lactic acid will contribute to the local fatigue of the muscle, it is the only metabolic pathway that can keep up with the high demand for ATP resynthesis and, thus, allow muscle to continue contracting at high intensities. The total capacity of anaerobic glycolysis to sustain maximal contractions is approximately 30 seconds.

When adequate oxygen is present (aerobic), pyruvate (the end-product of glycolysis) undergoes decarboxylation (a chemical reaction that removes a carboxyl group and releases CO_2) in the presence of **coenzyme** A (CoA) to produce acetyl CoA.

Acetyl CoA then enters the **Krebs cycle** (also known as the citric acid cycle or TCA cycle), which is the central pathway in oxidative metabolism and the first stage in cellular respiration (Figure 2.2).

Lactic acid
A by-product of anaerobic glycolysis that contributes to fatigue of the muscle.

Coenzyme
A substance that works with an enzyme to initiate or assist the function of the enzyme. It may be considered a helper molecule for a biochemical reaction.

Krebs cycle
A series of biochemical reactions that generate energy from the breakdown of pyruvate (the end-product of glycolysis).

Cellular respiration

The Krebs cycle, in conjunction with oxidative phosphorylation, provides the vast majority (more than 95 per cent) of energy used by aerobic cells in humans. The Krebs

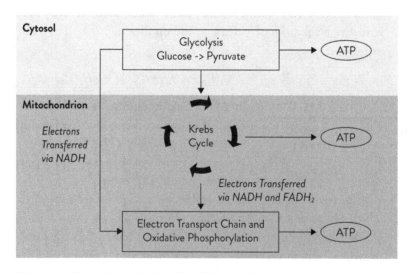

Figure 2.2. Metabolic pathways involved in ATP resynthesis

Box 2.1: Did you know? Aerobic vs anaerobic glycolysis

Before the 1980s, scholars and researchers referred to the complete oxidation of carbohydrate as 'aerobic glycolysis', as opposed to 'anaerobic glycolysis', which is often referred to now when pyruvate is converted to lactate (a temporary product formed when pyruvate combines with a hydrogen ion, H^+). The difference in terminology was based on the assumption that the extent of cell oxygenation was the primary determining factor for the complete oxidation of pyruvate via mitochondrial respiration or production of lactate. This is inconsistent with the biochemistry of glycolysis. We now know that if the intensity of the exercise is high enough, lactate is produced regardless of normal oxygenation, or even hyper-oxygenation such as with the breathing of pure oxygen. Terms—'lactic glycolysis' versus 'alactacid glycolysis' for intense and steady-state exercise conditions respectively—have been proposed as being more biochemically representative (Baker et al. 2010).

Electron transport chain
Electrons are passed through a series of proteins and molecules in the mitochondria to generate large amounts of ATP.

Cellular respiration
A series of metabolic reactions within the cell that generate energy (ATP) from nutrients.

Electron
Negatively charged subatomic particles.

cycle is a series of eight reactions that break down pyruvate to produce reduced coenzymes $NADH^+ + H^+$ and $FADH_2$, carbon dioxide and guanosine triphosphate (GTP), a high-energy molecule (Figure 2.2).

Oxidative phosphorylation

The **electron transport chain** (ETC) is the next step in the breakdown of glucose and the final step in **cellular respiration**. Requiring oxygen to function, reduced coenzymes from the Krebs cycle and glycolysis are re-oxidised with their **electrons** transferred through the ETC to produce large amounts of ATP (Figure 2.2). Mitochondrial oxidative phosphorylation is the only source of ATP production that has the capacity to support prolonged exercise.

The total yield from the complete oxidation of a glucose molecule is 38 molecules of ATP. This comes from:

- a net gain of two ATP molecules from glycolysis

- an additional two molecules from the conversion of pyruvate to acetyl CoA and subsequent metabolism via the Krebs (citric acid) cycle
- the assumption that the oxidation of the reduced coenzymes, NADH+ + H+ and $FADH_2$, will produce three and two molecules of ATP respectively.

Both glycolysis and the Krebs cycle give rise to ten molecules of $NADH^+ + H^+$ and two molecules of $FADH_2$ combined. In the case where two molecules of $NADH^+ + H^+$ produced by glycolysis are unable to enter mitochondria directly from the cytosol, the total yield is 36. The pathways involved in glucose degradation also play a central role in the breakdown of other organic molecules (discussed further in Chapter 4), such as nucleotides, amino acids and fatty acids, to form ATP.

INTERACTION AMONG METABOLIC ENERGY SYSTEMS: INFLUENCE OF SPORT AND EXERCISE

The interaction and relative contribution of the three energy systems during different exercise intensities and sporting activities have been of considerable interest to exercise scientists and biochemists. The first attempts to understand these interactions appeared in the literature in the 1960s and 1970s, using incremental exercise and periods of maximal exhaustive exercise. Although energy systems respond differently in relation to the diverse energy demands placed on them during daily and sporting activities, we now know that virtually all physical activities derive some energy from each of the three energy-supplying processes. With this in mind, the energy system most suited (dependent on the energy demands of the exercise) will contribute sequentially, but in an overlapping fashion, to provide energy (see Table 2.3 for examples of which energy system is best suited for various sporting activities).

Compare the demands of a 100-metre sprint to a 42.2-kilometre marathon. The sprint is fast, with minimal oxygen breathed in during its ten-second duration, making the event almost exclusively anaerobic (Newsholme et al. 1994). The marathon, on the other hand, is primarily an aerobic event completed in two to two-and-a-half hours at 80–85 per cent of an elite athlete's maximal capacity (Newsholme et al. 1994). Despite the different demands of each event, all systems are activated at the start of exercise to maintain ATP levels and ensure adequate supply for maximal power output and intensity. The anaerobic (non-mitochondrial) systems, which are capable of support-ing extremely high muscle force application and power outputs such as those during a 100-metre sprint, would be the predominant energy system used at these times. During a marathon race, the anaerobic system, which is limited in its capacity, is unable to meet the energy demands required by extended periods of intense exercise. The aerobic energy system (oxidative metabolism) is the only system that can resynthesise ATP at

Table 2.3. Energy systems used to support select sporting activities

Phosphagen (ATP-PCr, alactacid) system	Anaerobic glycolysis (lactic acid) system	Oxidative phosphorylation (mitochondrial ATP production)
Sprinting—performance is determined predominantly by the capacity of the ATP-PCr system because of the short distance covered. However, events longer than 100 m would require greater input from anaerobic glycolysis.	Swimming—performance is determined predominantly by the capacity of the ATP-PCr and glycolytic system because of the short distance covered. However, events such as the 1500 m would require input from oxidative phosphorylation.	Marathon running—although all energy systems would be activated, performance is determined predominantly by the capacity of oxidative phosphorylation, with input from anaerobic glycolysis during periods of sprinting.
Golf—given the explosive nature of the sport (i.e. club swing), performance is determined predominantly by the capacity of the ATP-PCr system.	Fencing—performance is determined predominantly by the capacity of the ATP-PCr and glycolytic system because of the numerous short, powerful bursts that last around 5–10 seconds.	Basketball—basketball games typically last about 50 minutes, which means performance is determined predominantly by the capacity of oxidative phosphorylation. However, the game also requires short bursts of explosive power and thus would need input from the ATP-PCr and glycolytic systems.

a rate that can maintain the required power and work output needed during the race. The aerobic system also plays a significant role in performance during high-intensity exercise, with a maximal exercise effort of 75 seconds deriving approximately equal energy from the aerobic and anaerobic energy systems (Baker et al. 2010).

QUANTIFYING ENERGY EXPENDITURE: APPLICATIONS IN SPORT AND EXERCISE

Regardless of which energy system predominates during exercise, all energy systems contribute to the supply of energy and thus have important implications for performance and recovery. Measurement of an athlete's energy expenditure helps determine the daily energy requirements for the athlete's training and competition, to inform dietary requirements to help them achieve body composition and performance goals. For example, a power lifter training to increase muscle mass would aim to consume more energy than is expended to increase his body mass. Alternatively, a boxer attempting to lose weight would aim to consume less energy than he expends. Of course, the composition of the diet can also impact on performance and body composition, as will be discussed in detail in other chapters.

Direct calorimetry
A direct measure of heat transfer to determine energy expenditure.

So, how do we measure energy expenditure? We know that the rate of energy metabolism is directly proportional to the amount of heat our whole body produces. As such, the rate of metabolism can be quantified by measuring heat produced by the body. This direct measurement method is known as **direct calorimetry**. This relationship is represented in Figure 2.3.

Direct calorimetry requires a person to be placed in an insulated chamber, which allows all heat production within the chamber to be measured. Although this method is highly accurate, building a calorimeter is expensive and requires a lot of space in a laboratory. Furthermore, heat that is produced by the exercise equipment when in use may complicate measurements. Therefore, a cheaper and smaller—but still accurate—method known as **indirect calorimetry** is more widely used for measuring energy expenditure. The most common approach to measuring oxygen consumption is by open-circuit spirometry. This involves collecting all exhaled gases into a mixing chamber, which is then processed and analysed by a metabolic cart (Figure 2.4). The metabolic cart analyses oxygen (O_2) consumed and carbon dioxide (CO_2) produced to calculate metabolic rate. Metabolic rate can be determined during rest (resting metabolic rate, RMR), or during submaximal or maximal intensity exercise. The maximal amount of oxygen that can be used by the body during high-intensity exercise is termed maximal aerobic capacity ($\dot{V}O_{2max}$), and is commonly used as an indicator of cardiorespiratory fitness (see Chapter 1 for more information about VO_{2max} and cardiorespiratory fitness).

Indirect calorimetry
A method of estimating energy expenditure by measuring oxygen consumption and carbohydrate production.

CO_2 produced and O_2 consumed can also be expressed as a ratio (CO_2/O_2) to obtain a number that is normally between 0.7 and 1.0. This number is known as the

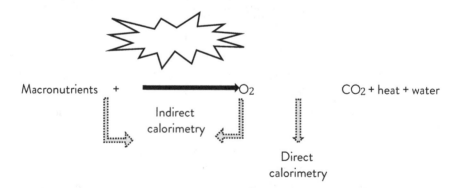

Figure 2.3. Aerobic metabolism pathway for macronutrients

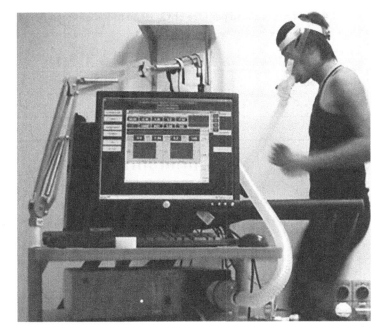

Figure 2.4. Indirect calorimetry using a mouthpiece connected to a metabolic cart

Photo courtesy of Sam Wu

respiratory exchange ratio (RER), and represents the composition of the mixture of lipids (fats) and carbohydrates oxidised through metabolism during submaximal exercise (Peronnet & Massicotte, 1991). These estimations are based on our knowledge of the exact amount of energy produced when metabolising carbohydrates, lipids and proteins with oxygen. Different types of macronutrients produce slightly different amounts of energy per litre of O_2 consumed (Table 2.4). However, as protein normally contributes negligible energy to exercise during aerobic exercise of less than two hours, a release of 4.82 kcal·L O_2^{-1} has been observed when burning a mixed macronutrient combination (Lemon & Nagle, 1981). For ease of calculation, 5 kcal of energy per litre of O_2 is generally used to calculate energy expenditure during aerobic physical activity. Therefore, a person utilising 3 L·min^{-1} of oxygen during a run would be expending approximately 15 kcal of energy each minute.

Ideally, tests to determine aerobic capacity and energy expenditure should be conducted in a controlled environment such as a laboratory to ensure accuracy and precision of results. Equipment specific to the athlete's sport, such as treadmills, bicycle ergometers, rowing machines and cross-country skis, is commonly used to

Respiratory exchange ratio
The ratio of carbon dioxide produced to oxygen consumed; used to indicate the relative contribution of substrates oxidised during submaximal exercise.

Table 2.4. Energy produced per litre of O_2 when metabolising different macronutrients

Macronutrient	kcal · L O_2^{-1}
Carbohydrate	5.05
Fat	4.69
Protein	4.49

*Note: 1 kcal = 4.186 kj

Source: Anonymous 1952.

Maximally exhaustive
Exercise that requires the participant to work at their maximal capacity until exhaustion.

maximise the relevance of results to the field. However, field tests are sometimes more appropriate, feasible and cheaper to conduct. Such tests, which are **maximally exhaustive** in nature, include the multistage shuttle run test (also known as the beep test), yo-yo endurance test, or 2.4-kilometre run test (see Table 2.5). At times where a maximal test is not appropriate due to the possible risks of maximal exhaustion, a health or fitness professional may choose to administer a submaximal test. A submaximal test requires a lower intensity of exercise and therefore is associated with a lower medical risk. Physiological data acquired during a submaximal test (commonly heart rate, blood pressure and ratings of perceived exertion) are then used to calculate and estimate the individual's maximal capacity.

RECOVERY FROM SPORT AND EXERCISE

During exercise, oxygen consumption increases to meet demands based on exercise intensity. Upon cessation of exercise, the increased oxygen consumption does not immediately return to pre-exercise levels, but gradually returns to baseline. This recovery period is known as **excess post-exercise oxygen consumption** (EPOC). Previously termed oxygen debt, it was hypothesised that the increased

Excess post-exercise oxygen consumption
An increased rate of oxygen consumption following high-intensity activity.

Table 2.5. Maximal tests of aerobic capacity and energy expenditure

The **multistage shuttle run** test, or beep test, requires participants to run repeats of 20 metres at increasing speeds every minute.
The **yo-yo endurance test** is a variation of the multistage shuttle run test with a higher initial running speed and different increments in speed.
The **2.4-kilometre run test, or Cooper 1.5-mile test,** involves running 2.4 kilometres on a hard, flat surface in the shortest time possible. VO_{2max} is calculated as (483/time in minutes) + 3.5.

Box 2.2: Estimating daily energy requirements

The daily energy expenditure for healthy adults can be calculated using the equations below, formulated based on adults 19–78 years of age. It is important to keep in mind that factors other than those accounted for within these equations can also influence resting energy expenditure. These factors include climate, body composition and surface area of the body.

Equations:

For females: resting energy expenditure (kJ/day)
= 9.99 × (weight in kg) +
6.25 × (height in cm) − 4.92 × age − 161

For males: resting energy expenditure (kJ/day)
= 9.99 × (weight in kg) +
6.25 × (height in cm) − 4.92 × age + 5

(Mifflin et al. 1990)

Resting energy expenditure calculated from the above equations can be multiplied by a factor according to the individual's physical activity level (PAL) for an estimated total daily energy expenditure. These factors are defined as:

1.0–1.39: Sedentary, activities of daily living, sitting in office

1.4–1.59: Activities of daily living plus 30–60 minutes of light intensity activity (e.g. walking)

1.6–1.89: Activities of daily living plus standing, carrying light loads, 60 minutes of walking

1.9–2.5: Activities of daily living plus strenuous work or highly active/ athletic lifestyle (Kerksick & Kulovitz 2014).

It is important to acknowledge that there is no clear classification for athletes of various fitness levels and training intensity. Therefore, using indirect or direct calorimetry should be encouraged for an accurate measurement of total daily energy expenditure.

oxygen uptake post-exercise was to repay the oxygen deficit created at the beginning of exercise, when energy production was not sufficient to meet a sudden increase in energy demands.

The energy required for EPOC is supplied primarily by oxidative pathways and is required to return the body to its resting, dynamically balanced level of metabolism (**homeostasis**). EPOC can be divided into two portions: a rapid component and a slow component. The metabolic processes that contribute to the rapid component of EPOC include increased body temperature, circulation, ventilation, replenishment of O_2 in blood and muscle, resynthesis of ATP and PCr, and **lactate shuttling**. The underlying mechanisms of the slow component of EPOC are much less understood. Apart from a sustained elevation of circulation, ventilation and body temperature, the slow component has been attributed to the storage of fatty acids as **triglycerides**, and a shift of substrate use from carbohydrates to lipids. The duration of EPOC depends on various factors, the most important being exercise intensity and duration. Short-duration and low-intensity exercise has been shown to produce short-lasting EPOCs, while high-intensity exercise clearly elicits a more substantial and prolonged EPOC lasting several hours (Borsheim & Bahr 2003). Several hormones released during physical activity also contribute to EPOC and would gradually return to baseline levels (Borsheim & Bahr 2003).

Homeostasis
Processes used by living organisms to maintain steady conditions needed for survival.

Lactate shuttling
Lactate produced at sites of high glycolysis can be shuttled (moved) to other muscles where it can be used as an energy source.

Triglycerides
The main type of fat in our bodies and our diets. They are made up of a glycerol backbone with three fatty acids attached.

SUMMARY AND KEY MESSAGES

Energy systems provide the human body with a continual supply of chemical energy in the form of ATP. Exercise increases the demands for this energy, but it is the intensity and duration of the exercise that ultimately determines the use of ATP and the fuel sources required for its resynthesis.

Key messages
- The two major forms of energy are kinetic energy and potential energy. Energy is the capacity to perform work and power is the rate of work completed.
- Chemical energy within the bonds of a fuel source can be extracted via a series of complex reactions specific to one of three energy systems: the phosphagen system (ATP-PCr, alactacid), anaerobic glycolysis (lactic acid) and oxidative phosphorylation (mitochondrial ATP production).
- The phosphagen system is the quickest of our energy systems, with the capacity to resynthesise ATP for up to six to ten seconds. It is predominantly used during very short, explosive movements.
- Anaerobic glycolysis is second fastest, with the capacity to resynthesise ATP for up to 30 to 60 seconds. It is predominantly used in short-duration, high-intensity 'speed' events such as the 400-metre track sprint.

- The aerobic energy system has the slowest rate of ATP resynthesis. Its advantage over the anaerobic energy systems is that it has a much larger capacity and is able to supply energy for hours rather than seconds.
- All activities require an energy contribution from at least two energy systems. Under maximal-effort conditions, all three systems are activated at the beginning of exercise, but one energy system will predominate.
- Metabolic rate and energy expenditure can be assessed by determining heat production from the body or by measuring an individual's oxygen consumption and carbon dioxide production for a given period.
- EPOC is necessary to return the body to a dynamically balanced resting state and is influenced mainly by exercise intensity and duration.

REFERENCES

Anonymous, 1952, 'Method of calculating the energy metabolism', *Acta Pædiatrica*, vol. 41, pp. 67–76.

Baker, J.S., McCormick, M.C. & Robergs, R.A., 2010, 'Interaction among skeletal muscle metabolic energy systems during intense exercise', *Journal of Nutrition and Metabolism*, vol. 13, doi:10.1155/2010/905612.

Borsheim, E. & Bahr, R., 2003, 'Effect of exercise intensity, duration and mode on post-exercise oxygen consumption', *Sports Medicine*, vol. 33, no. 14, pp. 1037–60.

Cooper, R., Naclerio, F., Allgrove, J. et al., 2012, 'Creatine supplementation with specific view to exercise/sports performance: An update', *Journal of International Society of Sports Nutrition*, vol. 9, no. 1, p. 33, doi:10.1186/1550-2783-9-33.

Kerksick, C.M. & Kulovitz, M., 2014, 'Requirements of energy, carbohydrates, proteins and fats for athletes,' in: Bagchi, D., Nair, S. & Sen, C.K., *Nutrition and Enhanced Sports Performance*: Amsterdam, Elsevier.

Lemon, P. & Nagle, F., 1981, 'Effects of exercise on protein and amino acid metabolism', *Medicine & Science in Sports & Exercise*, vol. 13, no. 3, pp. 141–9.

Mifflin, M.D., St Jeor, S.T., Hill, L.A. et al., 1990, 'A new predictive equation for resting energy expenditure in healthy individuals', *American Journal of Clinical Nutrition*, vol. 51, no. 2, pp. 241–7.

Newsholme, E.A., Leech, A.R. & Duester, G., 1994, *Keep on Running: The science of training and performance*, Chichester, UK: John Wiley & Sons.

Peronnet, F. & Massicotte, D., 1991, 'Table of nonprotein respiratory quotient: An update', *Canadian Journal of Sport Science*, vol. 16, no. 1, pp. 23–9.

Digestion and absorption of macronutrients in sport and exercise

Annie-Claude M. Lassemillante and Sam S.X. Wu

Our understanding of digestion began in 1822, when William Beaumont studied how food was digested by inserting and removing food from the stomach of Alexis St Martin, who had a hole in his stomach as a result of a shooting accident. This chapter will describe the various processes involved in digestion and explore our current knowledge on the impact of exercise on digestion and absorption and emerging evidence on training the gut.

LEARNING OUTCOMES

Upon completion of this chapter you will be able to:

- describe the role of the digestive tract, including accessory organs such as the liver, pancreas and gall bladder, in the digestion and absorption of nutrients
- identify and explain the role of key digestive enzymes and secretions in the digestion of nutrients

- explain how normal digestion and absorption processes are impacted by exercise
- identify and explain how common dietary practices among athletes affect normal digestion and absorption processes.

DIGESTION

Digestion is the process by which the body breaks down food into nutrients, which are essential for normal bodily functions. Digestion begins at the mouth, where food enters the body, and ends at the anus, where waste and undigested products leave the body.

During digestion, food is broken down mechanically and chemically. Mechanical processing involves breaking food into smaller pieces and mixing it with digestive

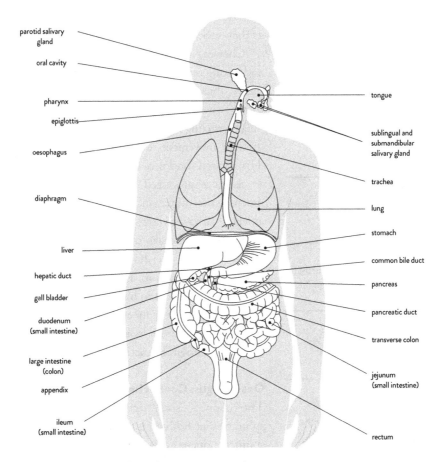

Figure 3.1. Components of the digestive tract and accessory organs

Source: Hodgson 2011, pp. 312–27.

Sphincters
Muscular rings that open or close to control passage of food along the digestive tract.

Peristalsis
The wave-like contractions of the longitudinal muscles of the digestive tract that propels food forward.

Segmentation
The contraction of the circular muscles of the digestive tract that leads to mixing and breaking up of food.

Macromolecules
Proteins (polypeptides), digestible carbohydrates, and fats (triglycerides) digested by humans.

Bolus
A portion, with respect to food, that is swallowed at one time.

Salivary amylase (or α amylase)
An enzyme in the saliva that breaks down amylose, a type of carbohydrate.

Lingual lipase
An enzyme secreted by the tongue that breaks down triglycerides, a type of fat.

Trachea
The tube leading to the lungs, more commonly known as the windpipe.

Hydrochloric acid (HCl)
An acid composed of hydrogen and chloride atoms that is produced by the gastric glands. HCl activates pepsinogen into the enzyme pepsin, which then aids digestion by breaking the bonds between amino acids.

secretions. Such breakdown includes chewing, opening and closure of **sphincters**, churning action of the stomach, **peristalsis** and **segmentation**. Chemical digestion involves breakdown of **macromolecules** by enzymes to form smaller molecules such as glucose, amino acids and fatty acids. These smaller molecules are then absorbed through the gastrointestinal lining and transported to the liver to be metabolised and redistributed to other parts of the body.

Mouth: The starting point of digestion

While digestion begins in the mouth, food is primarily broken down mechanically at this stage, with some chemical digestion of carbohydrates and fats (used mostly by infants as they suck on foods such as biscuits and rusks).

Chewing is the first stage of digestion, where the teeth and strong muscles of the jaw break food down into smaller pieces, thus increasing the surface area of the food exposed to digestive secretions. The tongue moves food around the mouth, mixing it with saliva that moistens and coats the food for easy movement down the oesophagus upon swallowing. The chewed food mixed with saliva is called the **bolus**.

Saliva is produced by the salivary glands and contains mucus, salts, water and digestive enzymes, namely salivary amylase (or α amylase) and lingual lipase. **Salivary amylase** begins the breakdown of specific bonds in starch molecules to produce maltose; however, this is only a small part of carbohydrate digestion. **Lingual lipase** begins the digestion of fats and is present in higher concentrations in the saliva of babies; its activity reduces with age due to reduced reliance on milk (and its fat content) for energy production and other physiological functions.

Oesophagus: Connecting the mouth to the stomach

The oesophagus connects the mouth to the stomach, with sphincters at both ends. Upon swallowing, the oesophageal sphincter opens, allowing the bolus of food to travel along the oesophagus. Peristalsis is responsible for the movement of food along this tube, allowing the bolus to reach the

Rugae
The folds of the stomach that occur when the stomach is empty.

Chyme
The mass of partially digested food that leaves the stomach and enters the duodenum.

Emulsification of fat
Involves formation of smaller fat droplets suspended in the aqueous digestive juices. This process increases the surface area of fat for more efficient digestion.

Gastric pits
Specialised cells in the gastric glands that secrete gastric juices.

Intrinsic factor
A glycoprotein produced in the gastric pits that binds with vitamin B12 to help in the absorption of vitamin B12.

Vitamin B12
An essential vitamin found in milk, eggs and meat. The active forms of this vitamin are methylcobalamin and deoxyadenosylcobalamin. See also Chapter 5.

Pepsinogen
Part of the zymogen enzyme family. These enzymes digest proteins and polypeptides (smaller proteins) in the body and are secreted in an inactive form to protect the digestive and accessory organ tissues themselves from being broken down. The enzymes can be activated by hydrochloric acid and other activated zymogens. The 'inactive' feature of these enzymes is very important to protect digestive and accessory organ tissues themselves from being broken down, as they are all made up of proteins.

stomach even if the person swallowing is upside down. The respiratory tract and digestive tract share the pharynx (between mouth and oesophagus); a small flap, called the epiglottis, closes during swallowing to prevent food from entering the **trachea.**

At the stomach end of the oesophagus, the gastro-esophageal sphincter opens for the bolus of food to enter the stomach. This sphincter also prevents the contents of the stomach from travelling up the oesophagus, hence protecting the oesophagus from the strong digestive secretions (**hydrochloric acid**) of the stomach. Gastroesophageal reflux disorder (GORD) is a condition in which this sphincter does not close properly for various reasons (for example, infection, long-term induced vomiting, pressure) resulting in a burning sensation caused by hydrochloric acid irritating the oesophageal lining.

Stomach: Where hydrochloric acid plays an important role

When the stomach is empty, it shrivels and forms internal folds, called **rugae.** This anatomical feature allows the stomach to increase its capacity from 50 millilitres to about 1.5 litres to accommodate food and/or beverages and gastric juices. The smooth muscles of the stomach (diagonal, circular, and longitudinal) contract and relax in many directions. This creates a churning action to mix the food with gastric juices to form **chyme.** This mixing is very important for breaking chewed food into smaller pieces, for **emulsification of fat** and for increased contact of digestive enzymes with their target macromolecules.

In the gastric glands (also called **gastric pits** due to their appearance), specialised cells secrete the gastric juices needed for digestion in the stomach. Hydrochloric acid and **intrinsic factor**, which is needed for the absorption of **vitamin B12**, are produced at the bottom of the gastric pits. Cells in the middle section of the gastric pits secrete the proteolytic enzyme **pepsinogen.** Towards the entrance of the gastric pits, alkaline mucus is secreted, which protects the stomach lining from the strong hydrochloric acid. The presence of partially digested proteins in the stomach triggers the release of the hormone gastrin, which in turn triggers the gastric juices.

Hydrochloric acid is responsible for the acidic environment (pH 2) in the stomach and is important for:

- neutralisation of slightly alkaline salivary amylase, hence stopping starch digestion
- **denaturation** of proteins
- activation of inactive enzymes, notably activation of pepsinogen to pepsin
- releasing vitamin B12 bound to proteins in food
- killing harmful bacteria that can cause infection or food poisoning.

Denaturation

The change that occurs in a protein's shape and structure and resulting in loss of function. This denaturation may occur due to external stressors such as chemicals, temperature, digestion or other factors.

In food, vitamin B12 is bound to a protein; hence, it is not available for absorption. During digestion, hydrochloric acid denatures the protein-bound form of vitamin B12, thereby releasing it. The free vitamin B12 then binds with intrinsic factor for transport to the small intestine, where it will be absorbed. The digestion of macronutrients from the mouth to the small intestine is outlined in Table 3.1.

Small intestine: The longest part of the digestive tract

Basic anatomy and physiology of the duodenum, jejunum, ileum and accessory organs

The small intestine is a long tube (4.5 to 7.5 metres) that comprises the duodenum, jejunum and ileum. The duodenum is a short section (30 centimetres) at the start of the small intestine, while the jejunum and ileum are the longer middle and end sections of the small intestine respectively. The pyloric sphincter controls the entry of chyme to the duodenum and prevents intestinal contents from travelling to the stomach. The ileocecal valve allows entry of intestinal contents into the colon.

Villi

Cells that form finger-like projections from the intestinal lumen and have microvilli protruding from them. This greatly increases the absorption surface of the intestine.

Enterocytes

Cells lining the intestine that are highly specialised for digestion and absorption.

Brush border

The microvilli-covered surface of the epithelial cells in the surface of the small intestine.

The small intestine coils around the peritoneal space, forming circular folds, and the intestinal lumen is covered with finger-like projections called **villi** (see Figure 3.2). Each individual villus is also covered with microscopic hair-like projections called microvilli, which extend from the plasma membrane of the **enterocytes**. The folds, villi and microvilli are responsible for the large surface area of the intestine; if these were all flattened, the small intestine would cover the surface of a tennis court. The **brush border** (the surface of the small intestine) gets its name from the collection of

Table 3.1. Action of digestive enzymes and their target nutrients

Region of digestive tract	Substrate	Enzyme	Secreted by	End-product
Mouth	Starch	Salivary amylase (α amylase)	Salivary glands	Shorter polysaccharide chains and dextrins
	Fat	Lingual lipase (minor contribution to fat digestion in adults)	Salivary glands	Diglycerides and fatty acids (see Chapter 4)
Stomach	Protein	Pepsinogen *Activated to pepsin by HCl*	Parietal cells of stomach	Polypeptides
Small intestine	Starch	Pancreatic amylase	Pancreas	Maltose
	Sucrose	Sucrase	Small intestine	Glucose and fructose
	Maltose	Maltase	Small intestine	Glucose
	Lactose	Lactase	Small intestine	Glucose and galactose
	Fat	Pancreatic lipase	Pancreas	Fatty acids and glycerol
	Polypeptides	Trypsinogen *Activated to trypsin by enteropeptidases*	Pancreas	Tripeptides, Dipeptides and amino acids
	Polypeptides	Chymotrypsinogen *Activated to chymotrypsin by trypsin*	Pancreas	Tripeptides, dipeptides and amino acids
	Polypeptides	Procarboxipeptidases *Activated to carboxypeptidases by trypsin*	Small intestine	Tripeptides, dipeptides and amino acids
	Tripeptides	Intestinal tripeptidases	Small intestine	Dipeptides
	Dipeptides	Intestinal dipeptidases	Small intestine	Amino acids

Glycocalyx
A protective mucus on the epithelial cells that is weakly acidic and consists of mucopolysaccharides.

villi, which look like the bristles on a brush. Many enzymes are secreted in the brush border and this is where macromolecules are broken down. Like the stomach, the brush border is covered by a protective layer of mucus with an additional layer of actin filaments, called the **glycocalyx.**

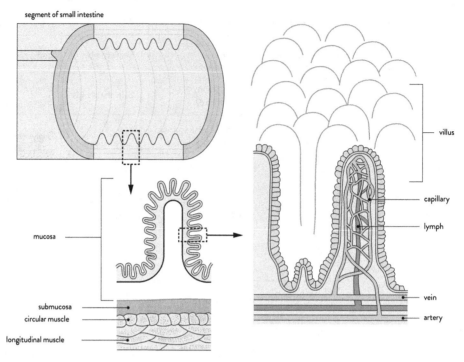

segment of small intestine

villus

capillary

lymph

mucosa

vein

artery

submucosa

circular muscle

longitudinal muscle

Figure 3.2. The intestinal folds and villi: important anatomical features that increase the surface area of the small intestine

Source: Hodgson 2011, pp. 312–27.

While some enzymes are secreted in the brush border, other enzymes and digestive juices are secreted by accessory organs and are transported to the small intestine. The pancreas and gall bladder are accessory organs to the digestive tract that are responsible for secretion and storage of digestive juices needed in the duodenum. See Table 3.1 for enzymes and their respective macronutrients and end-products of digestion.

The pancreas produces and secretes many enzymes used for the digestion of all three macromolecules (see Table 3.1) as well as bicarbonate for acid neutralisation. Secretin is a hormone released in the blood when the cells lining the wall of the duodenum sense the presence of chyme. This leads to the release of pancreatic juices in this region of the small intestine, to production of bile by the liver, and to inhibition of hydrochloric acid production in the stomach.

The gall bladder is a small pouch that concentrates and stores bile secreted from the liver. The presence of fat in the duodenum stimulates the release of the hormone cholecystokinin (CCK), which signals the gall bladder to contract and release bile in this region of the small intestine. Bile acids and salts are needed for the emulsification of fat and the formation of small fat droplets, which are key to the effective digestion and absorption of this macronutrient.

Movement of chyme along the small intestine

Upon leaving the stomach, the acidic chyme enters the duodenum via the pyloric sphincter. Upon sensing the acid, the sphincter closes until the pH rises and it relaxes again to allow the chyme to enter the duodenum. Here the pancreatic juices neutralise stomach acid and the digestion of macronutrients continues (see Table 3.1). The frequency of opening of the pyloric sphincter is governed by stomach content, volume and chyme consistency. For example:

- Gastric emptying is slower after a high-fat meal (hence high-fat chyme).
- Gastric emptying is faster after a large meal. The stretching and expansion of the stomach drives the opening frequency of this sphincter.
- Liquids pass through the small opening of the pyloric sphincter more easily than solid chyme.

Peristalsis propels the chyme along the small intestine, while the bi-directional flow of segmentation allows for mixing of chyme with pancreatic juices and bile for further emulsification of fat and mixing with other digestive secretions. By the time chyme reaches the **ileocecal valve**, digestion of nutrients is complete and most nutrients have been absorbed; only water and unabsorbed contents (such as fibre) remain. The latter serve as food for the gut bacteria residing in the small intestine and colon.

Ileocecal valve
The sphincter that separates the small and large intestine.

Table 3.2. Hormonal control of digestion—selected hormones

Hormone	Secreted by	Triggered by	Response
Gastrin	Stomach	Presence of food in the stomach	Stimulates release of hydrochloric acid and pepsinogen. Increases gastric and intestinal movement of chyme.
Secretin	Small intestine	Presence of acidic chyme in the duodenum	Stimulates secretion of pancreatic enzymes in the duodenum. Reduces intestinal movement of chyme.
Cholecystokinin (CCK)	Small intestine	Presence of fats and/or amino acids in the duodenum	Stimulates contraction of gall bladder to release bile into the duodenum. Secretion of pancreatic enzymes and juices into the duodenum.

Colon (large intestine)

The colon is larger in diameter than the small intestine and comprises five regions: the cecum and the ascending, transverse, descending and sigmoid colon. The small intestine is connected to the colon at the cecum; at the other end of the colon are the rectum, an internal anal sphincter and an external anal sphincter, which control defecation. The colon serves to absorb water and some minerals from intestinal content, to sustain fermentation of intestinal content by gut bacteria and to form stools. **Transit time** in the colon can range from 12 to 70 hours, during which colon content changes from liquefied form to semi-solid form due to absorption of water and digestive secretions. The colon is coated with mucus for protection and as a lubricant, and bicarbonate is also secreted to neutralise acids produced by bacteria.

Transit time
Duration of content movement through the colon. This can be affected by factors such as illness, infection and type and intensity of exercise. When transit time is accelerated there is not enough time for water and other macro- and micronutrients to be absorbed, resulting in their loss in stools.

Stools are generally composed of undigested food, some undigested nutrients, some water, sloughed intestinal cells, bacteria and indigestible fibre. When stools reach the rectum, defecation is stimulated and expulsion from the body is governed by strong muscle contractions in the sigmoid colon and rectum. The internal anal sphincter relaxes automatically, while the external anal sphincter is under voluntary control; therefore, a person can decide when to defecate.

ABSORPTION

The majority of nutrients are absorbed into the enterocytes of the duodenum, jejunum and/or ileum and transported to other parts of the body via the network of blood and lymphatic vessels in each villus (Figure 3.3). The nutrients move from the intestinal lumen into the enterocytes via different mechanisms:
- Passive diffusion is when small molecules, such as water and small lipids, are freely absorbed into the enterocytes across the concentration gradient.
- Facilitated diffusion occurs when a specific carrier is needed to transport nutrients (for example, water-soluble vitamins) through the enterocyte cell membrane.
- Active transport uses energy to transport some nutrients, against the concentration gradient, from one side of the enterocyte cell membrane to the other. Amino acids are absorbed through active transport, as is glucose, which is absorbed via the transporter sodium-glucose linked transporter I (SGLT-I).

Once the water-soluble nutrients and small lipids are absorbed through the enterocytes, they enter the bloodstream and are transported to the liver for further metabolism and distribution to other parts of the body. Larger lipids and fat-soluble vitamins are not water-soluble, and hence cannot be transported easily in blood. Instead, they are first absorbed into the enterocytes, where they are packaged with some proteins to form chylomicrons. These are then released into the lymphatic vessels for transport around the body.

SUMMARY AND KEY MESSAGES

The digestive tract includes the mouth, oesophagus, stomach, small intestine, large intestine and accessory organs, including the pancreas and gall bladder. Food is propelled along the digestive tract by peristalsis and enzymes are responsible for the breakdown of macromolecules into simple molecules. Many hormones regulate this process, which can also be impacted by exercise duration and intensity.

Key messages

- Digestion includes mechanical breakdown of food and mixing (chewing, opening and closing of sphincters, churning action of the stomach, peristalsis and segmentation) and chemical breakdown of nutrients.
- In the mouth, food is broken down into smaller pieces and salivary amylase begins the digestion of starch.
- In the stomach, hydrochloric acid activates pepsinogen for the digestion of proteins.
- The small intestine comprises the duodenum, jejunum and ileum.
- Intestinal digestive enzymes and secretions are produced by the pancreas, liver and brush border.
- In the colon, water and some minerals are absorbed.

REFERENCES AND FURTHER READING

Brouns, F. & Beckers, E., 1993, 'Is the gut an athletic organ?', *Sports Medicine*, vol. 15, no. 4, pp. 242–57.

Cermak, N.M. & Van Loon, L.J.C., 2013, 'The use of carbohydrates during exercise as an ergogenic aid', *Sports Medicine*, vol. 43, no. 11, pp. 1139–55.

Costa, R., Snipe, R., Kitic, C. et al., 2017, 'Systematic review: exercise-induced gastrointestinal syndrome—implications for health and intestinal disease', *Alimentary Pharmacology & Therapeutics*, vol. 46, no. 3, pp. 246–65.

De Oliveira, E.P., Burini, R.C. & Jeukendrup, A., 2014, 'Gastrointestinal complaints during exercise: Prevalence, etiology, and nutritional recommendations', *Sports Medicine*, vol. 44, suppl. 1, pp. 79–85.

Hodgson, J.M., 2011, 'Digestion of food', in Wahlqvist, M.L. (ed.), *Food and Nutrition: Food and health systems in Australia and New Zealand*, 3rd edn, Sydney, NSW: Allen & Unwin, pp. 312–27.

Jentjens, R.L. & Jeukendrup, A.E., 2005, 'High rates of exogenous carbohydrate oxidation from a mixture of glucose and fructose ingested during prolonged cycling exercise', *British Journal of Nutrition*, vol. 93, no.4, pp. 485–92.

Jentjens, R.L., Moseley, L., Waring, R.H. et al., 2004a, 'Oxidation of combined ingestion of glucose and fructose during exercise', *Journal of Applied Physiology*, vol. 96, no. 4, pp. 1277–84.

Jentjens, R.L., Venables, M.C. & Jeukendrup, A.E., 2004b, 'Oxidation of exogenous glucose, sucrose, and maltose during prolonged cycling exercise', *Journal of Applied Physiology*, vol. 96, no. 4, pp. 1285–91.

Jeukendrup, A.E., 2017, 'Training the gut for athletes', *Sports Medicine*, vol. 47, suppl. 1, pp. 101–10.

Murray, R., 2006, 'Training the gut for competition', *Current Sports Medicine Reports*, vol. 5, no. 3, pp. 161–4.

Peters, H., Wiersma, J., Koerselman, J. et al., 2000, 'The effect of a sports drink on gastroesophageal reflux during a run-bike-run test', *International Journal of Sports Medicine*, vol. 21, no. 1, pp. 65–70.

Pfeiffer, B., Stellingwerff, T., Hodgson, A.B. et al., 2012, 'Nutritional intake and gastrointestinal problems during competitive endurance events', *Medicine & Science in Sports & Exercise*, vol. 44, no. 2, pp. 344–51.

Wagenmakers, A., Brouns, F., Saris, W. et al., 1993, 'Oxidation rates of orally ingested carbohydrates during prolonged exercise in men', *Journal of Applied Physiology*, vol. 75, no. 6, pp. 2774–80.

Wallis, G.A., Rowlands, D.S., Shaw, C. et al., 2005, 'Oxidation of combined ingestion of maltodextrins and fructose during exercise', *Medicine & Science in Sports & Exercise*, vol. 37, no. 3, pp. 426–32.

CHAPTER 4

Macronutrients

Evangeline Mantzioris

The macronutrients—protein, fat and carbohydrate—are essential nutrients that supply energy and are required in relatively large quantities for the body. Protein and fat are also functional building blocks and have a diverse range of uses in the body, including growth and repair, as well as being the precursors for hormones and components of the immune system. While alcohol may be considered a macronutrient because it provides energy, it is in a unique category; it is not required by the body per se and it also has toxic properties, and for this reason it is not considered essential. Interestingly, all of these macronutrients are composed of the same elements: carbon (C), oxygen (O), nitrogen (N) and hydrogen (H). This chapter will outline their chemical and biological properties, the importance of each in the diet, and recommended intakes for good health. This chapter will also provide you with the foundation knowledge you will need to study the remaining chapters of this textbook, to build your knowledge on nutrition for exercise and performance.

LEARNING OUTCOMES

Upon completion of this chapter you will be able to:
- describe the chemical and biological properties of the macronutrients
- outline the physiological and biochemical uses of macronutrients in the body

- describe the health effects of under- and overconsumption of the macronutrients
- explain the synthesis and metabolism of the macronutrients
- outline the recommended intakes and dietary sources of the macronutrients.

PROTEIN

Proteins are essential nutrients, which provide 17 kJ/g (4 cal/g) of energy and are made up of single units known as **amino acids**. Amino acids are the building blocks of the human body and are used to synthesise cells, muscle, organs, hormones and immune factors, as well as acting as buffers to regulate the acidity or basicity of the body.

Chemical structure

Proteins are composed of amino acid chains, linked together by peptide bonds (chemical bonds between amino acids). Proteins vary according to the number and

Box 4.1: Calculating energy from macronutrients in food

To calculate the energy present in foods, you need to multiply the total amount of each of the macronutrients contained in the food (in grams) by the Atwater factors for protein, fat and carbohydrate. The Atwater factors provide the available energy for each of the macronutrients regardless of the food from which they are derived.

ATWATER FACTORS
- Protein: 17 kJ/g
- Fat: 37 kJ/g
- Carbohydrate: 17 kJ/g

For example, a food label might indicate that there is:
- Protein: 9.6 g
- Fat (total): 3.2 g
- Carbohydrate: 43.0 g

In this case, the energy in kilojoules that is provided by each nutrient is as follows:
- Protein: 9.6 x 17 = 163.2 kJ
- Fat: 3.2 x 37 = 118.4 kJ
- Carbohydrate: 43 x 17 = 731 kJ
- Total energy: 163.2 + 118.4 + 731 = 1012.6 kJ

sequence of amino acids, the folding of the protein and the interaction with other chemical groups in the protein to induce chemical change. All of this leads to unique individual proteins, reflecting the variety of roles they play in your body.

All amino acids have the same basic chemical structure: a central carbon to which is attached a hydrogen group (H), an amino group (NH_2), a carboxylic acid group (COOH) and a side chain group. It is the side chain group that makes each of the amino acids different (see Figure 4.1). There are 20 different amino acids; nine are essential and the remaining 11 are non-essential.

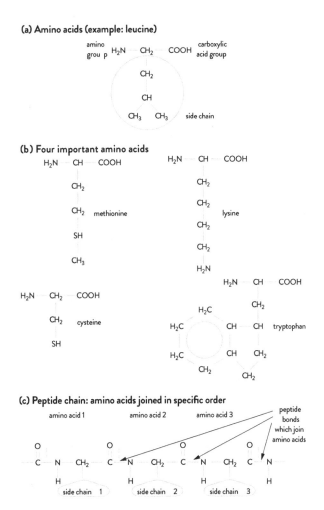

Figure 4.1. Chemical structure of amino acids

Source: Hodgson 2011, pp. 295–311.

Essential amino acids

There are nine amino acids that the human body requires but is unable to **synthesise**, and which therefore must be obtained from nutrients. As such, they are termed essential (or indispensable). These are histidine, isoleucine, leucine, lysine, methionine, phenylalanine, threonine, tryptophan and valine. Depletion of essential amino acids in the protein pool in the body will begin to limit the production of proteins essential for growth, repair, cell functioning and development.

Synthesise
To form a substance by combining elements.

Non-essential amino acids

There are 11 non-essential (or dispensable) amino acids that the body is able to synthesise, but that can also be provided by diet. In some conditions, a non-essential amino acid may become essential; in such cases the amino acid is referred to as conditionally essential (or conditionally indispensable). Tyrosine is a conditionally essential amino acid, as the body uses tryptophan to make tyrosine: if tryptophan is limited it is then unable to synthesise tyrosine.

Protein foods are often categorised in reference to their quality, both in terms of the mix and amount of amino acids that they contain. Complete protein sources often refer to animal-derived proteins that contain, in the required proportions, all the essential amino acids. Plant proteins are termed incomplete, as they are missing one or more of the essential amino acids, or have levels of an essential amino acid too low to meet requirements. Complementary proteins refer to the combination of two plant proteins to provide all the essential amino acids—for example, combining beans (lacking methionine) with grains (lacking lysine and threonine).

Uses in the body

Proteins have wide and varied roles in the human body: they are involved in the growth, repair and replacement of all cells (including blood, muscles, skeletal system, tissues and organs), and involved in regulating the homeostatic control and defence of the body (NHMRC et al. 2006).

One of the main functional roles of proteins in the body is as enzymes, which accelerate chemical reactions in the body. Enzymes are synthesised from amino acids as well as other dietary components (for example, zinc and selenium). They are used by every organ and cell to assist in the repair and growth of the body. Enzymes also contribute to the synthesis of proteins involved in the homeostatic control of the body, immune function, fluid balance regulation, transportation of nutrients and other molecules, and detoxification of the body. In addition to protein's critical role in growth and regulation of the body, protein can also be used as a source of energy if carbohydrate and fat intake is low (for instance, during times of starvation). If needed, muscle will be broken down to provide further energy if dietary intake of protein is also limited. Protein may also be metabolised for energy when energy demands are sustained over a long period of time in performance, such as in ultra-endurance events lasting 3–4 hours or more.

Box 4.2: Nutrient Reference Values (NRVs)

The National Health and Medical Research Council (NHMRC) has analysed and synthesised the data from many thousands of peer-reviewed journal articles (the evidence base) to formulate the Nutrient Reference Values (NRVs) (NHMRC et al. 2006). The NRVs are a set of recommended intakes for macro- and micro-nutrients that best support healthy Australians to maintain good health. Requirements are expressed in the following categories:

Estimated Average Requirements (EAR): This is a daily nutrient level that has been estimated from the evidence base to meet the requirements of half of the healthy individuals in a particular life stage and gender group.

Recommended Dietary Intake (RDI): The average daily dietary intake level that is sufficient to meet the nutrient requirements of nearly all (97–98 per cent) healthy individuals in a particular life stage and gender group. This is the recommended level of intake for individuals.

Acceptable Intake (AI): For some nutrients there is an inadequate evidence base to provide an EAR or RDI. In such cases an AI is recommended. This is defined as the average daily nutrient intake level—based on observed or experimentally determined approximations or estimates of nutrient intake of a group (or groups) of apparently healthy people—that is assumed to be adequate.

Estimated Energy Requirements (EER): The average dietary energy intake that is predicted to maintain energy balance in a healthy adult of defined age, gender, weight, height and level of physical activity, consistent with good health. In children and pregnant and lactating women, the EER is taken to include the needs associated with growth or the secretion of milk at rates consistent with good health.

Upper Level of Intake (UL): The highest average daily nutrient intake level likely to pose no adverse health effects to almost all individuals in the general population. As intake increases above the UL, the potential risk of adverse effects increases.

Acceptable Macronutrient Distribution Ranges (AMDR): Recommended ranges of macronutrient contribution to total daily energy intake to reduce chronic disease risk while still ensuring adequate micronutrient status: protein 15–25 per cent; fat 20–35 per cent; and carbohydrate 45–65 per cent.

The NRVs are expressed in different formats that reflect intakes recommended for individuals and groups, the level of evidence for a nutrient and, where relevant, the highest possible safe intake of a nutrient. It is important to realise that, like other biological characteristics of humans such as height or eye colour, each person is unique and will have different nutrient requirements, and the NRVs take that into account. For example, the RDI for men and women over 19 years of age for vitamin C is 45 mg/day, but not everyone will require that amount. In fact, 97.98 per cent of the healthy population will have their requirements met at this level of intake, meaning that only 2.02 per cent of the population will need more than this. The EAR for vitamin C is 30 mg/day, which indicates that half of the population will only need this amount.

Recommended intakes for non-athletes

Protein in the body is continuously broken down and resynthesised. This process is known as protein turnover, with small amounts of protein lost in the stools. Protein is required on a daily basis in the diet due to its ubiquitous role and limited storage in the body. It is recommended that protein intake provides about 10–15 per cent of the daily energy requirement. For the average adult who needs approximately 8700 kJ per day, this equates to about 50–75 g of protein per day. The NRV recommendations for protein are based on a g/kg of body weight for each gender and age group. The daily RDI for women aged 19–70 years is 0.75 g/kg and over 70 years is 0.94 g/kg of body weight. The RDI for men aged 19–70 years is 0.84 g/kg and over 70 years is 1.07 g/kg of body weight. Requirements for athletes may differ, dependent on their age and sport played, as discussed in Chapter 10.

Dietary sources

While animal products that are rich in protein are greatly valued for their high-quality protein (as they provide a complete set of amino acids), plant proteins provide a major source of protein for many millions of people around the world. Animal sources of protein also provide valuable additional nutrients that have limited presence in other foods, such as iron and zinc (present in meat), and calcium and vitamin B12 (present in dairy). Plant sources of protein (wheat, rice, pasta, legumes, nuts and seeds) also provide carbohydrates, B-group vitamins and fibre. This makes food sources of protein, compared to protein supplements, valuable for athletes and non-athletes who need to ensure that they are getting a balanced diet in regard to other macronutrients and micronutrients of importance in exercise and performance.

Health effects of protein

Protein is important for the maintenance and health of our bodies, and the majority of Western populations consume adequate intakes for this. However, in developing countries the health problems associated with protein deficiencies are devastating, and it is the leading cause of death among children in these places.

In most cases, protein deficiency occurs in combination with an energy deficiency, and is referred to as protein-energy malnutrition (PEM). Primary PEM occurs as the direct result of diets that lack both protein and energy. Secondary PEM arises as a complication of chronic illness, such as acquired immune deficiency syndrome (AIDS), tuberculosis and cancer, due to increased nutritional requirements, limited oral intake or malabsorption of nutrients. Acute PEM refers to a short period of food deprivation, as in the case of children who are often the appropriate height for age but underweight. Chronic PEM refers to long-term food deprivation that affects growth and weight, and is characterised by small-for-age children.

PEM presents clinically in two different forms: kwashiorkor and marasmus. Kwashiorkor typically represents a sudden and recent deprivation of food (protein and energy). In Ghanaian, the word refers to the illness an older child develops when the next child is born, as a result of being moved off the breast. Clinically, kwashiorkor has a rapid onset due to inadequate protein intake or following illness, with both weight loss and some muscle wasting. The characteristic clinical feature is oedema (swelling caused in the body as fluid leaks out of capillaries), which is evident from a child's swollen belly, enlarged fatty liver, dry brittle hair and the development of skin lesions. Apathy, misery, irritability and melancholy are also evident, with loss of appetite. Marasmus occurs with a severe deprivation of food (both in protein, energy and nutrients) for an extended period of time; the malnutrition develops slowly and children typically look small for their age. Unlike kwashiorkor, there is no oedema, no enlarged fatty liver and the skin is dry and easily wrinkles.

In developed regions, protein deficiency is more likely to arise due to chronic illness or poverty and, as such, it is unlikely an athlete will have a compromised protein intake—unless it reflects a philosophical or religious reason that limits their intake of animal products. Chapter 6 will discuss planning diets for people who choose to follow a vegetarian diet.

LIPIDS

Lipids (or fats) are a large and diverse group of naturally occurring molecules, both in the diet and in the human body. They include fats, waxes, sterols, fat-soluble vitamins, monoglycerides, diglycerides, triglycerides, phospholipids and esters, which we will cover in this chapter. Dietary fats provide a concentrated form of energy (37 kJ/g) and are also a vehicle in the diet for supplying fat-soluble vitamins (vitamins A, D, E and K) and essential fatty acids (alpha-linolenic acid and linoleic acid). Importantly, and often under-considered, dietary fat provides important **organoleptic** (taste and texture) properties to food that contains fats and to meals to which fats have been added. Lipids play critical roles in the body, including storing energy, cell signalling and as the major structural component of cell membranes. While the intake of certain dietary fats (saturated and trans fats) is associated with the development of chronic disease, dietary fats are an essential part of the diet, providing essential fatty acids, vitamins and other phytonutrients.

Organoleptic
The aspect of substances, in this case food and drink, that an individual experiences via the senses of taste, texture, smell and touch.

Chemical structure

All lipids are compounds that are composed of carbon, hydrogen and oxygen and are insoluble in water, but the different types of lipids that exist are structurally very diverse. There are four main categories: fatty acids, triglycerides, sterols and phospholipids (see Figure 4.2).

Fatty acids

Fatty acids are composed of a chain of carbon (C) atoms, attached by single bonds. Each C atom can have up to four H atoms attached. The carbon chain has a carboxyl group at one end and a methyl group at the other end. Fatty acids can be classified according to the number of C atoms in the chain. Short-chain fatty acids have 2–6 C atoms, medium-chain fatty acids 6–12 C atoms, long-chain 14–20 C atoms and, finally, very long-chain fatty acids more than 20 C atoms. Fatty acids are, however,

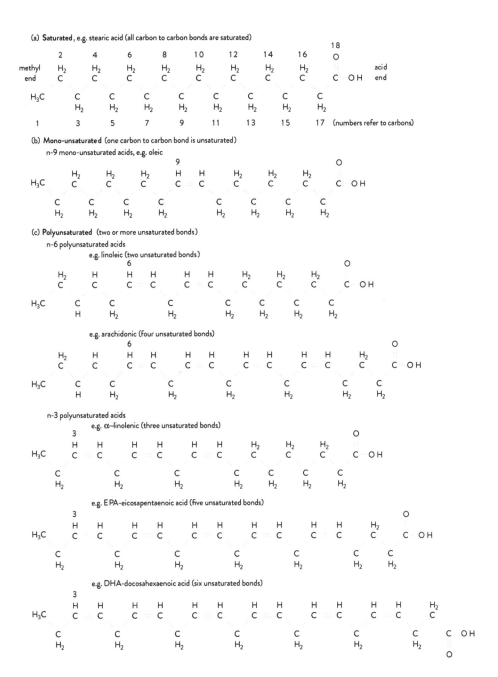

Figure 4.2. Structural relationship of some fatty acids

Source: Jones & Hodgson 2011, pp. 284–94.

more often classified according to the number of double bonds present between the C atoms—the more double bonds in the chain, the more unsaturated the fatty acid.

Saturated fatty acids

Fatty acid chains that contain no double bonds between the C atoms are referred to as saturated fatty acids. They are mostly found in animal food products, such as meat, cheese and butter, but are also present in some plant products, such as coconut and palm oils. Saturated fats are associated with an increased risk of cardiovascular disease; however, emerging research is beginning to show that their effect may not be as great as once thought (Dehghan et al. 2017). The research and scientific debate in this area is still continuing and as new high-quality evidence emerges this may lead to changes in dietary advice.

Monounsaturated fatty acids

Monounsaturated fatty acids contain one double bond in the C chain and are found in foods such as olives and olive oil, avocadoes and some types of nuts. Monounsaturated fats (from olive oil) are one of the main components of the Mediterranean diet, which has been shown in both **epidemiological studies** and **intervention studies** to reduce risk and provide benefits in cardiovascular disease. It is important to note that the other components of the Mediterranean diet (vegetables, fruit and grains) also play a role in good health.

Epidemiological studies
Studies that analyse the distribution (who, when and where) and determinants of health and disease in a defined population by observation. Epidemiological studies include ecological, case-control, cross-sectional and retrospective or prospective longitudinal cohorts study designs.

Intervention studies
Studies in which researchers make changes to observe the effect on health outcomes; in nutrition, this will include changes to diet.

Polyunsaturated fatty acids

Polyunsaturated fatty acids (PUFAs) contain two or more double bonds in the C chain. PUFAs are further subdivided according to the position of the first double bond in the chain. When the double bond occurs on the third C atom from the methyl end, they are referred to as n-3 (or omega-3) fatty acids. If the first double bond occurs on the sixth C atom from the methyl end they are referred to as n-6 (or omega-6) fatty acids. The parent fatty acids of the n-3 and n-6, alpha-linolenic and linoleic acid respectively, are the essential fatty acids. They are known as essential, as the human body is unable to synthesise them, and, as such, must be obtained from the diet.

n-6 polyunsaturated fatty acids

Linoleic acid (LA) is the parent fatty acid of the n-6 PUFA and, as it is essential, needs to be obtained from the diet. LA is found as a concentrated source in vegetable oils like safflower and sunflower oils, and salad dressings made from these oils. It is also present in some nuts and seeds. LA is important, as it can be metabolised through a series of reactions to form the longer-chain fatty acid, arachidonic acid (AA). AA can also be found in the diet (in meat). AA is the direct precursor of a diverse group of hormone-like substances known as eicosanoids, which play a critical role in the inflammatory process and in thrombosis (clot formation).

n-3 polyunsaturated fatty acids

Alpha-linolenic acid (ALA) is the parent fatty acid of the n-3 PUFA, and like LA, it needs to be obtained from the diet. ALA is found in concentrated sources in flaxseed (linseed) oil, and in smaller amounts in canola oil. Walnuts, chia seeds and green leafy vegetables also contain small amounts of ALA. ALA is metabolised through the same chain of reactions that converts LA to AA, to form the longer-chain fatty acids, eicosapentaenoic acid (EPA) and docosahexaenoic acid (DHA). EPA and DHA are found in fish, fish oil and breast milk. Like AA, EPA is important, as it is the direct precursor of a diverse group of hormone-like substances known as eicosanoids; however, eicosanoids derived from EPA are anti-inflammatory and anti-thrombotic, compared to those derived from AA.

This biochemical difference between the two classes of fatty acids and their eicosanoids has been used therapeutically in the management of inflammatory diseases such as rheumatoid arthritis and psoriasis. DHA is found in concentrated amounts in the cellular phospholipids of brain and neural tissue of humans and, as such, its role in foetal and early-life nutrition is critical.

Trans fatty acids

Trans fatty acids (TFAs) are a chemical variation of unsaturated fats. In the **cis-form** (the regular form), the C atoms that have double bonds and the H atoms are on the same side. In the **trans form**, the H-atoms are on opposite sides of the double-bonded C atoms, so that they look and act more like saturated fats.

Cis form
In a molecule, the C atoms that have double bonds and the H atoms are on the same side.

Trans form
In a molecule, the C atoms that have double bonds and the H atoms are on opposite sides.

TFAs naturally occur in dairy products and beef. In the food industry, manufacturers can produce TFAs by mixing H atoms with the unsaturated fatty acids, using a mixture of heat and pressure. This results in liquid oils being transformed into a solid state, making them very useful for the production of certain foods, such as spreads and vegetable shortening for baking. However, these TFAs have been shown to be worse for cardiovascular disease compared to the equivalent amounts of saturated fat. The WHO has recommended that no more than one per cent of our dietary energy be derived from TFAs. In many countries, including Australia, Denmark and the United States, there has been a reduction in TFA use in the food supply, either through voluntary initiatives or legislation (FSANZ 2017).

Triglycerides

Triglycerides are the main constituents of body fat (adipose tissue) in animals, including humans. They are made up of a glycerol backbone with three fatty acids attached. All triglycerides are composed of different types of fatty acids, from short-chain to long-chain. Triglycerides are also the main type of fat we consume in our food, from both vegetable and animal sources.

Sterols

Sterols are complex lipid molecules, having four interconnected carbon rings with a hydrocarbon side chain. The most familiar type of sterol is cholesterol, which is a critical component of cell membranes and a precursor to vitamin D, the sex hormones (oestrogen and testosterone) and the adrenal hormones (cortisol, cortisone and aldosterone).

Cholesterol can be synthesised in the body, and hence is not essential in the diet. Dietary cholesterol is only found in animal products. Cholesterol in the body can be classified as either high-density **lipoprotein** cholesterol (HDL-C) or low-density lipoprotein cholesterol (LDL-C) depending on whether it is part of a low-density lipoprotein (LDL) or high-density lipoprotein (HDL) molecule. LDL-C is referred to as 'bad' cholesterol, as LDL takes cholesterol to the blood vessels where it can form into atherosclerotic plaques, which can lead to blockages and myocardial infarction (heart attack). HDL-C is referred to as 'good' cholesterol, as HDL takes cholesterol away from the blood vessels to the liver, hence reducing the risk of a myocardial infarction.

Lipoprotein
A cluster of lipids attached to proteins that act as transport vehicles for the lipids in the blood. They are divided according to their density.

Plants synthesise many types of sterols, as well as stanols, which are structurally similar to sterols. Sterols and stanols are poorly absorbed by the body and reduce the absorption of cholesterol from the gastrointestinal system, which can have beneficial effects for cholesterol reduction. The food industry has added plant sterols to some types of margarines, milks, yoghurts and cereals, which can lead to a reduction in cholesterol levels if at least 2–3 g/day of plant sterols or stanols are consumed.

Phospholipids

Phospholipids have a unique chemical structure; they are soluble in both water and fat. They are similar to triglycerides, in that they have a glycerol backbone, but have only two fatty acids attached to the glycerol—the third position is taken up by a phosphate and a 'head-group'. It is the combination of the head-group, phosphate group and glycerol backbone that makes phospholipids soluble in water, while the fatty acids (the tail group) makes them soluble in fats. This feature gives them a critical role, both in the body and in the food industry. Despite their importance, phospholipids make up only a small portion of the diet (<5 per cent) and are not essential, as they can be synthesised by the body.

Phospholipids are able to freely move around the body, which enables them to transport other fats such as vitamins and hormones. They are also a critical component of the cellular membranes, where they form a phospholipid bilayer. The phospholipids assemble into two layers, with the hydrophilic (water-loving) ends on opposite sides, and the hydrophobic (water-fearing) ends facing each other on the inside. This arrangement allows for the transport of substances through the cellular membrane. Interestingly, the fatty acids attached to the phospholipids in the cellular membrane will reflect the dietary intake of fatty acids.

In the food industry, phospholipids (such as lecithin) allow foods to be emulsified, as in the production of salad dressings, mayonnaise, ice-cream and chocolate. Lecithin is found in eggs, liver, soybeans, wheat germ and peanuts.

Recommended intakes for the general population

The Nutrient Reference Values from the NMHRC have no set RDI, EAR or AI for total fat intake. However, there are recommendations for the intake of the essential fatty acids (NHMRC et al. 2006).

In the latest version of the *Australian Guide to Healthy Eating*, which provides qualitative guidelines on healthy eating (discussed in Chapter 6), the recommendation is now to 'avoid saturated fat', which has changed from the previous recommendation to 'decrease total fat' (NMHRC et al. 2009). The AMDR from the NRV states that fat should contribute 20–35 per cent of your total energy intake (NHMRC et al. 2006). This highlights the importance of reducing the intake of foods that contain saturated fats in our diet and replacing them with monounsaturated oils and foods (olive, canola

Table 4.1. Recommendations for the intake of the essential fatty acids

Fatty acid	Men 19+ years	Women 19+ years
LA	13 g/day	8 g/day
ALA	1.3 g/day	0.8 g/day
Total LC n-3 (DHA+EPA+DHA)	160 mg/day	90 mg/day

Source: NHMRC et al. 2006.

oil, avocado, almonds) or polyunsaturated oils and foods (nuts, fish, polyunsaturated vegetable oils).

CARBOHYDRATES

Carbohydrates, like fats and proteins, are molecules composed of C, H and O atoms. They are ubiquitous in the diet—present in breads, cereals, grains, legumes, rice, pasta, vegetables and fruit, although dairy is the only animal source of carbohydrates. Carbohydrates deliver the key source of fuel (energy) for the muscles and body, providing 17 kJ/g. Glucose, which is a monosaccharide (simple) sugar, is the exclusive source of energy for red blood cells and provides a significant portion of the energy that is required for the brain. Excess glucose in the blood is converted to the storage form of glucose, glycogen. The average person stores about 5000 kilojoules worth of glucose in the form of glycogen, which can be easily converted to glucose again to be used by the body when blood glucose levels begin to drop.

Carbohydrates have numerous biological functions in the body. Aside from their important role in providing energy, they also have a structural role. Ribose, which is a component of coenzymes and the backbone of RNA, is a five-C atom monosaccharide, and the closely related deoxyribose is a component of DNA. Carbohydrates also play key roles in the immune system and in blood clotting.

Chemical forms of carbohydrate

There are a wide variety of carbohydrates in the diet. They include simple carbohydrates (the sugars) and complex carbohydrates (the starches and fibre). Regardless of the length or complexity of the carbohydrate, they are all composed of sugar units (see Figure 4.3).

Monosaccharides

Monosaccharides are composed of a single unit of sugar and are the most basic units of carbohydrates. There are three monosaccharides or 'sugars': glucose, fructose and galactose. The monosaccharides all have the same number of C, H and O atoms but differ in their chemical structure. Monosaccharides are the building blocks of disaccharides and polysaccharides.

Glucose

Glucose ($C_6H_{12}O_6$) serves as the essential energy source for our body; when people talk about blood sugar levels, they are referring to glucose in the blood. Most of the polysaccharides in our diet are composed of chains of glucose, with starch being the most common polysaccharide.

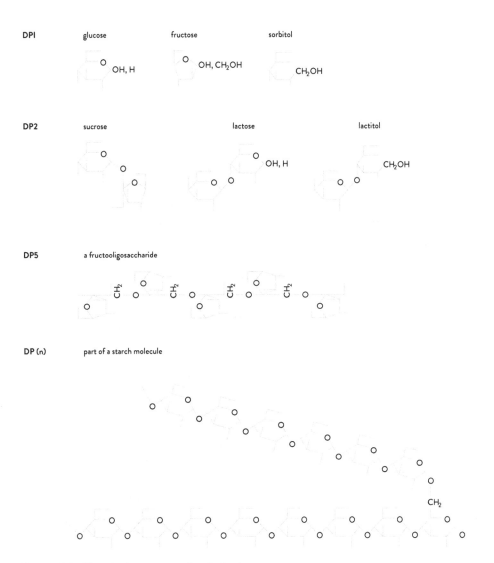

Figure 4.3. Chemical structure of carbohydrates

Source: Jones & Hodgson 2011, p. 268–83.

Fructose

The slightly different chemical structure of fructose results in it being the sweetest-tasting monosaccharide. Fructose occurs naturally in some fruits and honey. Fructose may be added to some foods, such as soft drinks, ready-to-eat breakfast cereals and desserts, and biscuit and cake mixes, through the use of high-fructose corn syrup.

Galactose

Galactose is found in dairy products and sugar beets, and is the least sweet-tasting monosaccharide.

Disaccharides

Disaccharides are composed of two glucose units and can be formed as pairs of any of the three monosaccharides. There are three disaccharides, and each contains glucose as one of the monosaccharide components. Sucrose, which is common table sugar refined from cane sugar, is made up of glucose and fructose. Lactose is found in milk and is composed of galactose and glucose. Maltose, also known as malt sugar, is the disaccharide that is produced when amylase, an enzyme, breaks down starch.

Lactose intolerance is fairly common, with only about 30 per cent of adults worldwide being able to digest lactose. Intestinal cells produce an enzyme called lactase, which breaks lactose down into galactose and glucose. When lactase activity is low in people, the lactose remains undigested in the intestinal tract and leads to a high concentration of contents in the intestine, which in turn draws fluid into the intestinal lumen and, in combination with the proliferation of bacteria that digest the lactose, leads to painful bloating, wind and diarrhoea.

Lactose intolerance
A condition that leads to the inability to digest lactose which results in bloating, abdominal discomfort, gas and diarrhoea.

Artificial sweeteners

Artificial sweeteners are chemicals, found naturally (Stevia) or synthesised industrially (aspartame, saccharin), or are **sugar alcohols**, that have a sweet taste with either no kilojoules or reduced kilojoules compared to sugar. This allows the food industry to replace sugars with artificial sweeteners without adding kilojoules to the product. It was assumed that this would lead to significant weight loss in the community due to the decreased consumption of kilojoules, but research shows a lack of the predicted effect. Whether this is due to people increasing their consumption of other foods or the artificial sweeteners affecting metabolism in other ways is still being debated among researchers (Fowler et al. 2008).

Sugar alcohols
Carbohydrates that have been chemically altered. They provide fewer kilojoules as they are not well absorbed and may have a laxative effect. They include sorbitol, mannitol and xylitol. While they have fewer kilojoules they can still lead to elevation in blood glucose levels and, hence, can have an impact on blood glucose control in people with diabetes; as such they need to be considered in the diet.

Complex carbohydrates

Complex carbohydrates include oligosaccharides, which contain between three and nine monosaccharide units, and polysaccharides, which contain ten or more monosaccharide units.

Oligosaccharides

Oligosaccharides are found in a variety of foods. Starch, which is found in a wide variety of foods, such as wheat, maize potato and rice, contains the α-glucan oligosaccharide maltodextrin. Maltodextrin is used in the food industry as a sweetener, fat substitute and to modify the texture of food through its thickening properties.

The oligosaccharides that are not α-glucans include raffinose, stachyose, verbascose, inulin and fructan, and are found in legumes, artichokes, wheat and rye, and in the onion, leek and garlic family. The fructans (including inulin) have unique properties in the gastrointestinal system and are referred to as **prebiotics**. Prebiotics remain undigested in the gastrointestinal system and promote the growth of select bacteria that improve human health. Consumption of these foods leads to alteration in the flora of the gut, with a domination of bifidobacteria and lactobacillus, and the production of short-chain fatty acids (SCFAs). SCFAs, also referred to as volatile fatty acids (VFAs), are important for colonic health as they are the primary energy source for colon cells and have anti-carcinogenic and anti-inflammatory properties.

Prebiotics
Food components that are not digested in the gastrointestinal system but are used by the bacteria in the colon to promote their growth.

Polysaccharides

Glycogen

Glycogen is found in limited amounts in food, with a small amount found in meat. However, it is its role in the body that is critically important and of interest to nutritionists, including sports nutritionists. Glycogen is a secondary form of energy storage (~5000 kJ in the average person). When blood glucose levels increase following a meal, insulin is released, which stimulates the uptake of glucose into cells and storage as glycogen. Conversely, when blood glucose levels decrease due to lack of dietary intake of carbohydrates or depletion of blood glucose levels from exercise, the pancreas releases glucagon, which stimulates the liver and muscles to release and break down glycogen and release glucose (known as glycogenolysis). Glucose can also be derived through gluconeogenesis, which is a metabolic pathway that leads to glucose formation from substrates such as lactate, glycerol and glucogenic amino acids.

Glycogen is a highly branched structure, containing up to 30,000 glucose units that surround a protein core. Glycogen in the muscle, liver and fat cells is stored in a hydrated form with three or four parts of water per part of glycogen. This explains the dramatic weight loss that is seen with low-carbohydrate diets. In this scenario, as blood glucose levels decrease, glycogen is converted back to glucose to supply the brain and muscles with fuel, which also releases the water, hence contributing to the weight loss observed.

Starch

Starch is the form in which plants store glucose to use for energy. Some common starches include amylopectin and amylose. Both of these contain hundreds to thousands of glucose units linked together, as is the case with glycogen. Starch is found in many different foods including wheat, rice, lentils, maize, beans and the tuber vegetables. Starch forms the most common carbohydrate in our diet.

Resistant starch is one type of starch that resists digestion in the small intestine and is fermented in the large intestine by bacteria into short-chain fatty acids. These SCFAs are important as they protect the bowel against cancer and are also absorbed into the bloodstream and may be involved in lowering blood cholesterol. Resistant starch is found in unripe bananas, potatoes and lentils. In Australia, resistant starch is also commonly added to 'high-fibre' breads and cereals. It is also considered to be a form of insoluble fibre, which is discussed below.

Fibre

While there are many definitions of fibre, most simply, dietary fibre is a carbohydrate that is not digested by our body. Fibre is the parts of the edible portions of plants that are not digested or absorbed in the small intestine, that go on to be partially or completely fermented in the large intestine and that promote beneficial physiological effects. These beneficial effects include laxation of bowel movements, reduced blood cholesterol and beneficial modulation of blood glucose levels. Dietary fibre can include polysaccharides, oligosaccharides and lignin (scientific definition paraphrased from NHMRC et al. 2006, p. 45). The recommended intake from the NHMRC for dietary fibre is 30 g/day for men and 25 g/day for women. As there is a variety of types of fibre in food, researchers and nutritionists classify them into two different groups according to their physiological actions in the body.

Soluble fibre

Soluble fibre dissolves in water to form gels. The process of dissolving into a gel slows down digestion. Soluble fibres are found in oat bran, barley, nuts, seeds, legumes, and in some fruits and vegetables. Soluble fibre is commonly linked with reducing the incidence of cardiovascular disease and protecting against diabetes, by reducing blood cholesterol levels and lowering blood glucose levels.

Insoluble fibre

Conversely, insoluble fibre does not dissolve in water and is found in wheat bran, some vegetables and wholegrains. Insoluble fibre absorbs water and expands, adding bulk to stools and speeding its transit through the intestines, thereby promoting bowel movements and ameliorating constipation.

Dietary recommendations for carbohydrates

The Nutrient Reference Values do not provide specific recommendations (in grams per day) for carbohydrates, as there is limited data on which to base EAR, RDI or AI requirements for most age and gender groups, except for infancy (0–12 months) where values are based on what the infant receives from breast milk. This lack of recommendations regarding carbohydrates for the majority of age groups does not reflect the value carbohydrates have in the diet for providing glucose as a direct energy source for the brain, as well as being a carrier for many micronutrients and fibre, as discussed above. There is a mounting body of evidence for the role of carbohydrates in relation to chronic disease, and as such, an acceptable range of intake between 45 and 65 per cent of energy is recommended (NHMRC 2013). The recommendation is that carbohydrates should predominantly be derived from wholegrain, low-energy dense sources and/or from low glycaemic index foods (see below). This is supported by more recent evidence-based nutrition advice from the World Health Organization (WHO) (WHO 2015), which recommends limiting intake of added sugars to ten per cent of total energy intake.

Glycaemic response, index and load

Glycaemic response

The glycaemic response is defined by the length of time it takes for glucose to be absorbed from foods that have been consumed, regardless of whether the foods contain disaccharides or polysaccharides. A low glycaemic response indicates that the glucose is slowly absorbed over a longer period of time, resulting in a steady and modest rise in blood glucose levels after consumption of the food. A high glycaemic response indicates that the glucose is absorbed more quickly and that there is a sharp immediate rise in blood glucose levels. Other factors in food that will affect the glycaemic response, through their ability to delay or enhance the absorption of glucose, include:

- fat content (delays gastric emptying)
- acid content (delays gastric emptying)
- protein content (delays gastric emptying)
- amount and types of fibre (soluble fibre has lower glycaemic index than insoluble fibre)
- type of starch (depending on the structure of the molecule, which affects the rate of enzyme digestion)
- level of processing (wholegrain bread has a lower glycaemic index than wholemeal bread)
- sugar type (fructose and lactose have lower glycaemic index than glucose).

Glycaemic index

The glycaemic index (GI) is a system that ranks foods according to their potential to increase blood glucose levels, relative to the reference food of white bread (which is given a GI rank of 100). Foods are considered high GI if they rank above 70, and low GI if they rank below 55. The GI of foods is also affected by the level of fat, protein and fibre in them and, in drinks, the amount of carbonation. As such, it is important to appreciate that the GI does not always correlate with the overall healthiness of foods, as it does not consider the level of other micronutrients, sugar and saturated fat. For example, some cola-based soft drinks and sweetened chocolate hazelnut spread have a lower GI than pumpkin, white rice and couscous.

Glycaemic load

Glycaemic load (GL) is a measure that takes into account the amount of carbohydrate in the portion of food consumed, together with the GI of the food. A large intake of a food with a low GI could result in a high glycaemic response, compared to consuming a small portion of a high-GI food, which will cause a smaller glycaemic response.

$$Glycaemic\ load = \frac{(GI \times amount\ of\ available\ carbohydrate)}{100}$$

As foods are rarely consumed in isolation or in set quantities, the use of the glycaemic load will describe the glycaemic response more accurately. While general health recommendations for the population focus on the selection of foods with a lower GI to promote **satiety** and confer health benefits, for the athlete, knowledge of the GI of foods is also important for implementing nutrition plans to optimise performance. Meals before exercise focus on consuming low-GI foods to enable a sustained release of glucose in the blood. However, during and after exercise, high-GI foods are preferred to promote a quicker glycaemic response, allowing the absorbed glucose to be utilised for performance and to replace lost glucose respectively.

Satiety
The feeling of fullness and satisfaction after consuming food which inhibits the need to eat.

Recommended intakes and health effects of sugars

The NHMRC recommends that the percentage of energy derived from carbohydrates (CHO) should be in the range of 45–65 per cent of total energy (NHMRC et al. 2006). For an average person consuming 8700 kJ/day, this equates to 230–330 grams of CHO per day. This recommendation is not, however, used to determine the requirement for fuelling exercise and performance for athletes, which will be discussed in Chapter 10.

In 2015, the WHO recommended that free sugar intake should be less than ten per cent of total energy intake, and that further health benefits could be attained with a reduction to less than five per cent of dietary energy for adults and children (WHO 2015). For adults, this equates to about 20–25 g/day for the average person. Free sugars refers to the monosaccharides and disaccharides added to foods and drinks by the food industry, as well as those incorporated in food preparation at home. It is important to note that this does not include foods that naturally contain these sugars, such as milk, fruit and some vegetables.

Sugars have been enjoyed in the diet for many centuries, as they provide sweetness and palatability (taste) to many foods; however, in recent years the intake of free or added sugars has increased significantly, leading to excessive intake and undesirable health outcomes. The impact of **hyperglycaemia** (high blood glucose levels) on cells and tissues in the body is also cause for concern. It is often difficult for the consumer to ascertain which foods contain sugars, as they assume various names on food labels, including brown sugar, raw sugar, corn sweeteners, corn syrup, dextrose, glucose, maltose, molasses, honey, or high-fructose corn syrup. An indirect impact of eating large amounts of added sugars is that they may replace other nutrient-rich foods and result in nutrient deficiencies. Foods such as lollies, cakes, biscuits, doughnuts, muffins and chocolate, and drinks such as sports drinks, soft drinks and fruit drinks, all have high amounts of added sugar with few other nutrients in them, so they are referred to as **nutrient-poor**. Of particular concern for the athlete is the quantity of sports drinks they may consume to enhance exercise performance, in terms of both general and dental health. Even, if they are 'rinsing and spitting', the sugar will stay in contact with their teeth for a period of time and can have a direct impact on the development of dental cavities.

Hyperglycaemia
Elevated blood glucose levels.

Nutrient-poor
A food or meal that has low content of nutrients relative to energy content.

ALCOHOL

Although consumed by some in the diet, alcohol is defined as a drug since it affects brain function. While alcohol can have some potential health benefits at low to moderate intakes, the harmful effects of alcohol, including accidental deaths, violence and motor vehicle accidents, generally outweighs any benefit. Alcohol causes on average 15 deaths and 430 hospitalisations every day in Australia and, in 2010, its misuse was estimated to cost Australia $36 billion (Manning et al. 2013). Therefore, any potential health benefit of alcohol has to be considered against the risk it poses to individuals and society. It is included in this chapter as it is a macronutrient, providing energy to the body (29 kJ/g); however, it is not necessary to include when planning diets and nutritional intakes for people, including athletes, due to the negative health and performance effects (discussed below).

Chemistry of alcohol

From the chemist's perspective, alcohol refers to compounds containing a hydroxyl group (–OH), which include methanol, ethanol, isopropyl alcohol, glycerol, butanol and pentanol. However, for most people the term 'alcohol' is used to describe alcoholic beverages containing ethanol.

Alcohol (ethanol or ethyl alcohol) is a two-carbon compound, with five hydrogen and one hydroxyl group attached (C_2H_5OH). Alcohol, which provides 29 kJ/g, is normally consumed in alcoholic beverages, and the addition of any added sugars and fats along with the percentage of alcohol must therefore be taken into account when determining the kilojoules consumed. A standard drink—regardless of the concentration of ethanol it contains—is defined as containing 10 grams of alcohol.

Metabolism of alcohol

Ethanol is readily absorbed in the jejunum and is one of the few substances that is absorbed from the stomach. It is distributed evenly throughout the body fluids, as it moves across cellular membranes, including the blood–brain barrier, breast and placenta. As such, blood and all organ systems (including the brain, breast milk and the foetus) reach a peak concentration of alcohol very quickly after consumption. The majority of alcohol is metabolised in the liver, although a small percentage is metabolised as it passes through the stomach wall, which is known as first-pass metabolism. A small amount of alcohol is passed through the urine and some is excreted in the breath, which is why breath testing can be used to detect blood alcohol levels.

Alcohol can be metabolised via three pathways (Zakhari 2006). The major pathway is through alcohol dehydrogenase in the liver. Ethanol is converted to acetaldehyde, followed by the conversion of acetaldehyde to acetic acid by aldehyde dehydrogenase. The lack of this enzyme in some people leads to alcohol flush reaction (Asian flush), which is characterised by facial flushing, light-headedness, palpitations and nausea.

The second pathway for ethanol metabolism occurs in the smooth endoplasmic reticulum (ER) system, and is referred to as the microsomal ethanol-oxidising system (MEOS) with cytochrome P450. The microsomes are induced on the ER after chronic alcohol consumption and, like alcohol dehydrogenase, ethanol is converted to acetaldehyde.

The third pathway for metabolism of ethanol to acetaldehyde is through an enzyme called catalase; however this is a very minor pathway, unless alcohol is consumed in a fasted state.

Health effects of alcohol

Ethanol is a depressant of the brain and nerve tissues (central nervous system) and affects a number of neurochemical processes, leading to an increased risk of suffering mental health problems, including alcohol dependence, depression and anxiety. Alcohol also impacts on other physiological processes in the body. Alcohol increases the risk of developing several chronic diseases (high blood pressure, cardiovascular disease and liver disease) as well as certain cancers (mouth, throat, oesophageal, liver, colorectal and breast). Importantly, if consumed as part of after-game celebrations, alcohol can limit athletes' ability to adhere to nutrition recovery plans (see Chapter 11).

Alcohol recommendations

Since alcohol does not provide any essential nutrients, and because it is also a drug, it is not listed in the NRVs (NHMRC 2009). However, the NHMRC has provided guidelines for consumption, which balance the health risks with any benefits.

Guideline 1: For healthy men and women, drinking no more than two standard drinks on any day reduces the lifetime risk of harm from alcohol-related disease or injury.

Guideline 2: For healthy men and women, drinking no more than four standard drinks on a single occasion reduces the risk of alcohol-related injury arising from that occasion.

Guideline 3: Parents and carers should be advised that children under 15 years of age are at the greatest risk of harm from drinking and that for this age group, not drinking alcohol is especially important. For young people aged 15–17 years, the safest option is to delay the initiation of drinking for as long as possible.

Guideline 4: For women who are pregnant or planning a pregnancy, not drinking is the safest option. For women who are breastfeeding, not drinking is the safest option.

SUMMARY AND KEY MESSAGES

The macronutrients, protein, fat and carbohydrate, play a key role in nutrition. They are metabolised to provide energy for the body and act as building blocks for cells, tissues and organs, and/or are precursors to essential hormones, immune mediators and enzymes. Alcohol, which provides energy, is not strictly considered a macronutrient as it also has drug-like properties in the body and can negatively affect health as well as sporting performance. While this chapter provides the background on macronutrients, it is important to remember that people eat food, not nutrients; the application of this nutritional information to food is presented in Chapter 6.

Key messages

- Carbohydrates are an important source of glucose for exercise and performance, but also supply essential B-group vitamins and fibre.
- Both protein and fat contain essential elements required to sustain life: the essential amino acids and essential fatty acids respectively, as well as other essential vitamins.
- The importance of protein and fat in the diet is reflected by their inclusion in the Nutrient Reference Values, which provide recommended intakes for all apparently healthy Australians.
- For athletes (as discussed in Chapter 10) these requirements need to be modified according to the athlete's training and competition schedule.

REFERENCES

Dehghan, M., Mente, A., Zhang, X., et al., 2017, 'Associations of fats and carbohydrate intake with cardiovascular disease and mortality in 18 countries from five continents (PURE): A prospective cohort study', *Lancet*, vol. 390, no. 10107, pp. 20150–62.

Food Standards Australia and New Zealand, 2017, *Trans Fatty Acids*, Canberra, ACT: Food Standards Australia and New Zealand, retrieved from <www.foodstandards.gov.au/consumer/nutrition/transfat/Pages/default.aspx>.

Fowler, S.P., Williams, K., Resendez, R.G., et al., 2008, 'Fueling the Obesity Epidemic? Artificially sweetened beverage use and long-term weight gain', *Obesity*, vol. 16, no. 8, pp. 1894–1900.

Hodgson, J.M., 2011, 'Protein' and 'Digestion of food', in Wahlqvist, M.L. (ed.), *Food and Nutrition: Food and health systems in Australia and New Zealand*, 3rd edn, Sydney, NSW: Allen & Unwin, pp. 295–327.

Jones, G.P. & Hodgson, J.M., 2011, 'Carbohydrates' and 'Fats', in Wahlqvist, M.L. (ed.), *Food and Nutrition: Food and health systems in Australia and New Zealand*, 3rd edn, Sydney, NSW: Allen & Unwin, pp. 268–94.

Manning, M., Smith, C. & Mazerolle, P., 2013, *The Societal Costs of Alcohol Misuse in Australia*, Trends and Issues in Crime and Criminal Justice, No. 454, Canberra, ACT: Australian Institute of Criminology.

National Health and Medical Research Council, Australian Government Department of Health and Ageing, New Zealand Ministry of Health, 2006, *Nutrient Reference Values for Australia and New Zealand*, Canberra, ACT: National Health and Medical Research Council.

National Health and Medical Research Council, 2009, *Australian Guidelines to Reduce Health Risks from Drinking Alcohol*, Canberra, ACT: National Health and Medical Research Council.

National Health and Medical Research Council, 2013, *Australian Dietary Guidelines*, Canberra, ACT: National Health and Medical Research Council.

World Health Organization (WHO), 2015, *Guideline: Sugar Intake for Adults and Children*, Geneva: World Health Organization.

Zakhari, S., 2006, 'Overview: How is alcohol metabolized in the body?', *Alcohol Research and Health*, vol. 29, no. 4, pp. 245–54.

CHAPTER 5

Micronutrients and antioxidants

Gina Trakman

Micronutrients are substances that humans need in small quantities for normal physiological function. In fact, micronutrients have roles in almost every human body system. They are required for energy metabolism, nervous system function, bone and teeth health, blood health, eye health, fluid balance, and function as antioxidants. This chapter looks at the interactive roles (related to athletic training and performance) of micronutrients, athletes' micronutrient requirements, the effect of micronutrient deficiency on athletic performance and the relationship between oxidative stress, antioxidants and exercise.

LEARNING OUTCOMES

Upon completion of this chapter you will be able to:
- identify food sources of the micronutrients that are of concern for athletes
- describe the functions of B-group vitamins, vitamin D, calcium, sodium, potassium, chloride, iron, folate, magnesium and zinc that are relevant to health, athletic performance and training

- identify common micronutrient deficiencies among athletes and describe the impact of micronutrient deficiencies on athletic performance
- define and describe the implications of oxidative stress for athletic performance
- identify common antioxidants and determine whether athletes should use anti-oxidant supplements.

MICRONUTRIENTS

It is important to consume micronutrients in the correct amount through our diet (Figure 5.1), since both deficiencies and excesses in intake can negatively affect general health. There are two types of micronutrients—vitamins and minerals. The vitamins were given their name because they are 'vital' to life and were once thought to contain an amine group (we now know they do not). Vitamins are organic compounds—they are classed as **water-soluble** (B-group vitamins and vitamin C) or **fat-soluble** (A, D, E, K). The minerals are inorganic chemical elements (such as magnesium) or compounds of

Water soluble

Compounds that can be dissolved in water and are found in the aqueous parts of the body (or food). Water-soluble vitamins are not stored in the body; they are excreted in the urine.

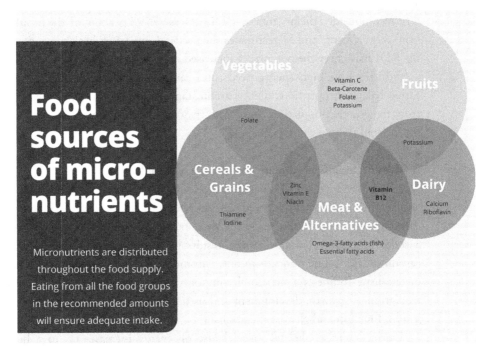

Figure 5.1. Food sources of micronutrients

Source: Gina Trakman.

Fat soluble
Compounds that can be dissolved in lipids (fats or oils) and are found in the lipids of the body (or food). Fat-soluble vitamins are stored in the body.

elements (such as sodium chloride). Minerals are grouped based on the quantities that they are required in by the body. The recommended intake for the macrominerals (calcium, chloride, magnesium, phosphorus, potassium, sodium, sulphur) exceeds 100 micrograms per day. Microminerals (copper, iron, zinc, molybdenum, manganese, selenium, fluoride) are needed in smaller amounts.

Determining micronutrient requirements

As described in Chapter 4, the Nutrient Reference Values (NRVs) are determined based on a variety of measures, including linking metabolic studies with dietary intakes of those nutrients in the population. Exercise can lead to increased micronutrient utilisation and degradation, as well as losses of minerals in sweat and urine. Athletes also often have high lean muscle mass and therefore may need extra micronutrients for muscle repair and maintenance (Woolf & Manore 2006). However, there is insufficient evidence to set specific NRVs for active individuals. As discussed in Chapter 4, the NRVs are intended to be used to assess populations and caution should be taken applying them to evaluate the adequacy of an individual's diet (athlete or otherwise). The recommended dietary intake (RDI) covers 97–98 per cent of the healthy population's requirements and overestimates the needs of almost all healthy people; therefore, the RDI may cover the potentially increased requirements of athletes.

Athletes have high energy needs and can usually avoid nutrient deficiencies by eating balanced, nutritious diets. Circumstances in which athletes' needs may differ from the general population, and where they are at risk of deficiency, are discussed in more detail throughout this chapter.

B vitamins, iodine, chromium and energy metabolism

Many of the B vitamins (thiamin, riboflavin, niacin, pantothenic acid, vitamin B6 and biotin) are needed for energy production, protein and fatty acid synthesis, and carbohydrate metabolism. Several of these nutrients are cofactors in the Krebs cycle, a series of chemical reactions that results in the release of chemical energy (and carbon dioxide). The minerals iodine, chromium and iron are also involved in energy metabolism. Iodine is a structural component of thyroid hormones, responsible for regulation of growth, development and metabolic rate, and chromium is required for insulin function and glucose metabolism.

During exercise, skeletal muscle's use of energy increases up to a hundredfold (Rodriguez et al. 2009). In fact, thiamin and riboflavin intake are sometimes reported as 'micrograms per 100 kilocalories', because of their importance in energy production

(Lukaski 2004). Since B vitamins are widely distributed throughout the food types (Figure 5.1), most athletes can achieve adequate intakes for meeting their energy needs provided they eat a balanced diet. However, deficiencies in riboflavin and vitamin B6 have been reported in female athletes who are vegetarian or have eating disorders.

Mild riboflavin and B6 deficiencies do not appear to lead to diminished aerobic capacity. Despite the lack of evidence for their efficacy, B vitamin supplements are often marketed to active individuals, with claims that they are required in 'times of physical stress' to support energy production and reduce fatigue. Supplementation is unlikely to be harmful because B vitamins are water-soluble and thus are excreted in urine. However, athletes should be aware that there is an upper level of intake (UL) set for B6, niacin and folate. Excess B6 intake via supplementation can lead to sensory neuropathy, which often presents as pain and numbness in the hands and feet. Symptoms of niacin toxicity include itchy, red or warm skin, dizziness, leg cramps, muscle pain and insomnia. The upper limit for folate is set because excesses in folic acid can mask vitamin B12 deficiencies.

Calcium, vitamin D and bone health

Calcium is a structural component of bone. It combines with phosphorus to form hydroxyapatite, a hard, crystalline structure that gives bones their strength. Vitamin D increases absorption of calcium and phosphorus from the gut. Magnesium and fluoride also play a role in mineralising bones. Finally, several proteins associated with bone turnover (for example, osteocalcin) require vitamin K for their synthesis. One of the best dietary sources of calcium is the dairy food group, such as milk, cheese and yoghurt. Phosphorus is found in most foods that are high in protein. Small amounts of vitamin D are also found in dairy, eggs, mushrooms and fortified margarine; however, to achieve adequate levels of vitamin D, appropriate exposure to sunlight is needed. Vitamin D exists on our skin as 7-dehydrocholesterol, which is activated upon exposure to ultraviolet B (UVB) rays. Sun exposure recommendations vary from six minutes per day (Cairns, Australia, summer) to 40 minutes per day (Christchurch, New Zealand, winter) (Nowson et al. 2012).

Physical activity does not appear to increase calcium or vitamin D losses or turnover. In fact, regular exercise (especially resistance activity) increases bone density by stimulating bone-building mechanisms. However, overtraining is known to decrease the production of the sex hormone oestrogen, which plays a vital role in maintaining bone mass, especially in females (Maughan 1999). Low bone mass and density will increase the risk of stress fractures and thus can have a detrimental effect on an athlete's ability to perform. Female athletes with eating disorders are at particular risk of stress fractures because their calcium intake is likely to be low, and it is probable that they have menstrual dysfunction, which is associated with decreased oestrogen production (Rodriguez et al. 2009).

Calcium status is difficult to measure, because the bone acts as a calcium reservoir and serum calcium levels are maintained within a relatively small window. Vitamin D status is measured based on circulating levels of 25-hydroxycholecalciferol (25(OH) D). Cut-off points for deficiency vary (see Table 5.1).

Vitamin D deficiency appears to be widespread among athletes and non-athletes (Rodriguez et al. 2009). In 2011–12 the estimated prevalence of vitamin D deficiency in Australian adults was 23 per cent. In New Zealand in 2008–09, the prevalence of individuals (aged 18 years and older) with vitamin D levels below the recommended average, including those with frank vitamin D deficiency, was 32 per cent. Data specifically on Australian and New Zealander athletes is limited. In general, the athletes at the greatest risk of vitamin D deficiency are those with dark skin, those who compete indoors, and those who live at high altitudes. All athletes with diagnosed deficiency should take a vitamin D supplement as prescribed by their doctor or dietitian (Powers et al. 2011). It is also recommended that (pending nutritional assessment) athletes with disordered eating and **amenorrhea** supplement their diet with 1500 micrograms of calcium and 400–800 International Units (IU) of vitamin D per day.

Amenorrhea
The absence or cessation of menstruation. Primary amenorrhea is defined as the delay of the first menstruation past 16 years of age. Secondary amenorrhea is defined as the absence of three to six consecutive cycles.

Calcium and vitamin D: other roles

Calcium has additional roles in muscle contraction, nerve conduction and blood clotting. Emerging evidence indicates that vitamin D also has a role in muscle tissue function. The discovery of a vitamin D receptor in skeletal muscle provided a

Table 5.1. Vitamin D status based on serum 25(OH)D (nmol/L) levels

Sports medicine (Powers et al. 2011)		General population (Nowson et al. 2012)	
Status	25(OH) D levels (nmol/L)	Status	25(OH) D levels (nmol/L)
Optimal	Not established	NR	NR
Sufficient	100	Adequate levels	>50
Insufficient*	50–80	Mild deficiency	30–49
Marginal deficiency	25–50	Moderate deficiency	13–29

biologically plausible explanation for observations that athletic performance improves in the summer and with exposure to UVB radiation. More recent research has shown that vitamin D status is correlated with jumping height and velocity, muscle strength and muscle power. However, at present there is insufficient evidence to set an 'optimal' level for Serum 25(OH) D for athletes, or to recommend vitamin D as an **ergogenic aid** (Powers et al. 2011).

Ergogenic aid
Any substance or aid that improves physical performance.

Iron, B12, folate and blood health

Iron is a structural component of **haemoglobin**, a protein in red blood cells that is responsible for the transport of oxygen to tissues. Iron is also a cofactor for enzymes that participate in the electron transport chain, a series of reactions that are needed for the synthesis of ATP, the body's energy carrier (see Chapter 2). Given its role in energy production and cell metabolism, it is clear that iron is an essential nutrient for athletes, especially endurance athletes. The iron needs of athletes can be more than 70 per cent higher than the recommendations for the general population (Rodriguez et al. 2009). Requirements, however, are often not met. **Iron deficiency anaemia** (IDA) is the most common nutrient deficiency among the general population and athletes. Athletes who are at particular risk of iron deficiency include:

Haemoglobin
The protein unit in the red blood cell that carries oxygen.

Iron deficiency anaemia
Depletion of iron levels in the blood that leads to low levels of haemoglobin and small pale red blood cells, which limits their capacity to carry oxygen.

Haemolysis
The rupture of red blood cells.

- athletes on energy restricted diets (most common reason)
- adolescent athletes (periods of rapid growth increase iron needs)
- vegetarian athletes (plant sources of iron are poorly absorbed)
- female athletes who are menstruating (iron is excreted through blood loss)
- athletes who undertake altitude training (increased production of red blood cells requires iron, along with other nutrients such as B12 and folate)
- endurance athletes, especially runners (pounding the pavement destroys red blood cells, often described as 'foot strike **haemolysis**')
- athletes who are injured (iron is needed for wound healing)
- athletes who donate blood.

There are a range of biomarkers used to assess iron status, including total iron binding capacity (TIBC), serum ferritin (SF), transferrin saturation, haemoglobin (Hb) and mean cell volume (MCV). Iron depletion occurs in three stages, as depicted in Figure 5.2.

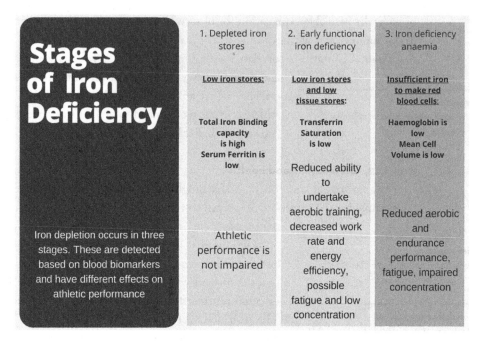

Figure 5.2. Stages of iron deficiency

Source: Image inspired by Deakin 2010.

Transferrin
An iron transport protein in the blood.

Iron is carried around the blood by a protein called **transferrin**; when blood iron stores are low, TIBC increases so that transferrin can bind to more of the available iron and, at the same time, SF levels drop. When transferrin saturation (serum iron/TIBC) is below 16 per cent, the body is experiencing early functional iron deficiency. If iron deficiency progresses further, the body is unable to make haemoglobin and the MCV of red blood cells decreases, leading to iron deficiency anaemia (IDA).

The final 'stage' of iron deficiency, IDA, has deleterious effects on athletic performance and also impacts concentration and, therefore, the ability to make tactical decisions during play (Deakin 2010). Correction of IDA with supplements increases **work capacity**, reduces heart rate and decreases lactate concentrations (Rodriguez et al. 2009). Supplementation in individuals with early functional iron deficiency (stage 2) may also improve work capacity, but research results regarding this are mixed. Reversing iron deficiency can take time (3–6 months) and requires supplementation. Unfortunately, iron supplements are often poorly tolerated by the gut. Therefore, at-risk athletes should be regularly screened (via blood test) and focus on

Work capacity
The total amount of work a person can sustain over a defined period of time.

Sports anaemia

Also referred to as dilutional anaemia or pseudo-anaemia, occurs when haemoglobin concentration is 'diluted' due to increased volume of the plasma (the liquid component of blood). Plasma volume generally increases in response to exercise; therefore, this 'anaemia' is transient and often fluctuates with training loads. Unlike the other anaemias described in this chapter, sports anaemia does not impair athletic performance or respond to nutritional changes.

preventing the development of IDA by obtaining adequate iron from foods. Red meat, chicken, fish and eggs are the best dietary sources of iron. Wholegrains, leafy greens, nuts and seeds also provide some iron. These vegetarian sources should be combined with vitamin C to increase absorption. Consumption of tannins (tea, coffee, wine) and calcium should be avoided when eating iron-rich foods because they inhibit iron absorption.

Vitamin B12 and folate are needed for the formation of red blood cells and have roles in protein synthesis, tissue repair and nervous system functioning. These nutrients are often low in the diets of vegetarians, females and energy restricting athletes. Inadequate intake of folate and vitamin B12 will lead to folate deficiency anaemia and B12 deficiency anaemia respectively. These anaemias are also associated with decreased endurance performance (Lukaski 2004). Folate is found in green leafy vegetables and wholegrains; B12 is found exclusively in animal foods—meat, chicken, fish, eggs and dairy.

Zinc and magnesium

Zinc and magnesium are cofactors for several enzymes involved in energy metabolism. Zinc also has roles in growth, building and repairing muscle tissue, and immune status—all relevant functions for athletes. Magnesium is needed for immune function, protein synthesis and muscle contraction. Athletes may experience magnesium and zinc loss through sweat, urine and faeces, but mineral losses are difficult to measure accurately. Studies comparing the magnesium status of athletes and non-athletes have concluded that they are similar. In contrast, endurance athletes have been found to have impaired zinc status in several studies (Lukaski 2004). Zinc and magnesium deficiencies occur predominantly among vegetarian, female and weight class athletes. Zinc deficiency can impair athletic performance by reducing cardiorespiratory function, muscle strength and endurance. Likewise, magnesium deficiency has been reported to increase oxygen requirements for performing submaximal activities (Rodriguez et al. 2009).

Magnesium supplementation to correct pre-existing deficiencies has been shown to improve performance. On the other hand, there is limited data to confirm a beneficial effect of zinc supplementation on performance. Zinc may have an indirect effect because it has been shown to enhance immune function and, therefore, could protect athletes' ability to train (Kreider et al. 2010). In general, however, single-dose zinc supplements are not recommended because they can interfere with absorption of iron and calcium and lead to zinc toxicity.

Potassium, sodium, chloride and fluid balance

Sodium is the main **cation** in extracellular fluid, potassium the main cation in intracellular fluid, and chloride the main **anion** in intracellular fluid. Together, these **electrolytes** maintain fluid balance. Sodium and phosphorus also act to ensure acid–base balance of body fluids and both sodium and potassium have additional roles in nerve-impulse transmission and muscle contraction. Athletes experience electrolyte losses through sweat and, therefore, have higher sodium and chloride needs than the general population (Rodriguez et al. 2009).

Sodium and chloride are often found together in foods as sodium chloride (salt). Table salt, soy sauce and other commercial sauces, processed foods, meat, milk and bread are all sources of sodium chloride. The mean sodium intake in Australians aged 19–30 exceeds the UL recommended for the general population (ABS 2014). Therefore, many athletes meet their increased salt needs incidentally. However, for athletes participating in endurance events, sports drinks containing electrolytes are frequently recommended. This is discussed in more detail in Chapter 11. Most athletes can meet their potassium needs through regular food intake by including potassium-rich foods such as fruit, vegetables and dairy.

Cations
Positively charged ions, which means they have gained electrons.

Anions
Negatively charged ions, which means they have lost electrons.

Electrolytes
Salts that dissolve in water and disassociate into charged particles called ions.

Antioxidants

Antioxidants prevent oxidative stress and have been extensively studied for their potential ability to reduce the **pathogenesis** of multiple chronic diseases. Antioxidants have received much media attention, and most people have heard of them at some time or another. Vitamin C (found in fruits and vegetables) and vitamin E (found in oils, nuts, seeds and wheat germ) have antioxidant functions. Vitamin E is fat soluble and, therefore, acts within cell membranes to prevent polyunsaturated fatty acids (PUFAs) and other phospholipids from being oxidised. Vitamin C regenerates vitamin E. After vitamin E has performed its antioxidant function, it will have an unpaired electron. Vitamin C regenerates vitamin E by donating an electron to (re) neutralise vitamin E. Several other compounds found in foods also have antioxidant functions, including:

Pathogenesis
The biological mechanism that leads to the development of diseases.

- lycopene (found in tomatoes)
- beta-carotene (found in orange and green fruits and vegetables)
- curcumin (found in turmeric)
- resveratrol (found in grapes and wine)

- quercetin (found in fruits and vegetables)
- isoflavones (found in soy).

Endogenous
Substances that originate or derive from within the body, in this case from body stores.

Free radicals
Also referred to as reactive oxygen species, free radicals are highly reactive chemical species that can damage cellular components, resulting in cell injury or death. They are usually produced by oxidation and contain an unpaired electron.

Antioxidants
Substances that decrease free radical damage by donating an electron to 'neutralise' free radicals.

Oxidative stress
Occurs when the body's production of free radicals occurs at a rate higher than the body's ability to neutralise them.

In addition to these food sources, the body has several **endogenous** antioxidant systems. Selenium and the amino acids cysteine and taurine have roles in these systems, as donors for thiol-based antioxidants.

Antioxidant supplements and antioxidant rich foods (for example, Montmorency cherry and exotic berries such as goji berries) are popular among athletes, but their use is controversial. The arguments for and against antioxidant supplementation in athletes are outlined below.

In addition to being studied for their potential to reduce oxidative stress, the effect of antioxidant supplementation on performance and recovery has been assessed. There is limited evidence to support their use in these situations.

Although antioxidant supplements are not (generally) recommended, a diet rich in antioxidants is encouraged. Practical tips for increasing antioxidants include the following.

- Go for 2&5—aim to have two servings of fruit and five of vegetables daily. Add fruit to breakfast cereals and

Table 5.2. Summary of functional roles of micronutrients related to athletic performance

Energy, macronutrient metabolism and macronutrient synthesis	Muscle contraction	Fluid balance	Bone health	Blood health	Immune function
Thiamin (B1) Riboflavin (B2) Niacin (B3) Pantothenic acid (B5) Biotin Pyridoxine(B6) Iodine Chromium Iron Zinc Magnesium	Magnesium Sodium	Sodium Potassium Chloride Phosphorus	Vitamin D Vitamin K Calcium Phosphorus Magnesium	Vitamin B12 Vitamin K Iron Folate	Vitamin C Iron Zinc

choose it as a snack. Add vegetables to main meals (grate into sauces, put on sandwiches) and snack on cherry tomatoes, carrots, celery and cucumber.
- Choose wholegrains over processed grains.
- Swap some meat/chicken/fish meals for tofu and lentils.
- Snack on nuts.
- Choose dark chocolate as a sweet treat.

SUMMARY AND KEY MESSAGES

Micronutrients (vitamins, minerals, antioxidants) are needed in small amounts for normal physiological functioning. They are distributed throughout the food supply and have roles relevant to athletic performance, including energy production, maintenance of bone health, control of fluid balance, muscle contraction and nerve impulse control.

Key messages
- There is insufficient evidence to set specific quantitative micronutrient recommendations for athletes which differ from the general recommendations.
- Athletes have increased needs for iron, sodium and potassium and may also have increased B vitamin, magnesium and zinc requirements, but this is yet to be demonstrated in research studies.
- Most athletes can meet their micronutrient needs by consuming a balanced diet that contains adequate energy (kilojoules).
- Certain athletes are at risk of nutrient deficiency. Common risk factors include being female, being vegetarian, participating in endurance activities, being on an energy restricted diet and disordered eating behaviours.
- The most common deficiency among athletes is iron deficiency; low serum levels of magnesium, zinc, vitamin D and low intakes of riboflavin and vitamin B6 are also reported among athletic populations.
- Deficiencies should be addressed by altering dietary intake. In most instances, micronutrient supplementation is also warranted and has been shown to improve performance. Supplementation should be based on blood test results and nutritional analysis and be supervised by qualified professionals.
- Micronutrient intakes (through food or supplements) above physiological requirements are very unlikely to have any ergogenic effects.
- Antioxidant nutrients (vitamins A, C, E and selenium) and food polyphenols have received much attention for their potential ability to enhance recovery from exercise by reducing oxidative stress. At present, the consensus is that antioxidant supplementation should be avoided due to lack of evidence and the potential adverse effects on adaptations to training.

REFERENCES

Australian Bureau of Statistics (ABS), 2014, *Australian Health Survey: Nutrition First Results—Foods and Nutrients 2011–12* [Online], Australian Bureau of Statistics, <http://www.abs.gov.au/ausstats/abs@.nsf/mf/4364.0.55.010>, accessed 20 July 2017.

Deakin, V., 2010, 'Prevention, detection and treatment of iron depletion in athletes', in Burke, L.M. & Deakin, V. (eds), *Clinical Sports Nutrition*, Australia: McGraw-Hill Education.

Kreider, R.B., Wilborn, C.D., Taylor, L. et al., 2010, 'ISSN exercise & sport nutrition review: Research & recommendations', *Journal of the International Society of Sports Nutrition*, vol. 7, p. 7.

Lukaski, H.C., 2004, 'Vitamin and mineral status: Effects on physical performance', *Nutrition*, vol. 20, no. 7-8, pp. 632–44.

Maughan, R.J., 1999, 'Role of micronutrients in sport and physical activity', *British Medical Bulletin*, vol. 55, no. 3, pp. 683–90.

Nowson, C.A., McGrath, J.J., Ebeling, P.R., et al., 2012, 'Vitamin D and health in adults in Australia and New Zealand: A position statement', *Medical Journal of Australia*, vol. 196, no. 11, pp. 686–7.

Powers, S., Nelson, W.B. & Larson-Meyer, E., 2011, 'Antioxidant and vitamin D supplements for athletes: Sense or nonsense?', *Journal of Sports Sciences*, vol. 29, suppl. 1, pp. S47–55.

Rodriguez, N.R., DiMarco, N.M. & Langley, S., 2009, 'Position of the American Dietetic Association, Dietitians of Canada, and the American College of Sports Medicine: Nutrition and athletic performance', *Journal of the American Dietetic Association*, vol. 109, no. 3, pp. 509–27.

Woolf, K. & Manore, M.M., 2006, 'B-vitamins and exercise: Does exercise alter requirements?', *International Journal of Sport Nutrition & Exercise Metabolism*, vol. 16, no. 5, pp. 453–84.

CHAPTER 6

Translating nutrition: From nutrients to foods

Adrienne Forsyth

The preceding chapters have provided us with an overview of the nutrients needed for good health and performance. We now understand why we need these nutrients; however, planning a nutritious diet is a complex task because we consume these nutrients as part of whole foods within the context of a diet influenced by a range of sociocultural, environmental and individual factors. The factors that influence our diet will be discussed in later chapters. In this chapter, we will explore how to meet our nutrient requirements through food and identify good food choices to meet the macro- and micronutrient requirements of athletes.

LEARNING OUTCOMES

Upon completion of this chapter you will be able to:
* understand the rationale for food-based dietary recommendations

- describe how whole food diets can be used to meet individual nutrient requirements
- identify food sources of macro- and micronutrients required by athletes
- recommend specific foods and food combinations to meet individual nutrient requirements.

FOOD IS MADE UP OF MORE THAN NUTRIENTS

Chapters 4 and 5 have described the role of a number of nutrients for health and performance. It is tempting to try to put together a magic bullet nutrient supplement to meet these needs. Indeed, we can obtain all of our micronutrient requirements from nutrient supplements. However, when we aim to consume our nutrient requirements in the form of food, we gain more than we would if we consumed supplements alone.

There are many benefits of consuming nutrients as part of whole foods rather than from supplements. To begin with, we know that some nutrients are absorbed better as part of a whole food. For example, the lactose in milk may assist with calcium absorption. Foods can also have a **synergistic** effect in promoting nutrient absorption and function. When plant sources of iron, such as beans, are consumed with a source of vitamin C, such as orange juice, the vitamin C assists with iron absorption and therefore increases its availability in the body. Many nutrients are also more effective when consumed as part of a whole food diet. Omega-3 fatty acids derived from eating fish are often found to be more effective in preventing conditions such as **ischaemic heart disease** than omega-3 supplements alone. Whole foods also often bundle nutrients in a convenient package. For example, dairy foods such as milk contain not only calcium but also magnesium and phosphorus, which work with calcium to help build and maintain strong bones. Alongside vitamins and minerals, foods provide a range of other compounds with beneficial actions, such as fibre and **phytonutrients**. Foods also often conveniently provide nutrients where they are needed. Wholegrains are good sources of B vitamins, and B vitamins are needed to help derive energy from the carbohydrates in wholegrains. Vitamin E is found in plant oils and helps to prevent oxidisation of the oil and minimise damage from **free radicals** in our bodies. Whole foods also have the added benefit of providing pleasure, creating an opportunity for

Synergistic
The interaction of two or more substances, in this case nutrients, to produce a combined beneficial effect that is greater than the sum of its individual effects.

Ischaemic heart disease
Also called coronary artery disease, a group of diseases including angina, myocardial infarction and sudden coronary death. The pathogenesis of this disease is due to the restriction of blood flow in the coronary arteries that results in reduced blood flow, and hence oxygen supply, to the heart muscle.

Phytonutrients
Substances found in plant foods that have a beneficial health effect, such as lycopene in tomatoes and anthocyanin in blueberries.

Toxicity
Occurs when nutrients are consumed in very high amounts and cause health problems. For example, very high levels of vitamin A consumed by pregnant women have been linked to birth defects. Toxicity is most likely to occur with overconsumption of fat-soluble vitamins and some minerals.

socialisation and promoting rest and relaxation during eating. On the other hand, supplements can be expensive, run the risk of **toxicity** with overconsumption, and may contain unwanted compounds or contaminants, which is particularly problematic for many competitive athletes.

Now, with an understanding of the importance of consuming our nutrients as part of a whole food diet, we need to learn what foods to consume to meet our nutrient requirements.

DIETARY GUIDELINES

Accredited Practising Dietitians
Health professionals who have completed a university degree in dietetics and have been accredited by the Dietitians Association of Australia to provide a range of nutrition-related services, including individualised medical nutrition therapy. In New Zealand, these professionals are known as Registered Dietitians.

Accredited Sports Dietitians
Accredited Practising Dietitians who have completed extra training and practical experience in sports nutrition and are accredited by Sports Dietitians Australia to provide nutrition services for athletes.

Australia and New Zealand each have their own evidence-based dietary guidelines designed to help the population make food choices that will meet their dietary requirements and promote good health. The Australian Dietary Guidelines (NHMRC 2013) and the New Zealand Eating and Activity Guidelines (Ministry of Health 2015) provide broad public health recommendations that have been developed by expert panels based on the analysis of data from published research. The advice in these guidelines is intended for healthy individuals to maintain good health. Individuals with medical conditions that require specialised medical nutrition therapy should seek advice from an **Accredited Practising Dietitian**. Athletes with specific dietary requirements may use the dietary guidelines as a starting point and should seek individualised advice from an **Accredited Sports Dietitian**.

Box 6.1: Australian Dietary Guidelines

GUIDELINE 1
To achieve and maintain a healthy weight, be physically active and choose amounts of nutritious food and drinks to meet your energy needs.
- Children and adolescents should eat sufficient nutritious foods to grow and develop normally. They should be physically active every day and their growth should be checked regularly.
- Older people should eat nutritious foods and keep physically active to help maintain muscle strength and a healthy weight.

GUIDELINE 2

Enjoy a wide variety of nutritious foods from these five groups every day:

- plenty of vegetables, including different types and colours, and legumes/beans
- fruit
- grain (cereal) foods, mostly wholegrain and/or high-cereal fibre varieties, such as breads, cereals, rice, pasta, noodles, polenta, couscous, oats, quinoa and barley
- lean meats and poultry, fish, eggs, tofu, nuts and seeds, and legumes/beans
- milk, yoghurt, cheese and/or their alternatives, mostly reduced fat (reduced fat milks are not suitable for children under the age of two years).

And drink plenty of water.

GUIDELINE 3

Limit intake of foods containing saturated fat, added salt, added sugars and alcohol.

a. Limit intake of foods high in saturated fat such as many biscuits, cakes, pastries, pies, processed meats, commercial burgers, pizza, fried foods, potato chips, crisps and other savoury snacks.
   - Replace high-fat foods which contain predominantly saturated fats such as butter, cream, cooking margarine, coconut and palm oil with foods that contain predominantly poly-unsaturated and monounsaturated fats such as oils, spreads, nut butters/pastes and avocado.
   - Low-fat diets are not suitable for children under the age of two years.
b. Limit intake of foods and drinks containing added salt.
   - Read labels to choose lower-sodium options among similar foods.
   - Do not add salt to foods in cooking or at the table.
c. Limit intake of foods and drinks containing added sugars such as confectionery, sugar-sweetened soft drinks and cordials, fruit drinks, vitamin waters, energy and sports drinks.
d. If you choose to drink alcohol, limit intake. For women who are pregnant, planning a pregnancy or breastfeeding, not drinking alcohol is the safest option.

GUIDELINE 4
Encourage, support and promote breastfeeding.

GUIDELINE 5
Care for your food; prepare and store it safely.

Source: NHMRC 2013.

Box 6.2: New Zealand Eating and Body Weight Statements

EATING STATEMENT 1
Enjoy a variety of nutritious foods every day, including:
- plenty of vegetables and fruit
- grain foods, mostly wholegrain and those naturally high in fibre
- some milk and milk products, mostly low and reduced fat
- some legumes, nuts, seeds, fish and other seafood, eggs, poultry and/or red meat with the fat removed.

EATING STATEMENT 2
Choose and/or prepare foods and drinks:
- with unsaturated fats (canola, olive, rice bran or vegetable oil or margarine) instead of saturated fats (butter, cream, lard, dripping, coconut oil)
- that are low in salt (sodium); if using salt, choose iodised salt
- with little or no added sugar
- that are mostly 'whole' and less processed.

EATING STATEMENT 3
Make plain water your first choice over other drinks.

EATING STATEMENT 4
If you drink alcohol, keep your intake low. Stop drinking alcohol if you could be pregnant, are pregnant or are trying to get pregnant.

EATING STATEMENT 5
Buy or gather, prepare, cook and store food in ways that keep it safe to eat.

BODY WEIGHT STATEMENT

Making good choices about what you eat and drink and being physically active are also important to achieve and maintain a healthy body weight.

Being a healthy weight:

- helps you to stay active and well
- reduces your risk of developing Type 2 diabetes, cardiovascular disease and some cancers.

If you are struggling to maintain a healthy weight, see your doctor and/or your community health care provider.

Source: Ministry of Health 2015.

In addition to these broad statements, the dietary guidelines provide practical tools to assist individuals in putting together a diet that is consistent with the dietary guidelines and meets their nutrient requirements. The Australian Guide to Healthy Eating and the New Zealand Serving Size Advice build upon the Nutrient Reference Values (NHMRC et al. 2006) to provide practical food selection advice. These food selection guides are developed based around groups of foods with similar key nutrient profiles, such as wholegrains. A food modelling system is then used to determine how much of each food group should be consumed to meet an individual's nutrient requirements and only enough energy to meet the needs of the smallest and least active person. This recommended eating pattern is called a **foundation diet**, and it meets one's minimum nutrient needs. Athletes often expend more energy and therefore have higher energy requirements, so they may need to consume more serves of each of the food groups to meet their energy and nutrient requirements. This complete diet is known as a **total diet**. Total diets should be developed for individual athletes based on their size, sex, body composition, activity levels, individual preferences and sport-specific requirements. For example, some athletes may prefer or require more carbohydrate-rich wholegrain foods, while others require more protein-rich meat and alternatives. The food selection guides can be found online at the Australian government's Eat for Health website (www.eatforhealth.gov.au/).

Many countries have their own dietary guidelines and food selection guides, based on their own best evidence and culturally appropriate foods. You will learn more about culturally diverse dietary patterns in Chapter 25.

Foundation diet
A food-modelling system that determines how much of each food group should be consumed to meet an individual's nutrient requirements and only enough energy to meet the needs of the smallest and least active person.

Total diet
The dietary pattern that is determined, using the Foundation Diet as the basis, to account for additional energy and nutrient needs for an individual.

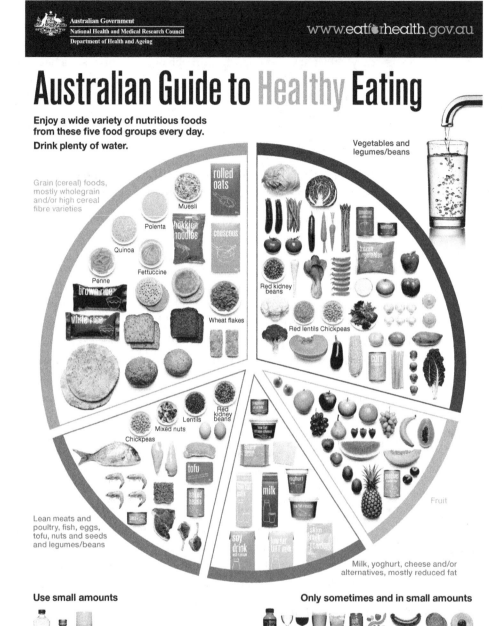

Figure 6.1. Australian Guide to Healthy Eating

Source: NHMRC 2013.

FOOD SOURCES OF MACRONUTRIENTS

Carbohydrates are found in foods in the form of starch or sugar. Starchy foods include:

- breads, rolls, wraps, bagels, muffins and crumpets
- breakfast cereals and porridge
- rice, pasta and noodles
- potato, sweet potato and corn.

Sugary foods include:

- lollies
- fruit (in the form of fructose)
- milk (in the form of lactose)
- table sugar, honey and maple syrup.

Some carbohydrate foods provide more nutrition than others. Lollies and added sugars can provide enjoyment and increase the palatability of foods, but are not health-promoting as they contain no or very little nutrition (these foods are referred to as **energy dense** and nutrient-poor). For good health, it is recommended that we consume foods that fit within the food groups in the food selection guides and choose the higher fibre options, such as wholegrain bread, brown rice and potatoes in their skins. For athletes, the timing of fibre intake is important; high-fibre foods should be avoided in the hours leading up to a training session to avoid gastrointestinal discomfort. Some people also experience unpleasant symptoms, such as gas, bloating, constipation and diarrhoea, after consuming some types of carbohydrates. Fermentable oligosaccharides, disaccharides, monosaccharides and polyols (FODMAPs) are poorly absorbed by some individuals and can cause these unpleasant symptoms. For others, these symptoms may occur following consumption of gluten-containing foods. Gluten is a protein contained in some carbohydrate-rich foods, such as wheat-based breads and cereals. Strategies for managing FODMAP intolerance and other gastrointestinal problems will be discussed in Chapter 23.

Energy dense
Foods that contain high levels of energy with little or no nutrients.

Protein is found predominantly in foods derived from animals. Meat, poultry, fish, eggs and dairy products are all good sources of protein. However, individuals may limit their intake of animal sources of protein due to the cost, or their personal preference to avoid animal food sources for ethical, environmental or religious reasons. Animal sources of protein may also contain high levels of saturated fats, but intake of these fats can be minimised by selecting lean cuts of meat, skinless poultry and reduced fat dairy products. Nuts, seeds and legumes such as beans, lentils and chickpeas are good options for vegetarian athletes and those looking for lower fat or less expensive sources of protein. It is important to keep in mind that vegetable sources of protein are considered incomplete (that is, they do not contain all of the essential amino acids) or limiting (that is, they contain very small amounts of the essential amino acids relative to requirements). So, vegetarians should aim to consume a variety of protein-containing foods to obtain all essential amino acids. See Table 6.1 for examples of complementary proteins.

These foods can be simply combined to make complete proteins—for example, peanut butter (legumes) on toast (grains), or beans (legumes) and rice (grains).

Leucine
An essential amino acid, which is required for muscle protein synthesis.

The amino acid **leucine** plays a role in stimulating muscle protein synthesis, making it an important part of the diet for athletes, especially masters athletes (Chapter 19) and those recovering from injury (Chapter 24). Whey protein, which makes up 20 per cent of the protein in dairy foods, is a good source of leucine, so dairy foods and whey protein supplements are popular among athletes.

To reduce their risk of developing chronic diseases, it is important for athletes and active people to limit their intake of saturated fats and consume moderate amounts of unsaturated fats. Saturated fats are found predominantly in animal products; they are in the fat on red meat, in chicken skin and in cream. Palm and coconut oils are also sources of saturated fat and are often found in commercially prepared baked goods and deep-fried foods. Where possible, these fats should be replaced with health-promoting mono- and polyunsaturated fats. Monounsaturated fats are found in olive oil and walnuts and are known to help reduce the risk of developing chronic diseases such as diabetes and cardiovascular disease. Omega-3 polyunsaturated fats are found predominantly in fish and help to reduce inflammation, which can support a number of healthy functions including joint health and circulation. For athletes with lower energy requirements, intake of fat may need to be minimised to limit total energy intake. Table 6.2. lists foods that are good sources of macronutrients.

Table 6.1. Food sources of complementary proteins

Food	Limiting amino acid(s)	Complementary food
Legumes	Methionine	Grains, nuts and seeds
Nuts and seeds	Lysine	Legumes
Grains	Lysine, threonine	Legumes
Corn	Tryptophan, lysine	Legumes

Source: Adapted from American Society for Nutrition 2011.

Table 6.2. Good food sources of macronutrients for athletes

Foods rich in carbohydrate	Foods rich in protein	Foods rich in healthy fats
Bread	Milk	Avocado
Rice	Eggs	Nuts
Pasta	Beef	Fish
Breakfast cereal	Chicken	Peanut butter
Porridge (oats)	Fish	Olive oil
Sweet potato	Tofu	Canola oil

FOOD SOURCES OF MICRONUTRIENTS

Every time we eat we have an opportunity to nourish our bodies. Athletes and active people should choose nutrient-dense foods as often as possible to support their bodies' increased nutrient requirements. Active people may have increased demands for calcium, iron, B vitamins and antioxidants, including vitamins C and E. With careful planning, these needs can be met with a whole food diet.

Some athletes may choose to take vitamin and mineral supplements in an effort to meet their nutrient needs. All athletes should be encouraged to consume a whole food diet that aligns with dietary guidelines to meet their nutrient needs; however, should they have concerns about their dietary intake, a multivitamin and mineral supplement may be considered. The supplement should not contain more than the recommended dietary intake of each nutrient unless advised by a doctor or dietitian.

It is important to understand that individual foods can be sources of many different nutrients. For example, milk contains protein, carbohydrate and calcium as well as other vitamins and minerals. You can use the table below to identify foods that will meet multiple nutrient needs. It is important to also consider that some foods that are good sources of some nutrients may also contain large amounts of unhealthy fats,

Table 6.3. Good food sources of select micronutrients for athletes

Foods rich in calcium	Foods rich in iron	Foods rich in vitamin C
Milk	Beef	Citrus fruit
Yoghurt	Lamb	Capsicum
Cheese	Beans	Berries

sugars or salt. For example, commercial peanut butter is a source of protein but is usually made with added fats, sugar and salt. When using Table 6.3, keep in mind that the nutrient values presented are per 100 grams of food, which may not correspond to the amount of food you actually consume.

COMBINING FOODS: MEALS FOR ACTIVE PEOPLE

Since we consume foods as part of meals and in the context of a whole diet, it is important to consider how different foods may fit together to create a healthy eating pattern for athletes and active people. Recreational athletes may focus on developing a healthy eating plan to promote good health, while highly competitive athletes may follow carefully designed eating plans to maximise performance and attain optimal body composition. There are a number of issues that should be considered when creating an eating plan for athletes.

- The amount and timing of carbohydrate and protein intake should be adjusted based on energy expenditure and sport-specific requirements (see Chapters 9 and 10 for more details).
- Fat intake should be adjusted to support appropriate energy intake and body composition goals (see Chapters 13 and 17 for more detail).
- Fibre should be avoided prior to a training session to minimise gastrointestinal disturbances (see Chapter 23 for more detail).
- Special dietary requirements and personal preferences should be considered as part of an individualised dietary plan to maximise satisfaction with and adherence to the diet.
- A variety of enjoyable flavours and textures should be used to encourage consumption.
- Food safety should be considered, especially for athletes eating on the go or travelling in foreign countries (see Chapter 21 for more detail).
- Convenience is important for busy athletes and active people juggling training, work and family commitments.
- Meal planning and time management are important skills to develop to support individuals to make time for healthy eating.
- Cooking skills may need to be taught to support athletes and active people to prepare their own healthy meals.

An example of a one-day eating plan that meets the Australian Dietary Guidelines and the Eating and Activity Guidelines for New Zealand Adults is provided in Box 6.3. This eating plan is just a starting point and may not meet all of an individual's macronutrient or energy requirements. It may also need to be modified to meet individual athletes' personal preferences and dietary requirements.

Table 6.4. Nutrient composition of foods commonly consumed by athletes

Food	Average serving size (g)	Energy (kJ/100 g)	Carbohydrate (g/100 g)	Dietary fibre (g/100 g)	Protein (g/100 g)	Total fat (g/100 g)	Saturated fat (g/100 g)	Monounsaturated fat (g/100 g)	Omega-3 polyunsaturated fat (g/100 g)	Calcium (mg/100 g)	Iron (mg/100 g)
Banana	98 (one medium)	385	19.6	2.4	1.4	0.3	0	0	0	5	0.29
Red apple	164 (one medium)	247	12.4	2.4	0.3	0.4	0	0	0	5	0.21
Orange	162 (one medium)	175	8.0	2.4	1.0	0.1	0	0	0	25	0.37
Strawberry	15 (per strawberry)	108	3.9	2.5	0.7	0.2	0	0	0	18	0.58
Sweet potato (cooked)	344 (one medium)	362	17.2	3.7	2.3	0.1	0	0	0	33	0.61
Broccoli (cooked)	67 (1/2 cup)	114	1.3	2.9	3.3	0.4	0	0	0	30	0.7
Kale	60 (1/2 cup)	70	1.1	1.9	1.6	0.2	0	0	0	78	2.5
Corn (cooked)	89 (1/2 cup)	438	12.8	4.8	4.2	2.8	0.3	0.6	0	3	0.6
Wholemeal bread	64 (two slices)	982	39.7	6.3	9.0	2.9	0.5	1.0	0	92	2.1
White bread	66 (two slices)	1027	45	2.8	9.7	2.1	0.3	0.7	0	62	1.48

Food	Average serving size (g)	Energy (kJ/100 g)	Carbohydrate (g/100 g)	Dietary fibre (g/100 g)	Protein (g/100 g)	Total fat (g/100 g)	Saturated fat (g/100 g)	Monounsaturated fat (g/100 g)	Omega-3 polyunsaturated fat (g/100 g)	Calcium (mg/100 g)	Iron (mg/100 g)
Pasta (cooked)	155 (one cup)	584	28.4	2.1	4.2	0.3	0.1	0	0	8	0.46
Rolled oats (cooked)	260 (one cup)	273	10.2	1.7	2.0	1.4	0.2	0.6	0	9	0.9
Beef rump steak, fat trimmed (cooked)	171 (medium steak)	742	0	0	31.7	5.5	1.9	2.5	0.1	6	3.25
Skinless chicken breast (cooked)	112 (small breast)	598	0	0	29.8	2.5	0.8	1.2	0	5	0.4
Tinned tuna	95 (1/2 cup)	518	0	0	24.8	2.6	0.9	0.5	0.7	12	1.3
Peanut butter	20	2470	12	5.8	22.2	50	8.7	34.7	0	55	1.77
Baked beans	275 (one cup)	355	10.1	5.2	4.9	0.3	0	0	0	40	0.95
Walnuts	30 (one handful)	2904	3	6.4	14.4	69.2	4.4	12.1	0	89	2.5
Full-cream milk	250 (one cup)	293	6.3	0	3.5	3.5	2.3	0.9	0	107	0.04
Skim milk	250 (one cup)	147	5	0	3.7	0.1	0.1	0	0	121	0.01

Food	Average serving size (g)	Energy (kJ/100 g)	Carbohydrate (g/100 g)	Dietary fibre (g/100 g)	Protein (g/100 g)	Total fat (g/100 g)	Saturated fat (g/100 g)	Monounsaturated fat (g/100 g)	Omega-3 polyunsaturated fat (g/100 g)	Calcium (mg/100 g)	Iron (mg/100 g)
Chocolate flavoured reduced fat milk	250 (one cup)	266	8.8	0	3.5	1.8	1.2	0.4	0	120	0.11
Plain Greek yoghurt	130 (1/2 cup)	367	5	0	6	4.4	2.8	1.3	0	193	0.08
Tasty cheese	30	1663	0.5	0	24.6	32.8	21.6	7.7	0.1	763	0.14
Sports supplement powder (for protein shakes)	45	1533	65.6	0	24	2	Data not available	Data not available	Data not available	775	21.4
Sports drinks	624 (one bottle)	113	7	0	0	0	0	0	0	7	0

Source: NUTTAB 2010 (Food Standards Australia New Zealand); The University of New South Wales; Professor Heather Greenfield and co-workers at the University of New South Wales; Tables of composition of Australian Aboriginal Foods (J Brand-Miller, KW James and PMA Maggiore). There are limitations associated with food composition databases. Nutrient data published in NUTTAB 2010 may represent an average of the nutrient content of a particular sample of foods and ingredients, determined at a particular time. The nutrient composition of foods and ingredients can vary substantially between batches and brands because of a number of factors, including changes in season, changes in formulation, processing practices and ingredient source. While most of the data contained in NUTTAB 2010 are generated from analysed values, some of the data are borrowed from overseas food composition tables; supplied by the food industry; taken from food labels; imputed from similar foods; or calculated using a recipe approach.

Box 6.3: A one-day eating plan

SUPER-START BREAKFAST

200 g plain reduced fat Greek yoghurt
¼ cup rolled oats or store-bought muesli
15 g walnuts (about 6 nuts)
15 g almonds (about 10 nuts)
¼ cup frozen raspberries
1 orange

This super-start breakfast provides good serves of protein and carbohydrate, and moderate amounts of monounsaturated fats. It combines the convenience of store-bought muesli with added nuts for additional fibre, protein and monounsaturated fats. The berries and citrus fruit provide antioxidants and boost the flavour.

This provides: 1 serve milk and alternatives, 1 serve grains, 1 serve meat and alternatives, 1.5 serves fruit, 46 g CHO, 15 g fibre, 27 g protein, 29 g total fat, 5 g saturated fat, 2420 kJ.

LUNCH-TO-GO

2 slices of wholegrain bread
40 g shredded cooked chicken breast
1 tbsp avocado
2 tsp reduced fat mayonnaise
1 slice Swiss cheese
10 baby spinach leaves
½ sliced tomato
¼ sliced red capsicum
¼ sliced cucumber
⅛ sliced red onion
1 red apple

This convenient lunch on the go can be prepared the night before and refrigerated or stored in a cooler bag with an ice pack until you are ready to eat. The simple chicken sandwich gets a flavour and nutrient boost with generous serves of a variety of salad vegetables. The amount of chicken or cheese can be increased if more energy or protein is required. To save time preparing food, chop up whole vegetables and place the unneeded portions in containers in the refrigerator ready for lunch the next day.

This provides: 2 serves grains, 0.5 serves milk and alternatives, 0.5 serves meat and alternatives, 2 serves vegetables, 1 serve fruit, 54 g CHO, 13 g fibre, 50 g PRO, 17 g total fat, 6 g saturated fat, 2163 kJ.

POWER-PACKED DINNER
150 g oven baked salmon fillet + 2 tsp lemon juice
1 medium boiled potato (skin on) + 2 tsp olive oil and 2 tsp chopped
    fresh parsley
½ cup steamed green beans
½ cup cooked carrots
1 wholemeal dinner roll

This simple dinner can be prepared with minimal cooking skills and packs in good amounts of carbohydrate, protein and omega-3 fats. The generous serves of vegetables are ideal for a meal that is consumed at the end of the day when you have time to sit down and enjoy time with friends or family. Vary the vegetables or the type of fish to suit your tastes, and make an extra portion so you have a meal ready to reheat for dinner tomorrow night. For a more budget-friendly option, try preparing salmon patties using tinned salmon.

This provides: 1 serve grains, 1.5 serves meat and alternatives, 4 serves vegetables, 29 g CHO, 7 g fibre, 51 g PRO, 39 g total fat, 8 g saturated fat, 2862 kJ.

SIMPLE SUPPER
1 cup mixed grain breakfast cereal
1 cup skim milk

Breakfast cereal is a great staple to keep on hand for a quick snack any time of the day. Check the labels to choose one that contains wholegrains and is low in sugar.

This provides: 2 serves grains, 1 serve milk and alternatives, 59 g CHO, 4 g fibre, 15 g PRO, 1 g total fat, 0 g saturated fat, 1321 kJ.

SUMMARY AND KEY MESSAGES

After reading this chapter, you should understand the importance of consuming whole foods and be familiar with food selection guides. You have identified some foods that can help you meet your dietary goals, and can use the resources listed in the Australian Dietary Guidelines <https://www.eatforhealth.gov.au/> and the Sports Dietitians Australia website <https://www.sportsdietitians.com.au/factsheets/>.

Key messages

- A whole food diet provides more benefit than can be gained by consuming nutrients alone.
- The Australian and New Zealand governments have used the best available evidence to develop dietary guidelines and food selection guides to help the general population maintain good health.
- Athletes may benefit from additional individualised dietary advice from an Accredited Sports Dietitian.
- Carbohydrate-rich foods can be selected to maximise performance and minimise gastrointestinal discomfort.
- Protein can be obtained from a number of plant and animal sources to meet an athlete's protein requirements.
- Athletes can meet all of their vitamin and mineral requirements with a whole food diet.

REFERENCES

American Society for Nutrition, 2011, *Protein Complementation*, <https://nutrition.org/protein-complementation/>, accessed 29 March 2018.

Food Standards Australia New Zealand, 2010, *NUTTAB 2010—Australian Food Composition Tables*, Canberra, ACT: Food Standards Australia New Zealand.

Ministry of Health, 2015, *Eating and Activity Guidelines for New Zealand Adults*, Wellington, NZ: Ministry of Health.

National Health and Medical Research Council, Australian Government Department of Health and Ageing, New Zealand Ministry of Health, 2006, *Nutrient Reference Values for Australia and New Zealand*, Canberra, ACT: National Health and Medical Research Council.

National Health and Medical Research Council, 2013, *Australian Dietary Guidelines*, Canberra, ACT: National Health and Medical Research Council.

CHAPTER 7

Dietary assessment

Yasmine C. Probst

The preceding chapters have provided us with an overview of the nutrients needed for good health and performance. In order to understand where these nutrients come from when we eat foods as part of our daily lives, we need to collect information about what people eat. Dietitians and nutritionists use many different types of tools, referred to as dietary assessment methods, to collect this information. To translate the food information into nutrient outcomes, we also need to use tools called food composition databases. In this chapter, we will explore some of the most common dietary assessment tools and address some considerations we need to be aware of when using food composition databases.

LEARNING OUTCOMES

Upon completion of this chapter you will be able to:

- describe common methods of dietary assessment, with particular focus on their strengths and limitations
- understand how food information can be translated to nutrient outcomes
- appreciate how dietary guidelines and nutrition policies can be used with dietary assessment information
- describe aspects of dietary assessment important in sports, including the timing of snacks or meals relative to training and competition.

WHAT IS DIETARY ASSESSMENT?

Dietary assessment is the process by which we find out what a person or group of people are eating and drinking. This is fundamental to the skills of a dietitian but may also be important for other health and fitness professionals to gain an understanding of people's food habits. Dietary assessments can be obtained at the time foods and drinks are consumed, or they can be performed retrospectively, after foods and drinks have been eaten, often relying heavily on a person's memory. To help capture the required information, a range of assessment methods have been developed and refined over time, each with their own advantages and disadvantages. These factors are unique to the situation in which the assessment method is being used and the individual or group with whom it is being used. Capturing dietary information for a five-year-old child, for example, will have many different considerations than capturing dietary information from an adult who lives alone and does all their own cooking and shopping. Not only will the types of tools used need to be considered but the impact of other factors will also need to be thought through. These other factors include things such as bias and literacy, which will be addressed below in relation to each of the specific assessment methods. The assessment methods vary in terms of how they are undertaken but also in relation to the form in which the food information is collected. This form can be pen and paper, or it can be in various digital formats. After the food information has been collected, careful consideration needs to be given to how the information will be used. Is nutrient information needed from the foods that were reportedly eaten or will these foods be related to dietary guideline recommendations? These two options will be discussed later in this chapter.

DIETARY ASSESSMENT METHODS

The types of dietary assessment methods that are commonly used include those based on recall and memory, such as the 24-hour recall (National Cancer Institute; Salvador Castell et al. 2015), the diet history interview (Tapsell et al. 2000) and the food frequency questionnaire (National Cancer Institute; Perez Rodrigo et al. 2015). Other assessments capturing intake at the time of consumption—namely, the food record or food diary—may also be used in isolation or in parallel with the other methods. These tools are then further categorised into whether they are capturing actual intake or usual intake information. The food record or food diary is the most suitable tool to capture actual food intake information. This assessment method requires a person to write down the names and brand names of all foods and beverages consumed by meal occasion and to quantify the amount consumed. The way in which this quantity is determined creates the differentiating factor

Estimated food record
A form of dietary assessment in which a person records all the food and drink they have consumed by estimating the weight or serving size of the food.

Weighed food record
A form of dietary assessment in which a person records with weights and volumes all the food and drink they have consumed.

between an **estimated food record** and a **weighed food record**. As the name suggests, an estimated food record only requires an estimate of portion size in terms the person recording the foods can relate to. A weighed food record, on the other hand, requires the person recording the foods to accurately measure and weigh all items to be consumed. This includes a breakdown of ingredients required for a food that is cooked as part of a recipe and requires the person to take the measuring equipment with them to all eating occasions. As a result, although the accuracy of the recorded food items *should* be higher than an estimated record, often subconscious or conscious changes to the types of food eaten occur and the actual intake is distorted. To reduce the impact of this bias, digital food records have been developed whereby the user takes photographs of the food being consumed before and after eating. Using images to capture the food items also reduces the burden related to the number of days of recording. Having more days required often results in less detailed information being provided, which also substantially affects the accuracy. As a result, the most common duration is the three-day estimated food record, which includes at least one weekend day.

A 24-hour dietary assessment follows a structured approach to dietary assessment by capturing information about foods and beverages consumed during the previous day or 24-hour period. Often administered by an interviewer, this form of assessment alone cannot capture usual intake information about the diet unless it is repeated over a number of occasions. During a 24-hour recall the interviewer follows a multiple pass approach to guide the interviewee's recall of their food and beverage intakes. This approach begins with a free-flowing recall of all items in the order they were consumed. The process is uninterrupted to allow the interviewee to recall an unprompted food list. This list is then addressed from the beginning to obtain further detail about the food item types, accompanying foods and commonly forgotten items, as well as the portion size of each of the foods and beverages recalled. The recalls often follow a meal-based format, although the eating occasion, timing and location may also be collected depending upon the requirements.

Like the 24-hour recall, the diet history interview is based on the memory of the person recalling their food and beverage consumption, but the process is largely interviewer-led and addresses usual intake. This usual intake period generally covers a one-month period but can vary substantially, from one week up to one year. The diet history interview follows a similar format to the 24-hour recall; however, its open-ended nature lends itself to recall of foods that are eaten less frequently, during particular seasons or at eating occasions such as birthdays. Guided by the interviewer, a diet history interview is a skill-based dietary assessment method traditionally undertaken by trained dietitians. Often followed up with a checklist of commonly forgotten foods,

Table 7.1. Summary of common dietary assessment methods

Assessment method	Recording type	Strengths	Limitations
Food record	• Prospective (recorded as they are consumed) • Self-administered	• Actual intake information • Using images reduces burden	• Increased days are affected by burden • Social desirability bias creates changed intakes • Requires literate persons
24-hour recall	• Retrospective (reflects back on dietary intake) • Multiple pass method • Interviewer assisted	• Quick to administer • Repeated recalls can give usual intake information • Structured approach	• Affected by memory • Affected by social desirability bias
Diet history interview	• Retrospective • Interviewer prompted	• Usual intake information • Captures in-depth information	• Affected by memory • Affected by social desirability bias • Requires interviewer • Requires 30–60 minutes to complete
Food frequency questionnaire	• Retrospective • Self-administered • Can be interviewer-assisted	• Usual intake information • Can be completed over multiple attempts • Can be tailored to requirements, e.g. nutrient type	• Length of food list affects accuracy • May not be quantified

the diet history interview provides information about the foods eaten by a person, the frequency at which those foods are eaten and the portion size that is usually eaten. This portion size may be guided by household measures such as measuring cups and spoons, by pictorial portion guides or using food models. Both the diet history interview and the 24-hour recall have been automated; the structure of the 24-hour recall lends itself particularly well to this format, with the prompts provided by an avatar on screen rather than in person by the interviewer. This format allows large numbers of people to recall their intakes without the need for additional resources.

Usual intake information may also be collected using a food frequency questionnaire. The questionnaire includes a list of food items suited to the purpose of the information being collected. For example, if the purpose is to determine calcium intake then only calcium-containing foods need be included. The food list may comprise single food items or it may group foods with similar characteristics. The person completing the questionnaire identifies how often the food is consumed based on the frequency categories provided. Food frequency questionnaires may span wide time intervals, with some even referring to the previous year. Food frequency questionnaires can be quantified or semi-quantified, meaning that they may also require information about the portion size most often consumed for each item in the food list. The portion sizes can refer to a standard size that may relate to dietary guidelines, or they may be displayed as images or different size options for each food choice. Inclusion of portion size information may also result in improved response rates. Food frequency questionnaires are commonly self-administered, meaning they do not require an interviewer to ask the questions. This does, however, leave the tool open to interpretation by the person reporting their intake and may lead to missed sections or skipped food items.

TRANSLATING DIETARY INTAKES TO NUTRIENT OUTCOMES

The above section has outlined a number of methods used to find out what food and beverages are being consumed by a person. These methods all result in information related to specific foods and beverages, which may not be of practical use if someone needs to determine how much protein or energy they are consuming. To translate the food and beverage information to nutrient information, tools referred to as **food composition databases** are used. These databases contain a list of foods available in the food supply and their nutrient information, including both macronutrients and micronutrients. Each country has its own unique food composition database, as many foods are affected by local processing, harvesting, soil conditions, UV exposure, food regulatory environments and many other factors. There is specialised software available to make the use of food composition tables fast and efficient. Although the software is useful, it does require the user to have a basic understanding of which food composition database to choose. If many assessments need to be translated, as is common in research, the person or people using the software need to ensure they use it consistently and follow the same assumptions. It also needs to be appreciated that not every food item found on the supermarket shelf will appear in a food composition database, but generic versions of most foods do exist and therefore careful choices for the correct food match need to be made.

In Australia, and many other countries across the globe, we have two types of food composition databases: a **survey database** and a **reference database**. The survey

Food composition databases
Databases that contain lists of foods available in the food supply and their nutrient information including energy, macronutrients and micronutrients.

Survey database
Databases that are specifically developed for the analysis of all foods reported in national nutrition surveys. For example, in Australia, AUSNUT was developed for the Australian Health Survey 2011–12.

Reference database
Databases developed from a wide range of foods that are primarily analysed in the laboratory. For example, in Australia, NUTTAB is the reference database.

database contains a complete nutrient set for all the foods listed and is based on the food items reported in the national nutrition survey for which it was developed. Some of this nutrient information is calculated or borrowed from overseas databases but the majority is based on the reference database. The reference database contains fewer food items, although a higher proportion of the items have been analysed in the laboratory to identify the amounts of nutrients in the foods. As a result, some foods may not include the same number of nutrient values and the database is therefore considered incomplete. The survey databases in Australia are referred to as AUSNUT (Australian Nutrient) databases and the reference databases as NUTTAB (Nutrient Tables) databases. The most recent AUSNUT database contains over 5700 food and beverage items, while the most recent NUTTAB database contains slightly more than 2500 food and beverage items (Probst & Cunningham 2015).

> ## Box 7.1: National Nutrition and Physical Activity Survey 2011–13
>
> The National Nutrition and Physical Activity Survey 2011–13 was the largest and most comprehensive food- and physical activity-related survey conducted in Australia. It involved the collection of detailed physical activity information using self-reported and pedometer collection methods, along with detailed information on dietary intake and foods consumed from over 12,000 participants across Australia. The nutrition component is the first national nutrition survey of adults and children (aged two years and over) conducted in over 15 years. More information and data can be found at the Australian Bureau of Statistics Australian Health Survey webpage (ABS 2014) <http://www.abs.gov.au/ausstats/abs@.nsf/lookup/4364.0.55.007main+features12011-12>.

To translate food and beverage information to nutrient information the survey, or AUSNUT, database should be used. As this contains a complete set of nutrient values, it will result in better quality nutrient outcomes with less incomplete data (Sobolewksi et al. 2010). The NUTTAB database can also be used, but is more useful when working out how much of a particular nutrient is in one or a few food items or when developing a specialised menu plan. Using NUTTAB ensures the nutrient values are primarily analysed in the laboratory and therefore more accurate. Where no matching food information is available, food label information may be used, but this is considered lower quality data as it is often based on calculations and limited to the nutrients required to be listed under the various regulatory codes and policies.

USING DIETARY GUIDELINES AND POLICIES IN PRACTICE

By now you will have read about the Australian Dietary Guidelines and how they were developed (Chapter 6). Armed with food information from a dietary assessment, and nutrient information obtained by using food composition databases, we now need to think about how we can use this information with our clients. The most common approach relates the food consumed to the Australian Dietary Guidelines (NHMRC 2013). These guidelines are designed to maximise intake from core food groups and limit consumption of foods known as discretionary sources. This comparison can be made using data collected through any of the assessment methods described in this chapter, although care needs to be taken that any recommendations based on this comparison are relevant for the individual client. For this reason, readily available and consumer-friendly resources, such as the Australian Guide to Healthy Eating, can be used to guide discussions with clients around portion sizes and the balance and types of foods being consumed, using the suggested serves per day for each of the food groups. Conversations based on the Australian Dietary Guidelines are considered to be within the scope of practice for trained nutrition, exercise and fitness professionals. However, more specific and personalised dietary planning is the speciality of dietitians; hence, when working with athletes it is best to refer to a dietitian if you are not specifically trained as one (https://daa.asn.au/find-an-apd/).

Other useful tools that can be aligned with dietary assessment outcomes are the Nutrient Reference Values (NRV) (NHMRC 2006) discussed in Chapter 4. After translating food and beverage information to nutrient intakes, the appropriate NRV can be used as a comparator to determine adequacy of intake. A person consuming insufficient amounts of important nutrients may need to increase or balance the foods that they are eating. Given that insufficient intake of some nutrients can result in deficiency symptoms, while overconsumption can result in toxicity symptoms, adjustments based on nutrient concerns are best supported by a trained dietitian. The dietitian will be able to consider the medical, lifestyle and exercise-related factors relevant to the individual and identify any possible medication interactions or underlying concerns as to why the nutrient levels are outside of the normal ranges. It is important to note that nutrient information taken directly from a dietary assessment method and translated using a food composition database can be affected by bias (see limitations in Table 7.1). For this reason, if the dietitian expresses concern he or she will likely suggest further medical intervention via a general practitioner.

Applying dietary assessment to sports

Although the Australian Dietary Guidelines are developed for the general population, the messages are applicable to many sporting practices as well. It should be noted, however, that the level and types of training undertaken by sporting professionals or athletes may require additional or modified guidance to optimise health and wellbeing. The long or intensive training sessions and competitive events require athletes to be at optimum performance for a given time period. The timing of such events may last for a season or for shorter intermittent periods of time throughout a year. Not only does the food eaten need to be taken into consideration but beverages and their amounts are also crucial to allow the athlete to perform at their best.

Following a dietary assessment, each of the above factors needs to be addressed with the athlete. Are they in an off-season period? Are they training or are they competing? The type of sport being undertaken, whether it is primarily strength- or endurance-focused, and the athlete's age, health status and sex should also be addressed. Many sports require careful timing of athletes' fluid intake, snacks and meals relative to their training schedule and intensity and their competitive games or events. The composition of these meals needs to be managed. Too much or too little of key nutrients, such as protein, carbohydrate and fat, which all provide energy to the body, can disrupt optimal performance and result in an athlete feeling lethargic or bloated or experiencing stomach cramps. Dietary planning needs to ensure that the athlete follows a general healthy, balanced diet with personalised adjustments made to the above nutrients via key foods as needed.

For a dietary assessment of an athlete, a diet history interview will likely capture the most in-depth food and beverage information and also allow a history of subjective factors—such as mood and perceived effects on performance—to be obtained. The interviewer has the ability to focus on key training and periods in the lead-up to an event while also considering other lifestyle-related factors that may impact the individual. Variation in dietary assessments due to the variable lifestyles of many athletes should also be taken into account. On some occasions more detail may be required, and a food record or diary may be used as well. This provides accountability for the athlete if they have been asked to follow a very specific eating plan and also raises awareness of serving sizes in relation to recommended portion sizes. The food record can also capture the time of the meals and record time of training to allow for meal plans to be tailored based on feedback from the athlete. The food diary should also endeavour to capture fluid intakes, even though beverages are often more intermittently consumed.

In the lead-up to an event, a 24-hour recall may also provide useful insights. Common recommendations for some sports, such as the timing and composition of pre-game meals and snacks, can be monitored with a quick recall. The recall can also capture information about food intake following an event and allow adjustments to be made to the food choices if needed to promote recovery.

Some sports have specific guidelines developed for them, based on the Australian Dietary Guidelines but tailored to the specific needs of the athletes. Accredited Sports Dietitians should be consulted to ensure any meal plans being followed are tailored to the individual.

SUMMARY AND KEY MESSAGES

After reading this chapter, you should be familiar with a range of dietary assessment methods. You should be able to identify which tools are most appropriate to use in different circumstances, and be able to outline the limitations associated with those methods. You should also have a basic understanding of food composition databases and be able to select the appropriate database for use in a specific context.

Key messages

- Dietary assessment methods need to be carefully selected based on the person or group of people whose diet needs to be assessed.
- All dietary assessment methods have inherent advantages and disadvantages.
- When translating food information from a dietary assessment, the correct food composition database needs to be selected.
- Dietary guidelines and Nutrient Reference Values may also be used as comparative tools when analysing a person's dietary intake.

Assessing dietary intakes of an athlete requires consideration of the type of sport being undertaken, as well as lifestyle factors, which can all be addressed by an Accredited Practising Sports Dietitian.

REFERENCES

Australian Bureau of Statistics, 2014, *Australian Health Survey: Nutrition First Results—Foods and Nutrients, 2011–12* [Online], Australian Bureau of Statistics, <http://www.abs.gov.au/ausstats/abs@.nsf/Lookup/by%20Subject/4364.0.55.007~2011-12~Main%20Features~Key%20Findings~1>, accessed 29 January 2018.

National Cancer Institute, n.d., *Dietary Assessment Primer: 24-Hour Dietary Recall (24HR) at a Glance*, retrieved from <https://dietassessmentprimer.cancer.gov/profiles/recall/index.html>, accessed 5 December 2017.

—— n.d., *Dietary Assessment Primer: Food Frequency Questionnaire at a glance*, retrieved from <https://dietassessmentprimer.cancer.gov/profiles/questionnaire/index.html>.

—— n.d., *Dietary Assessment Primer: Food Record at a Glance*, retrieved from <https://dietassessmentprimer.cancer.gov/profiles/record/>.

National Health and Medical Research Council (NHMRC) 2006, *Nutrient Reference Values*, <www.nrv.gov.au/>, accessed 22 September 2017.

—— 2013, *Eat for Health: Australian Dietary Guidelines Summary*, retrieved from <www.nhmrc.gov.au/_files_nhmrc/publications/attachments/n55a_australian_dietary_guidelines_summary_131014.pdf>.

Perez Rodrigo, C., Aranceta, J., Salvador, G. et al., 2015, 'Food frequency questionnaires', *Nutricion Hospitalaria*, vol. 31, no. 3, pp. 49–56.

Probst, Y.C. & Cunningham, J., 2015, 'An overview of the influential developments and stakeholders within the food composition program of Australia', *Trends in Food Science and Technology*, vol. 42, no 2, pp. 173–82.

Salvador Castell, G., Serra-Majem, L. & Ribas-Barba, L., 2015, 'What and how much do we eat? 24-hour dietary recall method', *Nutricion Hospitalaria*, vol. 31, no. 3, pp. 46–8.

Sobolewksi, R., Cunningham, J. & Mackerras, D., 2010, 'Which Australian food composition database should I use?', *Nutrition & Dietetics*, vol. 67, no. 1, pp. 37–40.

Tapsell, L.C., Brenninger, V. & Barnard, J., 2000, 'Applying conversation analysis to foster accurate reporting in the diet history interview', *Journal of the American Dietetic Association*, vol. 100, no. 7, pp. 818–24.

CHAPTER

8

Introduction to diet planning

Adrienne Forsyth and Tim Stewart

One of the main roles of nutrition professionals working with athletes and active people is to help them develop and implement their nutrition plans. In this chapter, we will describe the steps involved in planning diets for individual athletes and for teams, and consider a range of factors that influence an athlete's nutrition plan. We will also consider strategies to use when working with athletes to increase engagement and participation in the diet-planning process. At the end of this chapter, you will find two case studies (see Box 8.4) to work through to help you practise your diet-planning skills.

LEARNING OUTCOMES

Upon completion of this chapter you will be able to:
- describe the steps involved in planning diets for individual athletes and teams
- understand why nutrition counselling skills are important to engage client athletes
- consider individual physiological and social factors, training and sport requirements when prioritising nutritional concerns
- develop simple nutrition plans for healthy athletes.

PLANNING DIETS FOR INDIVIDUAL ATHLETES

Developing a nutrition plan is a complex task. There are a number of factors that may influence dietary intake; these are described in more detail below. To help simplify the process, the following steps may be used as a guide to follow when developing a nutrition plan.

Step 1: Collect information

- Identify baseline physiological requirements. How much energy and nutrients are required at rest?
- Identify additional requirements related to training and competition. How much extra energy is needed to support training sessions and competition events? Should this energy be focused on any specific macronutrients?
- Determine when training, competition and recreational activity will take place. It is important to be able to time meals to effectively fuel training, competition and recovery (see Chapters 9 and 10 for more information).
- Assess current **body composition** and evaluate this against any required standards or goals. What information is currently available? Take additional measurements if trained to do so and relevant to the athlete's goals.
- Identify any dietary requirements related to allergies, intolerances, religious or cultural beliefs, or personal values. Are there any foods that the athlete cannot consume?
- Identify personal preferences and food likes and dislikes. It is important to include favourite foods to develop a nutrition plan that the athlete will be willing to follow.
- Identify any factors that may influence access to food. Does the athlete have access to fresh food outlets? Can they afford to buy this food? Do they have facilities for food storage, preparation and cooking, and do they have the skills to do so?
- Identify social influences on dietary intake. Where does the athlete eat, and who do they eat with? Do they prepare their own meals? Are they cooking for other members of their household? How is their day scheduled? Do they have time to cook?
- Identify any nutrition-related health concerns. Does the athlete have any health issues that require input from a dietitian or other health professional?
- Identify any team requirements, restrictions or habits regarding food, beverages and supplements. What type of sport do they play? What is their position and what does it involve? How long do games/events run for? Will the athlete play for the entire game? Will they have access to food or fluid while they are playing or during breaks? Does the team or club eat meals together or provide food or supplements for athletes?

Body composition
The proportion of muscle, fat, bone and other tissues that make up the mass of an individuals' body weight.

- Collect and assess information about the athlete's usual diet and supplement use. What do they eat currently (what, when and how much)? Are they happy with this? What would they like to change and why?

Step 2: Identify priority areas

Ask the client what is important to them. Common goals include increasing lean (muscle) mass, reducing fat mass, or providing strategic fuelling suggestions to maximise performance in training or competition. There will be other important aspects to consider—for example, the athlete focused on fuelling a training session may also be interested in recovery strategies—but these do not all need to be addressed at the first appointment. Depending on the athlete's situation, you may also ask for input from a coach or trainer to help identify nutrition goals.

Step 3: Develop a plan

Put together a specific plan with detailed recommendations for when to eat, what to eat and how much to eat. Athletes will often like the structure of a rigid plan, but it is helpful to provide some flexibility to allow for changes in circumstances, preferences and access to foods. A flexible plan that includes options will also help to teach the athlete about the components of their dietary plan and enable them to make appropriate choices on their own.

Step 4: Trial the plan

Nutrition plans must be tailored to the individual athlete. As much as we can try to develop helpful nutrition solutions for athletes based on what we know about their needs and what we know about food, the only way to determine with any certainty whether a plan will be tolerated by an athlete and help to achieve their nutrition-related goals is to trial the nutrition plan. Ask the athlete to trial the plan at least once or twice before your next consultation with them. Nutrition plans that will be used in competition should be trialled in training as much as possible, to familiarise the athlete with the plan and to help train the gut (see Chapter 23 for more information).

Step 5: Assess the plan

Once the athlete has had some experience with the nutrition plan, it is important to meet and review how well the plan was tolerated and accepted by the athlete, and whether it is helping to achieve their nutrition-related goals. Did it cause any gastrointestinal discomfort? Did the athlete like the foods? Were the foods easy to access and prepare? Were foods planned for use during competition or training easy to consume during the activity? Were there any changes noted in performance at training, or in energy or mood through the day? Were there any barriers encountered in implementing the plan?

Step 6: Revise the plan

Based on the feedback provided by the athlete, make modifications to the plan. The new plan should also be trialled, assessed and revised as needed.

Following these steps should help you collect all of the information you require to work with an athlete to develop a nutrition plan. Take a look at Box 8.1 to see what information was collected for Janice, a recreational distance runner.

Box 8.1: Janice's baseline physiological requirements

Age: 26
Sex: Female
Height: 168 cm
Weight: 57 kg
Resting energy expenditure
= 9.99 x (weight in kg) + 6.25 x (height in cm) − 4.92 x age − 161
= 9.99 x 57 kg + 6.25 x 168 cm − 4.92 x 26
= 569.43 + 1050 − 127.92
= 1491.51 kcal/day
1491.51 kcal/day x 4.18 kJ/kcal = 6235 kJ/day
PAL 1.5 for activities of daily living plus 30–60 minutes of light intensity activity (e.g. walking)
6235 kJ/day x 1.5 = 9353 kJ/day

TRAINING AND COMPETITION ENERGY REQUIREMENTS
Trains 10 km/day five days per week.
- add 10 **METS** x 60 minutes = 2394 kJ
Trains or races 20–30 km/day one day per week.
- add 10 METS x 150 minutes (average time) = 5985 kJ
Has one rest day per week.
Races 40–50 km 2–4 times per year.
Total energy requirements on training days: 9353 kJ + 2394 kJ = 11,747 kJ
Total requirements on long training days: 9353 kJ + 5985 kJ = 15,338 kJ

TIMING OF TRAINING/COMPETITION/ACTIVITY
Trains after work (5 p.m.) during the week, and in the mid-morning on weekends.

BODY COMPOSITION
BMI = 57 kg/ (1.68 m)^2 = 20.2 kg/m^2 (considered to be within healthy range)

METS

Measures of energy expenditure typically used to describe the energy expended in physical activity. The standard resting metabolic rate is 1 MET, and is equivalent to 1.0 kcal/kg/hour, or 4.18 kJ/kg/hour (Ainsworth et al. 2000).

BMI

Body Mass Index, an index of a person's weight in relation to height. BMI = kg/m².

More detailed anthropometric measurements have not been performed. In recreational athletes of healthy BMI with no personal concerns about their body composition, there is no need to perform detailed anthropometric measurements.

DIETARY REQUIREMENTS

Nil allergies or intolerances.

PERSONAL PREFERENCES, LIKES AND DISLIKES

Prefers dairy, eggs and vegetable sources of protein to meat.

FACTORS INFLUENCING ACCESS TO FOOD

Works full time; is able to access shops on evenings and weekends. Shares a kitchen with one roommate.

SOCIAL INFLUENCES

Usually eats alone; occasionally eats dinner with her roommate. Eats lunch at her desk during the week. Works 8.30 a.m.–4.30 p.m. in an office close to home. Enjoys cooking, but not baking.

NUTRITION-RELATED HEALTH CONCERNS

Nil.

TEAM REQUIREMENTS, RESTRICTIONS OR HABITS

Long weekly training runs will require a source of carbohydrate, electrolytes and fluid while training.
Race-day nutrition strategies should be practised in training.

USUAL DIET

Breakfast (7 a.m.): 1 cup of cereal with skim milk and a glass of orange juice

Morning snack (9 a.m.): 2 slices of wholemeal toast with peanut butter and coffee with skim milk

Lunch (12 p.m.): 2 cups of salad using leftover vegetables from dinner plus 2 eggs, a small tin of tuna or crumbled feta with olive oil and vinegar to dress the salad plus an apple or pear

Afternoon snack (2.30 p.m.): chocolate bar or similar from the vending machine

Dinner (7 p.m.): pasta or rice with lentils, chickpeas or beans and vegetables, and fruit with ice cream or custard for dessert

Janice tells us that her nutrition priorities are to maintain her current body composition and to increase her energy levels at training. So, our plan will focus on providing an appropriate energy intake to maintain her current body composition, and timing her energy and macronutrient intake to increase her energy levels at training. We will also discuss non-nutritional strategies to increase energy levels, such as adequate amount and timing of sleep, and refer Janice to other health professionals where relevant.

An athlete's nutrition plan may cover a full week or even longer, to account for varied dietary requirements on different days of training, competition and rest. Here, we will present one day of a nutrition plan for Janice that focuses on nutrition for mid-week training. Look at how the plan is laid out for Janice in Box 8.2: you will see that the instructions are very specific. There are recommendations for when to eat, what to eat and how much to eat. These recommendations have been developed based on Janice's

Box 8.2: Janice's nutrition plan

7 a.m.	2 poached eggs on 2 slices of sourdough bread with 1 tomato and 6 mushrooms, grilled with 1 tsp olive oil 200 mL of orange juice
10 a.m.	2 slices of wholemeal toast with 1 tbsp peanut butter 250 mL coffee with skim milk
1 p.m.	1 cup of salad vegetables plus 95 g tuna, salmon or sardines and 30 g feta or ricotta cheese and ½ cup leftover cooked starchy vegetables with 1 tsp olive oil and 2 tsp vinegar and a dinner roll One piece of fruit
4 p.m.	1 cup of cereal (not a high-fibre option) with ½ cup skim milk
5 p.m.	Training
6 p.m.	1 piece of fruit with a 20 g slice of cheese
7 p.m.	1 cup cooked wholemeal pasta or brown rice with ½ cup cooked lentils, chickpeas or beans, ¾ cup tomato-based sauce, ½ cup cooked starchy vegetables (e.g. potato, sweet potato, corn) and ½ cup green vegetables (e.g. broccoli, green beans, spinach)
9 p.m.	200 mL yoghurt or custard with ¼ cup nuts and ½ cup berries

This plan provides 11,554 kJ, 132 g protein, 89 g fat and 328 g carbohydrate per day.

individual physiological and training requirements, as well as her personal preferences and social influences. This nutrition plan evolved over several iterations to include the right amount of energy and macronutrients at the right times throughout the day.

Did you note that this plan contains many elements from Janice's usual diet? We have moved the order and timing of some of the foods, but it is helpful to include as many foods as possible that are already familiar to and known to be tolerated by the athlete. You may also note that the total energy provided by the nutrition plan is not exactly what we calculated Janice's requirements to be. Remember that estimates of energy requirements are just that—estimates. It is more important to note Janice's usual intake and any changes in weight or body composition with dietary changes to inform fine-tuning of the nutrition plan. Estimated energy requirements are more likely to be used when an athlete requires a more substantial change to their diet, or when you have limited background information available to inform your plan.

Janice will now trial this plan on two training days and keep track of her experience in a **nutrition log (Box 8.3)**. She will record what she eats and when, as well as her energy levels and any gastrointestinal discomfort. After these two trial days, you meet with Janice to discuss her experience. Janice reports no concerns except that she felt hungry during training. Together, you adjust her lunch and pre-training snack to include more low-GI sources of carbohydrate, and you ask her to return with feedback after her next training day.

Box 8.3: Janice's nutrition log

Time	Food consumed	Mood and energy levels	Gastrointestinal symptoms
4 p.m.	1 cup cornflakes ½ cup milk	Energetic	Nil

NUTRITION COUNSELLING SKILLS

Many health professionals use a client-centred approach when working with their clients. This same approach can be applied to working with athletes. A client-centred approach means that any behavioural changes (such as changes to dietary practices) should be led by the client. The professional working with the athlete will focus on developing rapport, understanding the athlete's interests and motivations, providing nutrition education related to the athlete's goals, and helping the athlete identify changes that can be made to achieve these goals. In sports nutrition practice, the nutrition professional may need to provide more explicit advice than in general practice, since some foods, beverages and supplements used in sport are not commonly consumed as part of everyday diets. In some instances, there may be discrepancies between eating for health and eating for performance. Ultimately, nutrition recommendations for performance tend to support physical activity beyond normal daily levels, so foods recommended are in addition to, not instead of, a healthy diet that aligns with dietary recommendations. Athletes' goals and priorities can change over time, so it is important to revisit their goals, and ensure that their nutrition plan aligns with these goals, on a regular basis.

Nutrition professionals may draw upon theories and practices such as the **transtheoretical model of behaviour change** (Prochaska & DiClemente 1982; DiClemente & Velasquez 2002) and motivational interviewing (Rollnick & Miller 1995; Miller & Rollnick 2002) when supporting clients, including athletes, in adopting changes to their dietary practices. The transtheoretical model proposes five stages of change: (1) initial precontemplation, where clients are not currently considering change; (2) contemplation, where clients are evaluating the costs and benefits of changes to their behaviour; (3) preparation, where clients have committed to change and are making plans; (4) action, where clients are actively practising the changed behaviour; and (5) maintenance, where clients work towards sustaining the change in the long term. The approach a nutrition professional will take with an athlete may vary depending on their stage of change. An athlete in the contemplation stage may require more education and discussion about options and alternatives, while an athlete in the action stage and actively practising a changed behaviour may require encouragement and support to overcome unexpected barriers.

Transtheoretical model of behaviour change

An integrative theory that assesses an individual's readiness to act on new, healthier behaviour. It provides strategies and defines the processes of change to guide the individual.

Reflective listening

A practice used to develop rapport with clients. It involves listening carefully to what the client is saying, then paraphrasing their ideas back to them to confirm that you have understood them correctly. This reflection of their ideas is presented rather than any judgement or advice.

Motivational interviewing is a goal-directed, client-centred approach to behaviour change that incorporates and builds upon the transtheoretical model of behaviour change. The spirit of motivational interviewing suggests that motivation to change should come from the client, so it is the client's job to express and resolve their own uncertainty, while the nutrition professional supports them in this process rather than directly persuading them. Practitioners should build a relationship with their client by using **reflective listening** to understand their client's frame of reference; expressing acceptance and affirmation; eliciting motivational statements from the client and selectively reinforcing relevant concerns, desires, intentions and abilities to change; monitoring the client's readiness

Motivational interviewing
A goal-directed, client-centred approach to behaviour change that incorporates and builds upon the transtheoretical model of behaviour change. The motivation for change should come from the client, while the nutrition professional supports them in this process.

to change and working within the relevant stage of change; and reaffirming their freedom of choice. Miller and Rollnick (2002) highlight four general principles that underpin **motivational interviewing**.

1. Express empathy. Practice reflective listening and demonstrate acceptance of your client. Building a trusting relationship with your client is important to foster discussions that may lead to meaningful change.

2. Develop discrepancy. Clients are more likely to change when motivated by a perceived discrepancy between their personal goals and the outcomes of their current behaviour. Thoughtful conversation may help to point out these differences and allow the client to present their own arguments for change.

3. Roll with resistance. Arguing with clients is counterproductive. Avoid opposing their resistance to change, and instead try a different approach. Invite them to present their perspectives and to identify their own solutions.

4. Support self-efficacy. Clients will be responsible for identifying and implementing their own changes, so they need to believe that they are able to change. Affirming your belief in their ability to change can enhance clients' own beliefs and become a self-fulfilling prophecy.

If we think back to Janice, we can identify that she was at the contemplation stage of change and moving towards preparation. She had identified a problem with her diet (lack of energy for training), and engaged the services of a nutrition professional. In her case, making changes was fairly straightforward and she was able to identify what changes could be made based on some basic education provided at her first consultation. Individuals at the early stages of change, with complex nutrition requirements, with emotional attachment to food and eating habits, or with disordered eating patterns, are likely to require more support in a nutrition counselling session.

PLANNING DIETS FOR TEAMS

It is simply not possible to plan a single diet that will meet the needs of all athletes on a team. Given all of the individual factors that are considered when planning individual diets, it is logical to expect that there would be a variety of different dietary needs within a team. So, rather than planning for an individual athlete, we may instead provide a general nutrition plan that is suitable based on the requirements of the sport and provide advice on how to tailor the diet for individual requirements. For example, a soccer team that competes on Saturdays and trains three hours per day (two hours skills, one hour personal fitness) during the week will have consistent themes in their nutrition requirements. The timing and nutrient composition of meals and snacks will be similar for all athletes. However, depending on size, age, fitness level, playing time and individual body composition goals, the amount of food and beverages required will vary. The specific foods may also vary; for example, while all athletes will require a source of protein, some may prefer lean meats while others prefer dairy or vegetable sources. Advice for the team should be general, with a range of options provided. Athletes who require more support to develop an appropriate, individually tailored nutrition plan should seek the support of a nutrition professional. Those with nutrition-related health concerns should consult an Accredited Sports Dietitian. You can read more about the requirements of team sport athletes in Chapter 16.

Box 8.4: Case studies

Planning diets for athletes is a complex activity. In addition to all the considerations presented in this chapter, there are principles of sports nutrition and sport-specific dietary recommendations to consider. As you work through the remainder of this textbook, come back periodically to apply your new learning to the case studies below.

CASE 1: JONATHAN

Jonathan is a 44-year-old elite (age group) ironman triathlete. He recently raced in Ironman WA, where the weather conditions were hotter than expected with a temperature of 36°C and he suffered badly from cramps. This is the first time this has happened and he has been racing professionally for over ten years. Jonathon works full-time running his own coaching business.

Jonathan weighs 82 kg and is 186 cm tall. He previously had low iron levels but this was resolved with iron supplements. His training program is as follows:
- Monday—Swim session (1–2 km)—recovery session
- Tuesday—Bike (2–3 hours)—a.m., Run (60–90 minutes)—p.m.
- Wednesday—Long bike session (approximately 5 hours)
- Thursday—Swim (2–3 km)—a.m., Run (30–60 minutes)—p.m.
- Friday—Bike (1–2 hours), Run (off the bike)—30 minutes
- Saturday—Swim (open water) (3–4 km), Bike (3 hrs)
- Sunday—Run (3–4 hours)

Given his high energy expenditure and multiple days with two training sessions, energy intake and energy availability will be important considerations for Jonathan. He likes chocolate and prefers sweet foods over savoury. His usual diet is as follows.

Before activity (7 p.m.)
Coffee (latte, full-cream milk, no sugar), 2 slices of toast with honey

After activity (9–10 a.m.)
Muesli with dried fruit, 3 tbsp of natural Greek yoghurt and a handful of frozen berries

Lunch (12.30–1 p.m.)
Meat and salad roll with additional side salad with a light olive oil dressing OR
Leftovers from the previous dinner OR
Chicken burger (homemade with grilled chicken breast, lettuce, tomato, cheese, beetroot)

Afternoon snack (3 p.m.)/prep for afternoon session
2 pieces of fruit (prep for afternoon session) OR
1–2 x handfuls of mixed nuts (nil afternoon sessions)

Dinner (7–7.30 p.m.)
Pasta (spaghetti bolognese) OR
200–250 g meat (mainly chicken, fish and beef) with broccoli, cauliflower, carrot, potato OR
Beef stir-fry with rice noodles OR
Homemade pizzas (meat, tomato paste, cheese, olives)

Supper (8.30–9 p.m.)
Small piece of chocolate (dark)

Fluids
2–2.5 L water throughout the day
2.4–3.0 L during long ride sessions
2–3 x lattes/day

Consider the following points when working with Jonathan.
- Is he consuming enough energy, protein and carbohydrate to meet his needs?
- Is the timing and distribution of his meals appropriate to suit his training?
- Is he consuming enough iron to avoid another instance of iron deficiency?
- What are some strategies that could support Jonathan to consume more protein and carbohydrate without increasing the volume of food he is eating?

- How can Jonathan reduce the risk of cramping in the future?
- Is there any other information that you need to collect to help advise Jonathan?

CASE 2: JEREMY

Jeremy is a 23-year-old Australian football (AFL) player. He has recently commenced pre-season training and has been assigned a goal of increasing his muscle mass by 3–5 kg in the next three months. He currently weighs 83 kg and is 187 cm tall.

Jeremy tells you that he has been feeling sluggish and lacking energy. He is experiencing a low mood, is having difficulty making good food choices, and has had cold symptoms for the past three weeks. His training program is as follows.

- Monday—Running/skills session—a.m. (2–3 hours, likely to cover between 11 and 15 km), weight session (30–40 minutes, circuit-based session with individual programs)
- Tuesday—Weights (40 minutes, strength-based)—a.m., skills work (1 hour)
- Wednesday—Recovery day
- Thursday—Running/skills session—a.m. (2–3 hours, likely to cover between 11 and 15 km), weight session (30–40 minutes, circuit-based session with individual programs)
- Friday—Skills session (1–2 hours)
- Saturday—Weights (strength-based, 40 minutes)
- Sunday—Recovery day

Jeremy has modified his diet in an attempt to stay healthy and meet the goals set for him, and has attempted to reduce his carbohydrate intake to stay lean. Jeremy has limited cooking skills and does not enjoy cooking. His current diet is as follows.

Breakfast
2 poached eggs with ½ avocado and ½ slice of toast OR
½ cup muesli with 1 cup of natural Greek yoghurt

Morning snack
Handful nuts OR
Muesli bar OR
1–2 pieces of fruit (apple/banana/stone fruit/mango)

Lunch
Salad with grains (mainly quinoa or brown rice), tuna and vegetables including lettuce, tomato and carrot OR
Leftovers from dinner

Afternoon snack
Protein shake (post-weights), protein bar OR
Nil (on days off)

Dinner
Spaghetti bolognese OR
Beef stir-fry with black bean sauce (jar of sauce) OR
400 g steak/200 g salmon and vegetables (mainly ½ sweet potato, handful of beans, ½ carrot, ¼ cauliflower)

Supper/Dessert
Nil

Fluids
2–3 lattes with full-cream milk
Approximately 0.5–1 L during training sessions (mix of water and sports drink)
2–3 L water

Consider the following points when working with Jeremy.

- Is he consuming enough energy, protein, carbohydrate and fluids to meet his needs?
- Is the timing and distribution of his meals appropriate to suit his training?
- Are you concerned about Jeremy's energy levels? What nutrition-related strategies could you recommend to improve Jeremy's energy levels?
- What are some strategies that could support Jeremy to increase his muscle mass?
- Do you have any meal or snack suggestions for Jeremy that will require little or no cooking?
- Is there any other information that you need to collect to help advise Jeremy?

SUMMARY AND KEY MESSAGES

The development of a nutrition plan is a complex activity that requires consideration of a number of factors related to the athlete and the requirements of the sport. Adopting a client-centred approach can help to engage athletes and involve them to develop an individually tailored nutrition plan. Team nutrition plans can be developed based on the requirements of the sport, and athletes should be provided with advice on how to tailor the team plan to suit their individual requirements.

Key messages

- Nutrition plans for athletes should be individually tailored and take into consideration a number of factors related to the sport and the athlete's personal circumstances.
- Nutrition plans for teams can be sport-specific, and should provide options for individuals to be able to develop their own personalised nutrition plans.
- A client-centred approach will help nutrition professionals to effectively collaborate with athletes to develop realistic and successful nutrition plans.

REFERENCES

Ainsworth, B.A., Haskell, W.L., Whitt, M.C., et al., 2000, 'Compendium of physical activities: An update of activity codes and MET intensities', *Medicine & Science in Sports and Exercise*, vol. 32, no. 9, pp. S498–516.

DiClemente, C.C. & Velasquez, M.M., 2002, 'Motivational interviewing and the stages of change', in Miller, W.R. & Rollnick, S. (eds), *Motivational Interviewing: Preparing People for Change*, 2nd edn, New York, NY: The Guilford Press.

Miller, W.R. & Rollnick, S. (eds), 2002, *Motivational Interviewing: Preparing People for Change*, 2nd edn, New York, NY: The Guilford Press.

Prochaska, J.O. & DiClemente, C.C., 1982, 'Transtheoretical therapy: Toward a more integrative model of change', *Psychotherapy: Theory, Research and Practice*, vol. 9. no. 3, pp. 276–87.

Rollnick, S. & Miller, W.R., 1995, 'What is motivational interviewing?', *Behavioural and Cognitive Psychotherapy*, vol. 23, no. 4, pp. 325–34.

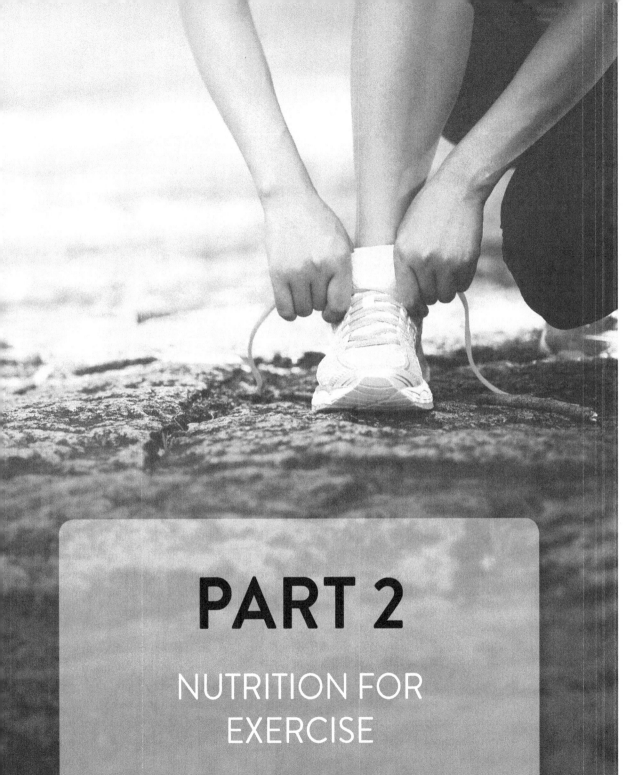

PART 2

NUTRITION FOR EXERCISE

Macronutrient periodisation

Louise M. Burke

Although most people now recognise that sports nutrition involves a personalised approach tailored to the specific needs of the event and the individual, there is still a perception that the athlete's goal is to develop an optimal meal plan (for example, a swimmer's diet or Swimmer X's diet), then carefully repeat it each day to provide consistent support for their training and competition goals. However, contemporary sports nutrition guidelines promote the benefits of a periodised approach to intake energy and macronutrient intake, with each athlete following a range of different dietary practices aligned to the different phases of their training cycles, competition calendars or career progress. Although there is no single or unified definition of the term 'dietary periodisation', Table 9.1 summarises four different themes that involve a strategic manipulation of nutrient intake between and within days to optimise athletic performance. Since the principles and practices of arranging nutrient intake around training/event sessions (intake pre-, during and post-session) are covered in Chapter 10, this chapter will review and summarise the evidence and application of the other three periodisation themes.

LEARNING OUTCOMES

Upon completion of this chapter you will be able to:

- understand that an athlete's training/competition schedule involves changes in the type, quantity and goals of exercise sessions, which should be supported by changes in energy and macronutrient intake
- appreciate that different dietary strategies can enhance the muscle's capacity to use different fuels (such as fat vs carbohydrate), which may play a role in enhancing competition performance
- understand the true meaning of 'metabolic flexibility' and some of the ways in which this concept is currently being used or misused
- be aware of an emerging theme in sports nutrition whereby nutrient support around training can be provided to promote performance/recovery or withdrawn to increase the training stimulus/adaptation.

THEME 1. PERIODISING NUTRITION TO TRACK THE PERIODISATION OF TRAINING AND COMPETITION

An athlete's peak performance is achieved over a number of years, during which they undertake various cycles of preparation and competition. Although many athletes may have a long-term program aimed at an Olympic cycle or the years of a college scholarship, the yearly training plan or annual competition calendar provides a useful snapshot of the concept of periodised training. Typically, the plan is centred around the major competition for which the athlete organises a performance peak. Depending on the logistics of the event and the culture/philosophies of the sport, the coach and athlete may plan for a single or double peak for the year (for example, two major competitions, or qualification for a national team then competition in the international event). The yearly training plan varies considerably between sports according to the athlete's level (developmental, elite, recreational), the type of competition (weekly fixtures, tournaments, single events spread over a season) and the type of event (how much recovery is needed). However, there are some common elements. These include:

- a generalised preparation phase
- a period of training that is more specific to the competitive event
- competition itself
- transition between phases, including an off-season or rest period.

Simplistic overviews of the typical yearly training plans of a team sport and an individual sport are presented in Figures 9.1 and 9.2 respectively, noting differences in the exercise load and goals across each phase that create differences in nutritional needs and strategies. The basic unit of each phase is the training microcycle (typically,

Table 9.1. Examples of themes in which nutrients are periodised to enhance performance

Theme	Description	Explanation or examples
General tracking of energy and nutrient goals	Changing energy and nutrient intake (between days, microcycles, macrocycles, etc.) to meet different needs or goals, according to the specific phases of the training and competition plan.	Athletes undertake a carefully periodised calendar involving different training phases that prepare them to meet short-term and long-term competition goals. Changes in the exercise load, physique-management goals, environmental conditions and many other factors change the energy cost and nutrient needs. The athlete should manipulate their dietary patterns to meet these changes in needs.
Nutrient timing	Arranging nutrient intake over the day, and in relation to training sessions, to enhance the metabolic interaction between exercise and nutrition.	Carbohydrate intake before and during exercise may provide fuel to allow the athlete to train harder or perform better in competition. Provision of nutrients after exercise may enhance recovery or adaptation; for example, optimal spread of protein includes intake soon after exercise and every 3–5 hours over the day. See Chapter 10 for more detail.
'Fat adaptation'	Exposure to a high-fat diet for a period, to increase capacity to use it as a muscle fuel for exercise, before returning to usual diet or competition diet.	Hypothetically, capacity for enhanced fuel utilisation during exercise might occur if adaptations allowing increased fat use can be added to scenarios of high carbohydrate availability and utilisation, leading to enhanced endurance performance.
'Training low' to enhance adaptation	Integrating specific sessions into the training program in which the standard practice of providing nutritional support to promote optimal performance is replaced by deliberate withholding of nutritional support for the session.	There is evidence that the absence of some nutrients around exercise leads to an increased training stimulus and/or an enhanced adaptation. At present, this theory is mostly applied to the theme of carbohydrate availability.

a seven-day rotation), in which a series of workouts (and in some sports, competition) are sequenced to integrate a range of training stimuli that aim to achieve the various physiological, biomechanical, technical, tactical and psychological characteristics needed for success. Typically, the microcycles are manipulated to gradually increase the important loading characteristics (type, volume, intensity) then allow for a lighter

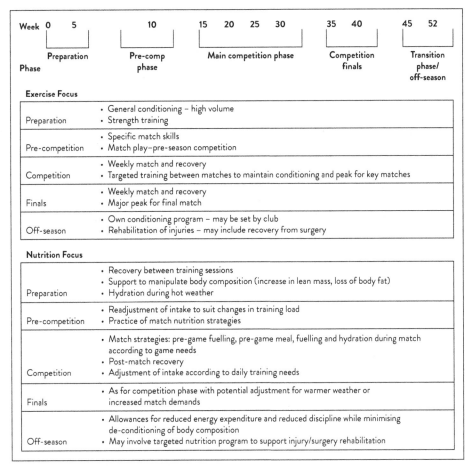

Figure 9.1. Example of a yearly training plan for a team sport (football) with a weekly match fixture

Source: Adapted from Burke and Jeacocke 2011.

'recovery' cycle before continuing to build. At times, an athlete might undertake a special training block, such as altitude or heat training, either to acclimatise to the environmental conditions in which a competition might be held or to gain the benefits of the additional training stimulus provided by thermal or hypoxic exposure. In the precompetition phase, the increased specificity of training will include opportunities to practice and fine-tune nutritional strategies that are important to performance in the event—for example, fluid and carbohydrate intake during exercise. The taper period prior to competition varies across sports, but typically involves a reduction in training volume to allow the athlete to reduce their fatigue levels and reach a performance peak.

The periodisation of training clearly can be improved by a careful periodisation of nutrient intake and dietary practices. Different phases of training—from day to day, within a training block or over the year—will have different requirements for energy and muscle fuel support, as well as differences in the focus on the manipulation or maintenance of physique (for example, to lose body fat, increase lean mass or meet weight division targets), competition practice, or importance of key nutrients (for example, adequate iron status during altitude training). Some of the high-level differences and changes in dietary focus are included in Figures 9.1 and 9.2. Here, the annual training plan for a team sport shows the conditioning phase of the pre-season, with a gradual increase in match-specific skills and practice matches; the main competition season, with a cycle of weekly matches culminating in finals; and an off-season (Figure 9.1). Meanwhile, in Figure 9.2, a swimmer undertakes base training in which 3–4 week cycles of training are integrated, with race-specific training and short race meets being increased towards the major competition. Altitude training may be included in the pre-competition peaking plan, and a significant taper leads into the multi-day swimming meet. In the case where a second competition peak is planned (often the most important competition), there is a short transition leading into a truncated preparation cycle. In this sport, there are major differences in the energy and fuel requirements of training, taper and racing, requiring major changes in food intake.

Within the training microcycle/week, different approaches to the optimal nutritional support for each individual training session should lead to changes in daily energy intake, as well as different emphases on the amount and timing of intake of special macronutrients (such as carbohydrate and protein) around a workout according to their role in 'training harder/better' or 'training smarter'. Some of these issues will be discussed further in Theme 3 and are illustrated by the summary of a typical week of periodised carbohydrate availability in a training study. It is often useful to create an athlete's periodised nutrition plan using an 'inside out' approach to build up a series of layers.

- Identify each key training session for the week and the specific goals of each session. Organise a targeted intake of the most important nutrients before, during and/or after each workout.
- Add the next layer by organising eating occasions for the rest of the day to continue to support these key sessions, also bearing in mind the athlete's 'bigger picture' nutritional needs such as energy (does the athlete need to be in energy balance, or to increase or reduce energy intake to manipulate body composition?), key micronutrients (does the athlete need to increase iron intake? Calcium intake?) and other special issues (for example, food preferences, finances, food availability, intolerance).

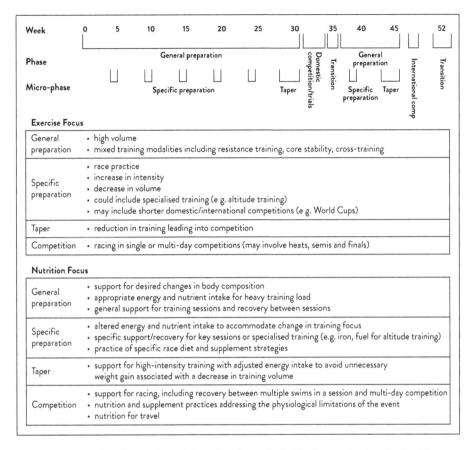

Figure 9.2. Example of a yearly training plan for an individual sport (swimming) with a double peak

Source: Adapted from Burke and Jeacocke 2011.

- Continue to organise eating for days with less important sessions, focusing on the bigger picture nutrition issues. Note that there may be less need to focus on fuelling for these sessions, and even an opportunity to undertake some 'train low' sessions where workouts are deliberately matched up with low-carbohydrate eating strategies (see Theme 3). On the other hand, there may be a need to use low-key training days to fuel up for the next day's important workouts.

The sophistication of this approach is likely to lead to day-to-day differences in intake or, on occasion, similar total intakes that are spread differently between and within days.

Practice of event fluid and fuel intake strategies is an important activity to build into the periodised programs of endurance, ultra-endurance and some team sports. This allows the athlete to individualise and fine-tune a nutrition plan to defend homeostasis and sustain fuel for optimal performance when it is most needed. However, in addition to familiarising themselves with competition eating and drinking behaviours or identifying the foods and drinks that best suit the scenario, targeted intake during training sessions can help to 'train the gut' (Jeukendrup 2017). For example, several adaptations may be needed to help the athlete meet the newer targets for aggressive carbohydrate intake during prolonged exercise; these involve increasing gut tolerance or comfort to allow intake of greater volumes of fluid and food as well as enhancing intestinal absorption of glucose via an increase in the number of **SGLT-1 transporters**.

SGLT-1 transporter
A sodium-dependent glucose transporter. Transport protein found on the walls of cells lining the small intestine, responsible for the transport of glucose and galactose from the small intestine into the circulation.

THEME 2. 'FAT ADAPTATION'

In many events, competitive success is determined by the muscle's ability to optimise the production of adenosine triphosphate (ATP) to meet the requirements of the exercise task. This reflects both the size of the available fuel stores and the muscle's ability to efficiently integrate their use, a concept termed **metabolic flexibility**. Depletion of the body's relatively limited carbohydrate stores is a common cause of fatigue or suboptimal performance during endurance sports (typically defined as events involving prolonged (>90 minutes) continuous exercise). Therefore, it has been proposed that strategies that improve the athlete's capacity to make better use of their larger fat stores will spare the muscle glycogen stores and increase metabolic flexibility. Although training achieves this outcome, the use of fat as a muscle fuel can be further (and more substantially) increased by adapting to a low-carbohydrate, high-fat diet (LCHF). Indeed, short-term (~5 days) exposure to a diet providing <20 per cent energy from carbohydrate and >60 per cent from fat while undertaking both high-volume and high-intensity training sessions achieves a robust retooling of the muscle to increase the mobilisation, transport and oxidation of fat during exercise (Burke 2015).

Metabolic flexibility
The ability of the muscle to integrate and transition between fuel sources in response to exercise or hormonal stimuli. This is enhanced by training.

Two different tactics are possible, and both have been proposed in lay and scientific literature to 'increase metabolic flexibility'. The first protocol involves switching chronically to such a diet to promote the use of fat as the predominant muscle fuel. If this high-fat diet is further carbohydrate-restricted (<50 g/day carbohydrate plus ~80 per cent energy from fat), additional benefits from exposure to high levels of circulating ketone bodies are also claimed; this ketogenic LCHF diet has recently resurfaced in popular interest (Volek et al. 2015). Despite considerable discussion about this diet being 'the future of elite endurance sport' in lay and social media, there is no evidence that it enhances the performance of competitive sports of this type. There is no doubt that chronic (>3–4 weeks) adaptation to the ketogenic LCHF substantially increases the muscle's capacity for fat oxidation during exercise, providing effective fuel support for moderate-intensity exercise (Phinney et al. 1983). However, a recent study from the Australian Institute of Sport, in which elite race walkers were adapted to the LCHF, provided recognition of an important biochemical fact: that the oxygen cost of oxidising fat to produce a given amount of ATP is greater than that of carbohydrate (Burke et al. 2017). Although the group of highly trained to world-class athletes was observed to achieve the highest rates of fat oxidation ever reported in the literature across a range of speeds relevant to the races on the Olympic program, this was associated with a loss of **economy** (that is, a greater amount of oxygen was required to walk at the same speed). In contrast to a control group of walkers who undertook the same training on a diet with high carbohydrate availability, the LCHF walkers failed to improve their 10,000-metre race times at the end of the training block, despite improving their aerobic capacity to a similar extent. This was attributed, at least partially, to reduced walking economy—that is, a reduction in ATP production during high-intensity exercise when oxygen becomes limiting in the support of fat oxidation. This suggests that adaptation to LCHF may be suited to athletes who compete in events conducted entirely at moderate intensities, but provides a disadvantage in endurance sports and ultra-endurance sports involving critical passages of higher-intensity work, where success is determined by the ability to exercise as economically as possible at the highest sustainable intensity.

However, a second strategy involves the sequential optimisation of the two main muscle fuel sources around a competitive event. Specifically, undertaking adaptation to a high-fat diet, before re-establishing high carbohydrate availability via 24 hours of glycogen super-compensation and carbohydrate intake before and during the event, might improve performance if it could combine high carbohydrate stores with an ability to use them more slowly due to increased fat utilisation (Burke 2015). This concept has been studied by several laboratories using the protocol of the shortest effective adaptation to a non-ketogenic LCHF diet (5–6 days) followed by a variety of strategies to restore glycogen and **exogenous carbohydrate availability** around an exercise challenge. However, these attempts failed to find that fat adaptation–carbohydrate restoration protocols enhance the performance of subsequent prolonged

Endogenous carbohydrate fuels
Carbohydrate fuel found inside the muscle cell (glycogen).

Exogenous carbohydrate fuels
Carbohydrate fuel taken up into the muscle from the circulation (blood glucose, which is greatly supplemented by the intake of carbohydrate during exercise).

Box 9.1: Exercise economy

In endurance sports, the term 'exercise economy' describes the oxygen cost of achieving a speed, power or intensity and is highly correlated with competitive performance. Although most high-calibre athletes have a high aerobic capacity (VO_{2max}), within a group of such athletes, economy of movement—being able to move quickly at a relatively low percentage of this capacity—often determines performance. This is especially important when the event, or critical parts of it, are conducted at intensities around the so-called anaerobic threshold.

exercise, despite achieving remarkable reductions in muscle glycogen use (for review, see Burke 2015). One of the apparent explanations for this outcome is that, rather than sparing glycogen utilisation, fat adaptation impairs the muscle's ability to use it as an exercise fuel. In addition to reducing rates of glycogen breakdown, fat adaptation has been shown to impair muscle carbohydrate oxidation via down-regulation of the activity of an important enzyme in the mitochondria—the **pyruvate dehydrogenase** enzyme complex. The consequences of reduced efficiency of carbo-hydrate oxidation are likely to manifest in a reduced ability to support the ATP requirements for exercise at higher intensities. Indeed, a study of the fat adaptation–carbohydrate restoration protocol on performance in a 100-kilometre cycling time-trial found a significant impairment of the cyclists' ability to complete a series of 1-kilometre sprints (>90 per cent peak power output or ~80 per cent VO_{2max}) embedded within the longer protocol (Havemann et al. 2006).

Although other combinations of fat adaptation with or without carbohydrate restoration are possible and merit further study, the current evidence suggests that strategies to chronically adapt to high-fat diets achieve a *reduction* rather than an improvement in metabolic flexibility. Indeed, even when glycogen is available, fat-adaptation strategies appear to interfere with the muscle's capacity to use it as an exercise fuel, particularly via oxidative pathways. This is likely to translate into reduced performance of shorter

Pyruvate dehydrogenase (PDH)
Mitochondrial enzyme complex that commits the breakdown products of glycolysis (the first step in glucose metabolism) into the citric acid (Krebs cycle) oxidation pathway. This step is irreversible and is the rate limiting step in carbohydrate oxidation.

Carbohydrate availability
Consideration of the timing and amount of carbohydrate (CHO) intake in the athlete's diet in comparison to the muscle fuel costs of the training or competition schedule. Scenarios of 'high carbohydrate availability' cover strategies in which body CHO supplies can meet the fuel costs of the exercise program, whereas 'low carbohydrate availability' considers scenarios in which endogenous and/or exogenous CHO supplies are less than muscle fuel needs.

endurance events conducted at these exercise intensities (for example, half marathon, 40-kilometre cycling time-trial), as well as an impaired ability to undertake the critical activities within most longer endurance/ultra-endurance sports events—the break-away, the tactical surge, attacking a hill, the sprint to the finish line—that determine the overall outcome. Therefore, the range of sporting events or scenarios to which they might be suited is small.

THEME 3. 'TRAINING LOW' TO ENHANCE TRAINING ADAPTATIONS

Scientific techniques now allow us to study the cellular responses to exercise and nutrient stimuli. Such techniques have provided the insight that, across many areas of sports nutrition, the processes related to muscle adaptation may be opposite to those that promote recovery/performance. Simply stated, many processes that promote recovery from exercise to restore homeostasis and exercise capacity are based on the provision of nutrient support. Meanwhile, the absence or deliberate withdrawal of nutritional support may increase exercise stress and/or promote signalling pathways that remodel the muscle and other physiological systems to enhance the training response. There-fore, the athlete may use some nutritional strategies to compete optimally or to complete key training sessions as well as possible ('train harder'). Conversely, they may implement the opposite strategy to stimulate greater adaptation to the same exercise stimulus (a 'training smarter' approach). There is evidence that although fluid intake enhances endurance performance in the heat (see Chapter 11), deliberate dehydration during training sessions may enhance the physiological and cardiovascular processes of acclimatisation (Garrett et al. 2014). Nevertheless, the area in which most investi-gation has been undertaken around the theme of strategic addition or withholding of nutritional support involves the manipulation of carbohydrate availability.

Dietary practices that promote high carbohydrate availability are recommended on days in which competition or high-quality/demanding training sessions will benefit from optimal fuelling of muscle and central nervous system function (for instance,. optimisation of work rates, perception of effort, skill and technique, concentration and mental processing). As outlined in Theme 1, carbohydrate intake should be inte-grated with other dietary goals to achieve adequate muscle fuel from glycogen stores supported by additional exogenous carbohydrate supplies as well as to support other body processes requiring carbohydrate (such as immune system support). Targets will consider both the total amount of carbohydrate and its timing of intake around the workout or event. Competition strategies will need to address the practical consider-ations for consuming nutrients around exercise (for example, event rules, opportunity to consume foods/drinks and availability of supplies). On days when training is of lower volume and/or intensity, it may be less critical to meet such targets or practice these strategies.

More recently, it has been shown that glycogen plays important roles in regulating the cellular activities that underpin the muscles' response to exercise. Specifically, undertaking a bout of endurance exercise with low muscle glycogen stores produces a coordinated up-regulation of key signalling and regulatory proteins in the muscle to enhance the adaptive processes following the exercise session (Bartlett et al. 2015). This can be achieved around targeted training sessions by doing two training sessions in close succession or with minimal carbohydrate intake between them, to enable the second bout to be commenced with depleted glycogen stores. Strategies that restrict exogenous carbohydrate availability (such as training in a fasted state) also promote an improved signalling response, although of a lower magnitude than is the case for exercise with low glycogen stores (Bartlett et al. 2015). These strategies enhance the cellular outcomes of endurance training, such as increased maximal mitochondrial enzyme activities and/or mitochondrial content and increased rates of lipid oxidation.

Studies in sub-elite athletes, in which these protocols have been superimposed on most workouts in a training block, have shown evidence of enhanced cellular adaptation. Somewhat curiously, however, these 'muscle advantages' have not transferred to superior performance outcomes compared with the improvements seen following training with high carbohydrate availability. Although there are always challenges in measuring small but important changes in sports performance, the most likely explanation for the 'disconnect' between mechanistic and performance outcomes in these studies is that training with low carbohydrate availability reduced the intensity of the training sessions. In other words, although metabolic benefits were achieved on one hand, they were negated by the sacrifice of training quality. This suggests that 'train low' strategies need to be carefully integrated into the periodised training program to carefully match the specific goal of the session and the larger goals of the training period. Indeed, a more recently identified exercise–nutrient interaction adds another strategy to the carbohydrate periodisation options to assist with this integration. Delaying glycogen resynthesis by withholding carbohydrate in the hours after a higher-intensity training session has also been shown to up-regulate markers of mitochondrial biogenesis and lipid oxidation during the recovery phase without interfering with the quality of the session.

A practical application of this new strategy is that it allows the sequencing of (1) a 'train high' high-quality training session, (2) overnight or within-day carbohydrate restriction ('sleep low') and (3) a moderate-intensity workout undertaken without CHO intake ('**training low**'). This series, demonstrated in two different styles in the case study, supports the important features of each training session while promoting enhanced adaptation. Studies have shown that the integration of several cycles of this sequence into the weekly training programs of sub-elite athletes achieved performance improvements which were not observed in another group who undertook similar training with a similar intake of carbohydrate evenly distributed within and between days (Marquet et al. 2016). Such an approach has been described in the real-life preparation of elite endurance athletes (Stellingwerff 2013). A summary of strategies that promote high or low carbohydrate availability is provided in Table 9.2.

Finally, it should be recognised that studies of elite athletes appear to show less responsiveness to periodisation of carbohydrate availability than seen in sub-elite athletes. Our investigation of the three-week program of intensified training in world-class race walkers failed to detect any difference in the immediate performance benefits achieved between the group that consumed a periodised carbohydrate diet and another group that consumed an evenly spread distribution of the same total carbohydrate intake to promote high carbohydrate availability for all training sessions (Burke et al. 2017). Another study of elite endurance athletes reported no benefits to training adaptation or performance gains from the integration of a within-day sequence of a 'train high'/'recover low'/'train low' protocol, three days a week during a training block, compared with a diet providing more consistent CHO availability (Gejl et al. 2017). It is uncertain whether the lack of benefits is systematically related to the calibre of the athlete. For example, it is possible that elite athletes have a reduced ceiling for improvements in which differences are harder to detect, or an ability to undertake training of such intensity and volume that the stimulus already maximises the adaptive response. Further investigation is merited, but it is likely that most highly trained athletes already integrate some form of periodisation of carbohydrate availability within their schedules, either by design or necessity. The challenge for sports science will be to improve on what athletes achieve through trial and error.

SUMMARY AND KEY MESSAGES

Many of the current frontiers in sports nutrition involve the periodisation of nutrient and energy intake—manipulating intakes between and within days to promote specific goals of adaptation, performance and recovery. Each athlete has unique nutritional goals and requirements, which change according to the specific time of their periodised training and competition calendar. The optimal sports nutrition plan will change from day to day to accommodate these changing goals. We await new knowledge about strategies to optimise the muscle's ability to integrate economical use of its available fuel sources and the potential for strategic withholding of nutritional support around some training sessions to increase the exercise stimulus and promote greater adaptation. Of course, there is often a disconnect between the hypothetical advantages of a single strategy and the overall effect on performance. Therefore, research must continue to evaluate the

Table 9.2. Dietary strategies that achieve specific goals with carbohydrate availability

Low carbohydrate availability: strategies undertaken to increase the exercise stimulus and/or to enhance the adaptive response to an exercise bout	
Protocol	**Strategy**
Chronic low carbohydrate availability (achieves low endogenous and exogenous carbohydrate availability)	Ketogenic LCHF diet (<50 g/day carbohydrate, ~80% energy as fat). Non-ketogenic LCHF diet (15–20% energy as carbohydrate, 60–65% energy as fat).
Acute low carbohydrate availability training ('train low')—endogenous	Undertaking prior bout of prolonged sustained or intermittent exercise followed by restricted intake of carbohydrate to limit glycogen resynthesis during recovery phase. Note that it is the second session that is done as a 'train low' session, and the between-session recovery phase can be brief (1–2 hours) or prolonged (overnight or full day).
Acute low carbohydrate availability training ('train low')—exogenous	Undertaking workout in the morning in a fasted state, and without any carbohydrate intake during the session. (Note: could also be done for a session later in the day with only water during the session.)
Acute post-exercise low carbohydrate availability ('recover low' or 'sleep low'—if overnight)	Restricting carbohydrate intake in the hours after a key workout to delay glycogen resynthesis.
High carbohydrate availability: strategies undertaken to provide adequate fuel for the exercise session, promoting optimal performance or practising event nutrition strategies	
Protocol	**Strategy**
Chronic high carbohydrate availability	Consuming enough carbohydrate in the everyday diet to consistently meet the fuel needs of training or competition, with intake organised around each exercise session to ensure optimal fuelling.
Active refuelling	Consuming carbohydrate in sufficient quantities, starting soon after an exercise session to optimise glycogen resynthesis after the session.
Training high—endogenous	Consuming adequate carbohydrate in the recovery between two sessions, including a pre-session snack or meal to provide adequate glycogen for the workout or competition event.
Training high—exogenous	Consuming carbohydrate in the pre-exercise meal to ensure high liver glycogen levels as well as carbohydrate during the session to provide an ongoing supply of blood glucose as an additional muscle fuel.
Carbohydrate loading	Organising an exercise taper in conjunction with high carbohydrate intake to supercompensate muscle glycogen stores prior to endurance or ultra-endurance competition.

overall significance of a strategy rather than focusing on a single perspective. Sports performance involves a complex mixture of whole-body physiology and central drive, as well as muscle characteristics. Although in many cases sports science merely explains or supports practices that athletes and coaches have already found to be valuable, advances in sports nutrition knowledge arising from investigations of cellular changes are likely to lead to new concepts and opportunities to enhance sports performance.

Key messages

- Modern sports nutrition promotes eating practices that are personalised, periodised and specific to the athlete and their event and training schedule.
- Just as athletes have a periodised program of training and competition, nutrition strategies should be strategically organised to maximise the interaction between exercise and key nutrients.
- Energy and macronutrient intake should change from day to day (and even within the day, according to the needs of each training session or competition schedule) according to the specific exercise load, the goals of each session and the athlete's overall nutrition goals.
- An outcome of an athlete's training—especially for endurance sports—is to increase the muscle's ability to store and use carbohydrate and fat fuels. This is known as metabolic flexibility and is particularly important in endurance and ultra-endurance events, where the fuel needs of the event may exceed the muscle's normal carbohydrate stores.
- Strategies to consume carbohydrate before, during and after exercise increase carbohydrate availability and are associated with enhanced capacity for prolonged moderate- to high-intensity exercise, including the ability to increase intensity for critical parts of the event.
- Although a high-fat diet can increase muscle capacity to use fat as an exercise fuel, the adaptations also seem to reduce capacity for carbohydrate utilisation and may decrease overall metabolic flexibility. Although fat can fuel exercise of moderate intensity, it is associated with reduced exercise economy (a greater oxygen cost to produce the same amount of ATP and, therefore, the same speed or power output). Compared to carbohydrate fuels, fat is less able to sustain higher-intensity exercise when the oxygen supply to the muscle becomes limiting.
- Despite the recent renewal of interest, low-carbohydrate, high-fat (LCHF) diets appear to be less suited to the needs of competitive endurance athletes who need to undertake all or critical parts of their events at high intensities supported by carbohydrate metabolism. They may be better suited to ultra-endurance events in which the athlete competes at a steady pace of moderate-intensity exercise.

- Endurance athletes may make use of the developing ideas around training protocols that integrate specific strategies of high carbohydrate availability around key training sessions (allowing them to 'train harder') alongside strategies that deliberately achieve low carbohydrate availability after or during other sessions to increase the training stimulus and adaptive responses (promoting 'a train smarter' outcome).

REFERENCES

Bartlett, J.D., Hawley, J.A. & Morton, J.P., 2015, 'Carbohydrate availability and exercise training adaptation: Too much of a good thing?', *European Journal of Sport Science*, vol. 15, no. 1, pp. 3–12.

Burke, L.M., 2015, 'Re-examining high-fat diets for sports performance: Did we call the "nail in the coffin" too soon?', *Sports Medicine*, vol. 15, suppl. 1, pp. S33–49.

Burke, L.M. & Jeacocke, N.A., 2011, 'The basis of nutrient timing and its place in sport and metabolic regulation', in Kerksick C. (ed.), *Nutrient Timing: Metabolic Optimisation for Health, Performance and Recovery*, Boca Raton, FL: CRC Press, pp. 1–22.

Burke, L.M., Ross, M.L., Garvican-Lewis, L.A., et al., 2017, 'Low carbohydrate, high fat diet impairs exercise economy and negates the performance benefit from intensified training in elite race walkers', *Journal of Physiology*, vol. 595, no. 9, pp. 2785–807.

Garrett, A.T., Goosens, N.G., Rehrer, N.J. et al., 2014, 'Short-term heat acclimation is effective and may be enhanced rather than impaired by dehydration', *American Journal of Human Biology*, vol. 26, no. 3, pp. 311–20.

Gejl, K.D., Thams, L., Hansen, M., et al., 2017, 'No superior adaptations to carbohydrate periodisation in elite endurance athletes', *Medicine & Science in Sports & Exercise*, vol. 49, no. 12, pp. 2486–97.

Havemann, L., West, S., Goedecke, J.H., et al., 2006, 'Fat adaptation followed by carbohydrate-loading compromises high-intensity sprint', *Journal of Applied Physiology*, vol. 100, no. 1, pp. 194–202.

Jeukendrup, A.E., 2017, 'Training the gut for athletes', *Sports Medicine*, vol. 47, suppl. 1, pp. 101–10.

Marquet, L.A., Hausswirth, C., Molle, O., et al., 2016, 'Periodization of carbohydrate intake: Short-term effect on performance', *Nutrients*, vol. 8, no. 12, pp. 755.

Phinney, S.D., Bistrian, B.R., Evans, W.J., et al., 1983, 'The human metabolic response to chronic ketosis without caloric restriction: Preservation of submaximal exercise capability with reduced carbohydrate oxidation', *Metabolism*, vol. 32, no. 8, pp. 769–76.

Stellingwerff, T., 2013, 'Contemporary nutrition approaches to optimise elite marathon performance', *International Journal of Sports Physiology and Performance*, vol. 8, no. 5, pp. 573–8.

Volek, J.S., Noakes, T., & Phinney, S.D., 2015, 'Rethinking fat as a fuel for endurance exercise', *European Journal of Sport Science*, vol. 15, no. 1, pp. 13–20.

CHAPTER 10

Exercise nutrition

Regina Belski

Athletes need to consume a diet that meets their energy, macronutrient and micronutrient requirements, and maximises their exercise outcomes and recovery. The optimal sports nutrition plan for each athlete will change from day to day to accommodate changes in training, goals and other factors impacting on the athlete. However, there are some broad recommendations for what to eat and drink before, during and following exercise, and these will be the focus of this chapter. The International Society of Sports Nutrition position stand (Kerksick et al. 2017) on nutrient timing was updated in 2017, and their position is considered in this chapter.

More specific recommendations, where available, are discussed in the following chapters, which focus on sporting categories: Endurance (Chapter 14), Strength and power (Chapter 15). Additionally, the emerging trends of macronutrient periodisation, 'training low' and fat adaptation are discussed in more detail in Chapter 9.

LEARNING OUTCOMES

Upon completion of this chapter you will:
- understand the current recommendations for nutrient intake and hydration prior to, during and following exercise
- be able to suggest practical meal and snack ideas to athletes suitable for before, during and after exercise

- appreciate that all individual athletes are different, and there is no one-size-fits-all approach to exercise nutrition.

GENERAL EATING FOR TRAINING AND EXERCISE

As discussed in previous chapters, it is critical that athletes consume appropriate intakes of energy, macro- and micronutrients for training and competition, to have appropriate energy and **substrate** availability for the exercise that they undertake and to enable tissue growth and repair. This means that it is important to consider their overall diet quality, and not solely what they eat before, during and after exercise. There are general macronutrient intake recommendations for athletes, which are summarised below.

Substrate

The substance, in this case the macronutrients carbohydrate, fat and protein, on which enzymes work.

Fat intake recommendations for athletes are consistent with public health guidelines and should be individualised based on training level and body composition goals.

Carbohydrate requirements vary greatly based on the type and intensity of sport/exercise (Burke et al. 2011):

- Light exercise: 3–5 g/kg of body mass (BM) per day
- Moderate intensity: 5–7 g/kg BM/day
- High intensity: 6–10 g/kg BM/day
- Very high intensity: 8–12 g/kg BM/day.

Protein requirements also vary, with current data suggesting that the level of intake necessary to support metabolic adaptation, repair, remodelling and for protein turnover in athletes is likely higher than previously recommended, as studies' previous recommendations were based on used methods which are now known to underestimate protein needs. The latest International Society for Sports Nutrition position stand on protein and exercise (Jäger et al. 2017) suggests that:

- Daily intakes of 1.4 to 2.0 g/kg/day should be the minimum recommended amount with higher amounts likely needed for athletes attempting to restrict energy intake while maintaining muscle mass.
- Meeting the total daily intake of high-quality protein (containing essential amino acids, especially leucine), preferably with evenly spaced protein feedings of 0.25–0.40 g/kg BM/dose, approximately every 3–4 hours during the day, should be viewed as a primary area of emphasis for exercising individuals. Higher doses may be needed to maximise muscle building for older/elderly individuals.

Casein protein

Casein is a family of related phosphoproteins, which are found in mammalian milk. About 80 per cent of the protein in cow's milk is casein.

- Consuming 30–40 grams of **casein protein** before sleep can lead to acute increases in muscle protein synthesis and metabolic rate without influencing fat breakdown.

EATING AND DRINKING BEFORE EXERCISE

The key goal of eating and drinking before exercise is to optimise fuel and hydration levels and to make an athlete feel well-prepared for the exercise ahead. There is also now evidence that the nutrients consumed prior to exercise may impact on muscle protein synthesis following exercise.

Timing of meals

The right time to consume foods before training or competition will vary depending on when the exercise is to take place. It is generally recommended that consuming a 'main' meal about 2–4 hours prior to exercise will prevent any gastrointestinal issues arising; however, if an athlete is training or competing early in the day, or planning a long exercise session, then a small meal or snack 1–2 hours before exercise may be advised.

When working with individual athletes it is important to listen to their feedback regarding their preferences and past experience, as some athletes have no digestive issues (see Chapter 23) related to eating even within 15 minutes of commencing exercise, while others struggle if less than two hours has passed since their last meal. This simply emphasises that individual gastric emptying rates, as well as the type of food consumed, play an important role in what the best pre-exercise timing may be for an individual athlete.

Content of meals

It is well recognised that carbohydrate intake before exercise may provide fuel to allow the athlete to train harder or perform better during training and competition. Therefore, a meal or snack high in carbohydrate is generally recommended, as this enables the body to top-up its blood glucose and glycogen stores.

Recommendations vary regarding the amount and type of carbohydrate to consume. Low glycaemic index (GI) carbohydrates (see Chapter 4) have been promoted as a good choice, since they would be more slowly absorbed and lead to a rise in blood glucose in time for, or during, exercise; however, while some early research suggested this outcome, it has not been consistently supported by research. It appears that athletes can select whichever form of carbohydrate they tolerate best, as long as the amount they can consume is appropriate. It is also recommended that foods consumed should be those easier to digest—namely, foods lower in fat and fibre. The reason for lower fat choices is to minimise the length of time the food sits in the stomach, while the lower fibre also allows for food to transition faster, minimising risk of gastrointestinal discomfort (see Chapter 23).

The recommended amount of carbohydrate to consume before exercise sessions lasting more than 60 minutes is 1–4 g/kg BM in the 1–4 hours beforehand. However, generally speaking, for training or events lasting less than 90 minutes, the consumption of a high-carbohydrate diet incorporating 7–12 g/kg BM of carbohydrates in the 24 hours beforehand should be adequate to meet the needs of most athletes (Thomas et al. 2016).

What about protein?

While the benefits of consuming protein immediately after exercise are well known, the benefits of consuming protein prior to exercise are less clear. Recent research suggests that protein consumption before and/or during exercise may further stimulate post-exercise muscle growth. Researchers working in this space have also suggested that the consumption of protein before or during exercise may offer an even greater benefit during the early stages of recovery from more intense training sessions (van Loon 2014). The International Society of Sports Nutrition position stand on protein and exercise suggests that timing of protein ingestion should be based on individual tolerance, since benefits will be derived from intake before or after a workout (Jäger et al. 2017). Although it diminishes with time, the anabolic (muscle-building) effect of exercise lasts for at least 24 hours (Jäger et al. 2017).

Research also suggests that pre-exercise consumption of amino acids in combination with carbohydrate can achieve maximal rates of muscle protein synthesis (Jäger et al. 2017).

Fluid

As discussed in detail in the chapter on hydration (see Chapter 11), being well hydrated prior to commencing exercise is important. The current recommendation is to aim for 5–10 ml/kg BM in the 2–4 hours prior to exercise. Depending on the length of the planned exercise session, and whether food is also being consumed, water or sports drink may be the best options.

Pre-exercise meals and snacks

Some suggestions of suitable pre-exercise meals and snacks are listed in Box 10.1. These are just ideas and may not be suitable for all athletes. Athletes should be supported in developing individualised plans based on personal preferences, and these should be trialled during training.

Common problems reported by athletes

Nerves

While being nervous is not uncommon in athletes before exercise, nerves can be particularly problematic prior to competition as they can impact on the athlete's ability to fuel

Box 10.1: Examples of suitable pre-exercise meals/snacks

PRE-EXERCISE MEAL (2–4 HOURS PRIOR)
- Breakfast cereal with low-fat milk
- Pancakes with jam/fruit and fruit yoghurt
- Sandwiches/rolls with meat filling
- Pasta dish with low-fat, tomato-based sauce
- Low-fat rice dish

PRE-EXERCISE SNACK (1–2 HOURS PRIOR)
- Fruit
- Fruit yoghurt
- Low-fat fruit smoothie
- Sports bar/Cereal bar
- Toast with honey/jam
- Low-fat creamed rice

PRE-EXERCISE SNACK (<1 HOUR PRIOR)
- Carbohydrate gel
- Sports bar
- Sports drink
- Jelly lollies, e.g. jelly babies

up appropriately. Athletes often report lack of appetite, a feeling of butterflies in their stomach and nausea as common symptoms. It is clear that such issues can impact on an athlete's ability to consume a suitable meal or snack prior to training or competition. Athletes should seek support to develop specific strategies to manage and overcome these challenges. This may include finding foods that might be tolerated even with nausea, such as dry toast or plain pasta, or, if pre-exercise eating is not possible, planning the meal the night before an early session to maximise nutrition and hydration status.

Gastrointestinal discomfort
Gastrointestinal discomfort, which may include abdominal pain, flatulence and diarrhoea, can also be caused by nerves or by some of the foods/fluids being consumed by the athlete. This topic is discussed in more detail in Chapter 23. Athletes should never be encouraged to try a new type, amount or timing of food/supplement/sports drink during a competition, and should experiment with new foods and fluids only

during training sessions where they have control over the environment and situation. The drinks/foods/gels that will be provided at competitions should be identified and trialled well in advance. If these options are not well tolerated by the athlete, individual nutrition provision needs to be planned, practised and brought to the competition.

EATING AND DRINKING DURING EXERCISE

Generally speaking there are two key approaches to food and fluid provision during exercise; one aims to replace as much of the fuel and fluid used during the exercise session as possible with the aim of maximising exercise performance, and the other focuses on the concept of 'training low' to enhance adaptation.

Replacing nutrient and fluid loss

For exercise sessions up to 90 minutes, it is generally sufficient to simply replace fluid losses. For most athletes, water will be sufficient; however, for those athletes who are big or 'salty' sweaters, beverages containing **electrolytes** may be a better choice, particularly as sweat rates can vary considerably (from 0.3 to 2.4 L per hour). Furthermore, if athletes are training without having consumed an appropriate meal or snack containing carbohydrate leading up to the session, the consumption of carbohydrates via sports drinks is also often advised.

For longer sessions, especially those focused on endurance-type exercise, it is important for athletes to consider their likely fluid and nutrient losses and plan suitable drinks/snacks to maintain their fuel and hydration levels and optimise the exercise session.

Electrolytes
Salts that dissolve in water and disassociate into charged particles called ions.

Stop-start sports
Sports in which the play is frequently stopped due to the ball going out of play or the referee stopping play because of violations of the rules. This includes sports like basketball and football.

The recommended amount of carbohydrate to consume during training/events varies based on length and intensity, with 30–60 grams per hour recommended for endurance sports and **stop-start sports** lasting 1–2.5 hours and as much as 90 grams per hour (mixed-substrate) for ultra-endurance sessions/sports lasting in excess of 2.5–3 hours (Thomas et al. 2016). More details on the needs of endurance athletes, and strategies for fuelling endurance events, can be found in Chapter 14.

There are also specific recommendations from the International Society of Sports Nutrition based on the latest research (Kerksick et al. 2017).

- For extended bouts of high-intensity exercise lasting over an hour, carbohydrate should be consumed at a rate of 30–60 grams of carbohydrate per hour in a 6–8 per cent carbohydrate-electrolyte solution every 10–15 minutes throughout the entire exercise session.

- When carbohydrate consumption during exercise is inadequate, adding protein (0.25 g of protein/kg body weight per hour of endurance exercise) may help increase performance, minimise muscle damage and improve glycogen resynthesis.
- Carbohydrate ingestion throughout resistance exercise has also been shown to promote steady blood sugar levels and higher glycogen stores.

It is important to consider what the athlete will tolerate best, as some athletes have no problems consuming sports drink and a sandwich during an event while others struggle even to drink water without experiencing gastrointestinal issues. Nutrition plans should be based not only on the type and length of exercise, but also on the individual needs and preferences of the athlete.

As discussed in detail in Chapter 11, the current recommendation is to aim to consume 400–800 mL/hour of fluid during exercise, with the aim of avoiding body-water losses of more than two per cent. Cold drinks are recommended for hot conditions.

It is important to note that during exercise sessions exceeding two hours in length, gastrointestinal tolerance and availability of fluids will restrict what fluids will be accessible and tolerable to athletes. This makes it unlikely that athletes will be able to match sweat fluid losses with fluid intakes (Garth & Burke 2013). Athletes should be encouraged to commence exercise well-hydrated and to replace fluid losses after exercise.

Suitable drinks and snacks during exercise

Some suggestions of suitable snacks to consume during exercise are listed below. These are just ideas and may not be suitable for all athletes. Athletes should be supported to develop individualised plans based on personal preferences.

Suitable snacks/drinks providing 30–40 grams of carbohydrate:

- 600 mL sports drink
- 1 sports bar
- 1.5 carbohydrate gels
- 40 g jelly lollies
- 1.5 cereal bars.

Training low

The concept of 'training low' to enhance adaptation generally refers to training with low carbohydrate availability, but may also be practised with other nutrients. The aim of this approach is to integrate specific sessions into a training program where the standard practice of providing nutritional support to promote optimal performance is replaced by deliberately withholding nutritional support prior to and during the session. There is some evidence to suggest that the absence of certain nutrients (for instance, carbohydrate) around exercise leads to an increased training stimulus and/or an enhanced metabolic adaptation to exercise. There are numerous different ways in which athletes can 'train low', with different metabolic outcomes. Refer back to Chapter 9 for more detail regarding the evidence and recommendations for training low.

EATING AND DRINKING AFTER EXERCISE

The key aim of eating and drinking after exercise is to replenish the body's fluid and fuel stores used during exercise and optimise recovery post-exercise. The provision of nutrients after exercise may also enhance metabolic adaptations to exercise.

Carbohydrates

One of the goals of post-exercise nutrition is to restore glycogen levels; this requires adequate carbohydrate intake and time. The glycogen resynthesis rate appears to be around five per cent per hour. The consumption of 1–1.2 g/kg BM/h of carbohydrate early in the recovery period (during the first 4–6 hours) has been shown to be effective in maximising refuelling time between workouts (Thomas et al. 2016).

Protein

Research has shown that the consumption of high-quality protein sources (0.25 g/kg BM or an absolute dose of 20–40 grams), rich in essential amino acids, within two hours of completion of exercise results in increases in muscle protein synthesis. (Jäger et al. 2017).

What about if rapid recovery is needed?

During times of intensive training or competition, rapid recovery and restoration of glycogen stores may be required. Where there is less than four hours of recovery time available, the following strategies—as recommended by the International Society of Sports Nutrition based on current research—should be considered (Kerksick et al. 2017).

- Intensive carbohydrate refeeding (1.2 g/kg BM/h) with high glycaemic index carbohydrates (see Chapter 4).
- Consumption of caffeine (3–8 mg/kg BM).
- Combination of carbohydrates (0.8 g/kg BM/h) with protein (0.2–0.4 g/kg BM/h).

Fluid

Hydration and rehydration are discussed in detail in Chapter 11. After exercise, it is recommended that athletes replace 125–150 per cent of fluid loss. For example, if

> **Box 10.2: Snack/meal options for after exercise**
>
> - Sports drink with low-fat fruit yoghurt
> - Low-fat chocolate milk
> - Liquid breakfast substitute drinks
> - Fruit smoothies made with low-fat milk/yoghurt
> - Pancakes with fruit and low-fat yoghurt

an athlete has lost 2 kilograms of weight during exercise, they should aim to consume 2.5–3 litres of fluid following exercise to replace the loss. Eating solid food at this time will help maximise fluid retention.

SUMMARY AND KEY MESSAGES

After reading this chapter, you should understand that the athlete's general nutrition is important for optimal health and wellbeing and poor general nutrition choices will impact on exercise performance. Making appropriate choices throughout the day, as well as optimising food and fluid intake around exercise, will help the athlete to undertake quality training sessions. The aim of food and drink consumption prior to exercise is to optimise fuel and hydration levels and enable an athlete to feel prepared for exercise. During exercise, the key objective is to try to manage the fluid loss and refuel with carbohydrate to maintain blood glucose levels and train harder or perform better. Following an exercise session, the aim is to refuel, rehydrate and enhance recovery or adaptation. Nutrition plans should be developed using the most suitable choices based on athletes' specific requirements and personal dietary preferences.

Key messages
- Athletes' general diets are most important for optimal health and exercise performance.
- Training and competition nutrition should be planned in accordance with the individual athlete's training, goals and preferences.
- Nutrition should be provided before exercise to be well hydrated with full glycogen stores.
- During exercise, athletes should aim to top-up as much lost fluid and carbohydrate as possible, or utilise appropriate 'train low' techniques.
- After exercise, athletes should aim to rehydrate and refuel in time for the next exercise session, as well as consume the appropriate type and amount of nutrients to support metabolic adaptation and muscle growth.

REFERENCES

Burke, L.M., Hawley, J.A., Wong, S.H. et al., 2011, 'Carbohydrates for training and competition', *Journal of Sports Sciences*, vol. 29, suppl. 1, pp. S17–27.

Jäger, R., Kerksick, C.M., Campbell, B.I. et al., 2017, 'International Society of Sports Nutrition position stand: Protein and exercise', *Journal of the International Society of Sports Nutrition*, vol. 14, suppl 2, p. 20.

Garth, A.K. & Burke, L.M., 2013, 'What do athletes drink during competitive sporting activities?', *Sports Medicine*, vol. 43, no. 7, pp. 539–64.

Kerksick, C.M., Arent, S., Schoenfeld, B.J., et al., 2017, 'International Society of Sports Nutrition position stand: Nutrient timing', *Journal of the International Society of Sports Nutrition*, vol. 14, suppl. 2, p. 33.

Thomas, D.T., Erdman, K.A. & Burke, L.M., 2016, 'American College of Sports Medicine Joint Position Statement. Nutrition and Athletic Performance', *Medicine & Science in Sports & Exercise*, vol. 48, no. 3, pp. 543–68.

van Loon, L.J., 2014, 'Is there a need for protein ingestion during exercise?', *Sports Medicine*, vol. 44, suppl. 1, pp. 105–11.

CHAPTER 11

Hydration

Ben Desbrow and Christopher Irwin

In this chapter, we explore the role of water as an essential nutrient and the physiological basis of hydration. Firstly, we discuss the importance of hydration and the effects of dehydration on performance. We then examine methods of hydration assessment, recommendations for staying hydrated and explore drinking strategies that promote rehydration during and after exercise. We also examine the role of beverage ingredients and how they influence rehydration. Finally, we explore the impact of drinking alcohol on hydration, recovery and performance.

LEARNING OUTCOMES

Upon completion of this chapter you will be able to:
- understand the fundamental roles of water in the human body
- describe the effects of dehydration on performance
- describe hydration assessment techniques and the strengths and limitations of various methods
- identify appropriate drinking strategies to optimise rehydration for athletes
- understand the interaction between food and fluid combinations on rehydration
- describe the effect of alcohol on recovery and rehydration.

THE IMPORTANCE OF HYDRATION

Water accounts for approximately 50–70 per cent of body weight (BW) in humans. However, this volume varies with body composition (lean and fat mass) and is therefore generally greater in males (60–70 per cent BW) compared to females (50–55 per cent BW) (Oppliger & Bartok 2002; Jequier & Constant 2010).

Hydrolytic reaction
When the addition of water to another compound leads to the formation of two or more products; for example, the catalytic conversion of starch to sugar.

Water has many important roles in the body. It serves as a chemical solvent, a substrate for **hydrolytic reactions**, a transport medium for nutrients and metabolic waste products, a shock-absorbent, lubricant (for example, to the gastrointestinal and respiratory tracts) and a structural component. Almost every biological process occurring in the human body is dependent on the maintenance of **total body water** (TBW) balance.

Total body water
The total sum of water in the body. It is the sum of water within the cells (intracellular) and outside the cells (extracellular).

Water loss occurs naturally in humans as part of daily living. The majority of daily losses occur through urine (~1–2 litres), faeces (~200 ml), respiration (~250–400 ml), and via the skin (~450–500 ml) (Maughan 2003). In general, this equates to about 2–3 litres per day ($L \cdot d^{-1}$) for a sedentary adult (Jequier & Constant 2010). However, these amounts are influenced by many factors, such as dietary intake, environmental conditions and physical activity levels. Individuals exposed to extremely hot climates, and those who are physically active, are likely to have increased losses. But these losses are usually corrected quite rapidly (within 24 hours) provided adequate fluid consumption occurs (Cheuvront et al. 2004).

Thermoregulation
The maintenance of the body at a particular temperature regardless of the external temperature.

For athletes, it is the cardiovascular and **thermoregulatory** functions of water that are most critical to performance (Murray 2007). The energetic demands of muscular activity (primarily, the demand for oxygen) are met via circulating blood, the major component of which is water. Circulating blood also contributes to thermoregulation, transporting excess heat generated via substrate oxidation from the body's core to the surface of the skin, where it can be lost to the environment. Thus, it is important that athletes are sufficiently hydrated to optimise these processes.

EXERCISE AND DEHYDRATION

During exercise the body cools itself by sweating, but this ultimately results in the loss of body fluid. If this fluid loss is not replaced, it can lead to dehydration. Generally, the body is capable of tolerating low to moderate levels of dehydration (<2% BW loss); however, as levels of dehydration rise (≥2% BW loss), performance (physical and mental) may become impaired (Murray 2007). Dehydration can cause:

- increased heart rate
- increased perception of effort
- increased fatigue
- impaired physical performance (for example, strength, endurance)
- impaired cognitive performance (for example, concentration, decision-making, skill and coordination)
- gastrointestinal issues, such as nausea, vomiting and diarrhoea
- increased risk of heat illness.

For that reason, current practical guidelines for athletes encourage consumption of sufficient volumes of fluid before, during and after exercise to minimise dehydration.

Exercise can also elicit high electrolyte losses (mainly sodium) through the sweating response, particularly in warm to hot conditions. While sweat sodium concentrations vary between individuals (depending on factors such as sweat rate, genetics, diet and acclimation), in the event of large fluid losses most athletes need to also consider replacing lost electrolytes.

HYDRATION ASSESSMENT

There is no general agreement on the most effective method of assessing an individual's hydration status at any single point in time. There are, however, a number of techniques commonly used for the assessment of hydration status. These typically involve either whole body, blood, urinary or sensory measurements. Some of these methods are only suitable for use in laboratory environments, while others can be used easily in the field. A number of novel techniques have also been developed in an effort to devise ways of accurately measuring changes in hydration status without the need to remove clothing or provide invasive biological specimens. However, these methods are still undergoing experimental testing to determine their validity.

Each method has its own specific strengths and limitations, and the process of selecting the most suitable technique is dependent on several factors that influence practicality, such as cost, the technical expertise required, portability and efficiency (Table 11.1). In addition, while some methods are able to provide valid assessments of hydration status across acute and chronic time points, others are only valid under specific conditions. For example, most urine markers are not considered to be a valid measure of current hydration status as these values are subject to large variations in response to rapid consumption of fluid (Sawka et al. 2007). However, they may be used after a standardised period (for example, on waking or after a period of restricted fluid consumption). Monitoring urine colour is a convenient hydration assessment tool and typically indicates prior fluid consumption behaviour. That is, when optimal

Table 11.1. Summary of commonly used hydration assessment techniques

Measure	Purpose	Practicality				Accuracy	Validity
		Cost	Analysis time	Technical expertise	Portability	Overall practicality		
Field measures								
Urine specific gravity	Fluid concentration	2	1	1	1	M/H	M	C
Urine colour	Fluid concentration	1	1	1	1	H	M	C
Body weight change	TBW change	1	1	1	1	H	M	A
Rating of thirst	TBW change	1	1	1	1	H	L	A
Laboratory measures								
Isotope dilution	TBW content	3	3	3	3	L	H	A & C
Neuron activation	TBW content	3	3	3	3	L	H	A & C
Bioelectrical impedance	TBW content	2	3	2	2	M	M	A

Measure	Purpose	Practicality					Accuracy	Validity
		Cost	Analysis time	Technical expertise	Portability	Overall practicality		
Field measures								
Haematocrit & haemoglobin	Plasma volume change	2	2	3	3	M	H	A
Plasma osmolality	Fluid concentration	3	2	3	3	M/L	H	A & C
Urine osmolality	Fluid concentration	3	2	3	3	M/L	M	C
Experimental measures								
Tear osmolarity	Fluid concentration	3	1	2	2	M	L	A & C
Salivary osmolality	Fluid concentration	3	2	3	3	M/L	L	A

Notes: TBW: Total body water; 1: Small/Little/Portable; 2: Moderate/Intermediate; 3: Great/Much/Not portable; A: Acute; C: Chronic; H: High; L: Low; M: Moderate

Source: Adapted from Sawka et al. 2007 and Armstrong 2005.

amounts of fluid are consumed, urine should be pale yellow or clear. If inadequate fluid has been consumed, urine will be dark yellow. Urine colour can be monitored easily by comparing against the eight-point urine colour chart (Armstrong et al. 1998). However, as with all urine markers of hydration status, urine colour is influenced by rapid consumption of fluid, which facilitates **diuresis**. Therefore, it is best used as an indicator of first morning hydration status, upon waking and prior to ingestion of any fluid.

Diuresis
Increased or excessive production of urine.

The precision, accuracy and reliability of the assessment techniques are particularly important and should be prioritised, within the constraints of technical expertise and cost, when selecting the most appropriate method to monitor the hydration status of athletes.

BEFORE, DURING AND AFTER SPORT FLUID CONSIDERATIONS

An athlete's choice of a beverage (and the volume they consume) can be influenced by many factors, such as availability, palatability, thirst, gastrointestinal tolerance, temperature, nutrition knowledge and cost. It is also important to recognise that while fluid consumption may offset the effects of dehydration, it may also facilitate the ingestion of other ingredients (for example, carbohydrate) known to enhance performance. The timing of consumption relative to the exercise bout has a significant influence on beverage recommendations given to athletes to optimise performance (see Table 11.2).

During exercise ≤120 min, gastrointestinal tolerance (see Chapter 23) and access to fluids restrict the beverages that are likely to be well tolerated by athletes. Water and

Table 11.2. Summary of fluid recommendations prior to, during and following exercise to optimise performance

	Recommendation	Other considerations
Prior to exercise	5–10 ml·kg⁻¹ BW 2–4 hrs before exercise	Use urine colour to guide volume. Avoid high-fat fluids.
During exercise	Typically 400–800 ml·h⁻¹ Avoid deficit <2% BW	Sweat rates can vary considerably (range 0.3–2.4 L·h⁻¹). Drink cold beverages in hot conditions.
Following exercise	Replace 125–150% of fluid deficit	Food consumption likely to improve fluid retention.

Source: Adapted from Nutrition and Athletic Performance: Position of Dietitians of Canada, the Academy of Nutrition and Dietetics and the American College of Sports Medicine 2016.

carbohydrate-electrolyte beverages (sports drinks) are commonly recommended for consumption during events involving high-intensity, short-duration competition (such as netball, football and basketball). While commercial sports drinks are specifically formulated to be well tolerated and utilised under conditions of physical exertion (containing 6–8 per cent carbohydrate and 10–25 per cent mmol·L^{-1} of sodium), during competition athletes are unlikely to match sweat fluid losses with beverage intakes (Garth & Burke 2013). This suggests that athletes need to ensure they commence competition well hydrated and/or aim to replace fluid deficits following exercise.

Effectiveness of different beverages on fluid retention

In hydration science, the effect of any beverage on body fluid status is judged by the balance between how much the body retains of any volume that is consumed. Accurately establishing retention rates of different beverages typically involves laboratory research and the prescription of a fixed volume of a beverage under standardised conditions, followed by a period of monitoring fluid losses. Recently, the 'beverage hydration index' (BHI) has been established to describe the fluid retention capacity of different beverages by standardising values to the retention of still water (Maughan et al. 2016). The BHI research findings indicate that many beverages are as effective at delivering fluid as water. Only milk beverages and oral rehydration solutions produced superior fluid retention to water (Table 11.3).

Beverage-hydration index
An index system that has been developed to describe the fluid retention capacity of different beverages by standardising values to the retention of still water.

One strength of the BHI is that it recognises that all beverages make a contribution to total fluid intake (ranking some as more effective than others). In contrast, many fluid recommendations focus on avoiding certain beverages (such as caffeinated

Table 11.3. Summary of fluid retention from commonly consumed beverages when consumed without food

Beverages with **inferior** fluid retention to water	Beverages with **similar** fluid retention to water	Beverages with **superior** fluid retention to water
Beer (>4 %ABV)	Sparkling water Sports drinks Cola Diet cola Tea (hot or iced) Coffee Beer (≤4% ABV)	Full-fat milk Skim milk Soy milk Milk-based meal replacements Oral rehydration solutions

Note: ABV = Alcohol by volume

Source: Adapted from Maughan et al. 2016, Desbrow et al. 2013, 2014.

beverages or drinks containing alcohol). However, individuals may respond to this by avoiding and not replacing these beverages, leading to a reduction in total fluid intake.

IMPACT OF FOOD

Since most fluid consumed by athletes is co-ingested with meals and/or snacks, the influence of food on rehydration has significant practical application. Consuming food may impact on rehydration in a number of ways. Firstly, food may provide nutrients (such as carbohydrate, protein or sodium) that directly assist with fluid recovery. In addition, the interaction of food and fluid may influence the volume of drink consumed, thereby impacting total fluid intake. To date, only four studies have investigated rehydration in settings where athletes were encouraged to consume food (Table 11.4). Collectively, these studies indicate that the ingestion of food is likely to facilitate rehydration following exercise. Two of these investigations allowed participants to self-select the volume of fluid they consumed (that is, voluntary rather than prescribed fluid intake), thereby allowing the interaction between food and the volume of fluid consumed to be explored.

Importantly, when drinking and eating voluntarily both males and females appear to achieve similar levels of fluid retention, irrespective of beverage type. However, the consumption of high-energy (kJ) beverages such as sports drinks or milk-based drinks is likely to result in greater total energy consumption and differences in nutrient intakes compared to the consumption of water with food (Campagnolo et al. 2017). Therefore, fluid choice post-exercise when food is available should be strategic and

Table 11.4. Studies investigating the interaction of food on rehydration

Study	Food provided	Beverage(s) (method)	Outcome
Maughan et al. 1996	Rice and beef meal	Sports drink (prescribed)	↑ Fluid retention (rehydration) with food
Pryor et al. 2015	Beef jerky	Sports drink (prescribed)	↑ Fluid retention (rehydration) with food
Campagnolo et al. 2017	Selection of foods/ snacks	Water Sports drink Milk-based supplement (voluntary)	Rehydration achieved with all beverages
McCartney et al. (under review)	Selection of foods/ snacks	Water Sports drink Milk-based supplements (voluntary)	Rehydration achieved with all beverages

considered. Selection should be influenced by immediate post-exercise nutrition requirements, as well as overall dietary intake goals.

IMPACT OF ALCOHOL ON HYDRATION, RECOVERY AND PERFORMANCE

Alcoholic beverages (particularly beer and champagne) have a long association with sport. In many countries, athletes commonly consume alcoholic beverages as part of their post-match routine. Clearly, large doses of alcohol have a number of effects (for example, impairing muscle synthesis, delaying muscle glycogen restoration and influencing sleep quality) that make it an undesirable recovery agent. However, considering beer may be consumed in large volumes after exercise, researchers have investigated beer's potential to influence rehydration.

Studies on the diuretic impact of beer suggest that the fluid loss associated with alcohol is less pronounced after exercise-induced fluid losses. Additionally, by reducing the alcohol concentration of beer (≤4 per cent alcohol by volume) and raising the sodium content, significantly greater fluid retention can be achieved compared to drinking a traditional full strength beer (Desbrow et al. 2013). A low-alcohol beer with added sodium may provide a compromise to the dehydrated athlete following exercise, in that it is a beverage with high social acceptance that avoids the poor fluid retention observed with full-strength beer.

SUMMARY AND KEY MESSAGES

After reading this chapter, you should understand the role of water in the human body, how fluid loss can lead to dehydration and the impact of dehydration. You should be able to identify different techniques for measuring hydration status, as well as the strengths and limitations of each method. You should be able to describe factors that influence fluid consumption and identify appropriate drinking strategies to optimise rehydration for athletes.

Key messages

- Cardiovascular and thermoregulatory functions of water are critical for athletes.
- During exercise the body cools itself by sweating, but this causes loss of body fluid.
- Performance impairment typically occurs when dehydration exceeds 2% BW loss.
- Timing of consumption relative to exercise has a significant influence on beverage recommendations.
- It is important to recognise that all beverages make a contribution to total fluid intake.
- Ingestion of food is likely to facilitate rehydration after exercise.

- Large doses of alcohol can have a number of negative effects that make it an undesirable recovery agent.
- Low-alcohol beer with added sodium may provide a beverage with high social acceptance that allows rehydration.

REFERENCES

Armstrong, L., Soto, J., Hacker, F. et al., 1998, 'Urinary indices during dehydration, exercise, and rehydration', *International Journal of Sport & Nutrition*, vol. 8, no. 4, pp. 345–55.

Armstrong, L.E., 2005, 'Hydration assessment techniques', *Nutrition Reviews*, vol. 63, suppl. 6, pp. 40–54.

Campagnolo, N., Iudakhina, E., Irwin, C. et al., 2017, 'Fluid, energy and nutrient recovery via *ad libitum* intake of different fluids and food', *Physiology & Behaviour*, vol. 171, pp. 228–35.

Cheuvront, S.N., Carter, R., Montain, S.J. et al., 2004, 'Daily body mass variability and stability in active men undergoing exercise-heat stress', *International Journal of Sport Nutrition & Exercise Metabolism*, vol. 14, no. 5, pp. 532–40.

Desbrow, B., Jansen, S., Barrett, A., et al., 2014, 'Comparing the rehydration potential of different milk-based drinks to a carbohydrate-electrolyte beverage', *Applied Physiology, Nutrition, and Metabolism*, vol. 39, no. 12, pp. 1366–72.

Desbrow, B., Murray, D. & Leveritt, M., 2013, 'Beer as a sports drink? Manipulating beer's ingredients to replace lost fluid', *International Journal of Sport Nutrition & Exercise Metabolism*, vol. 23, no. 6, pp. 593–600.

Garth, A.K. & Burke, L.M., 2013, 'What do athletes drink during competitive sporting activities?', *Sports Medicine*, vol. 43, no. 7, pp. 539–64.

Jequier, E. & Constant, F., 2010, 'Water as an essential nutrient: The physiological basis of hydration', *European Journal of Clinical Nutrition*, vol. 64, no. 2, pp. 115–23.

Maughan, R.J., 2003, 'Impact of mild dehydration on wellness and on exercise performance', *European Journal of Clinical Nutrition*, vol. 57, suppl. 2, pp. 19–23.

Maughan, R., Leiper, J. & Shirreffs, S., 1996, 'Restoration of fluid balance after exercise-induced dehydration: Effects of food and fluid intake', *European Journal of Applied Physiology and Occupational Physiology*, vol. 73, no. 3-4, pp. 317–25.

Maughan, R.J., Watson, P., Cordery, P.A. et al., 2016, 'A randomized trial to assess the potential of different beverages to affect hydration status: Development of a beverage hydration index', *American Journal of Clinical Nutrition*, vol. 103, no. 3, pp. 717–23.

McCartney, D., Irwin, C., Cox, G.R. et al., under review, 'Fluid, energy and nutrient recovery via *ad libitum* intake of different commercial beverages and food in female athletes', *Applied Physiology, Nutrition & Metabolism*.

Murray, B., 2007, 'Hydration and physical performance', *Journal of American College of Nutrition*, vol. 26, suppl. 5, pp. 542–48.

Oppliger, R.A. & Bartok, C., 2002, 'Hydration testing of athletes', *Sports Medicine*, vol. 32, no. 15, pp. 959–71.

Pryor, J.L., Johnson, E.C., Del Favero, J. et al., 2015, 'Hydration status and sodium balance of endurance runners consuming post-exercise supplements of varying nutrient content', *International Journal of Sport Nutrition & Exercise Metabolism*, vol. 25, no. 5, pp. 471–9.

Sawka, M.N., Burke, L.M., Eichner, E.R. et al., 2007, 'American College of Sports Medicine Position stand. Exercise and fluid replacement', *Medicine & Science in Sports & Exercise*, vol. 39, no. 2, pp. 377–90.

Thomas, D.T., Erdman, K.A. & Burke, L.M., 2016, 'Position of Dietitians of Canada, the Academy of Nutrition and Dietetics, and the American College of Sports Medicine: Nutrition and athletic performance', Dietitians of Canada, pp. 23–25, <https://www.dietitians.ca/Downloads/Public/noap-position-paper.aspx>, accessed 15 November 2018.

CHAPTER 12

Sports supplements

Michael Leveritt

The preceding chapters have provided an overview of how specific dietary patterns, foods and nutrients can enhance health and wellbeing as well as exercise performance and adaptations to training. We now understand that well-selected nutrition strategies can have a significant positive impact on an athlete's performance and overall wellbeing. While most of the nutritional benefits for an athlete are the result of thoughtfully selected foods and overall dietary patterns, some additional benefit can be gained from specific sports foods and supplements. This chapter will look more closely at the sports foods and supplements used by athletes to enhance performance, promote recovery and facilitate optimal training adaptation.

LEARNING OUTCOMES

Upon completion of this chapter you will be able to:
- define sports foods and sports supplements
- understand placebo and belief effects associated with sports supplements
- briefly describe the mechanism of action of specific supplements that have been shown to enhance exercise performance
- explain the recommended supplement intake protocols for specific supplements that have been shown to enhance exercise performance

- discuss emerging evidence associated with new and potentially beneficial sports supplements.

SPORTS FOODS

Research in sports nutrition over several decades has identified how different nutrients can enhance exercise performance, improve recovery and modulate training adaptation. This knowledge has subsequently led to the development of specific sports foods. Sports foods are specifically formulated with the aim of helping individuals achieve specific nutritional or sporting performance goals and are designed to supplement the diet of athletes rather than to act as the main source of nutrition. These products are regulated under Food Standards Australia New Zealand's Standard as 'Formulated supplementary sports foods'. It is important to note that this Standard allows the addition of substances that are not permitted or are restricted in other foods, as well as higher levels of some vitamins and minerals, meaning that most of these foods may not be suitable for children or pregnant women. Additionally, in New Zealand sports-related products may also be manufactured under the New Zealand Food (Supplemented Food) Standard 2010 and compliant products can be imported into Australia under the Trans-Tasman Mutual Recognition Arrangement (Food Standards Australia New Zealand 2018).

Foods which fall under this category include sports bars, carbohydrate gels and protein drinks. Over the last decade there has been a large increase in the type and variety of products available, and a huge surge in marketing, increasing the popularity and use of sports foods. The vast majority of these specialised sports foods are simply convenient packages of nutrients that might be easily accessible to an athlete when required. In fact, athletes can often receive the same benefits from consuming these nutrients in regular foods. In many instances, regular foods may actually provide a cheaper, albeit less convenient, alternative. Nevertheless, sports foods may have a role to play in an athlete's diet. For example, we know that consuming protein after resistance training enhances subsequent muscle protein synthesis. Many foods that are good sources of high-quality protein, such as meat, chicken, eggs and dairy foods, require refrigeration and can be difficult to access after a training session. A protein powder that can be mixed with water is an example of a sports food that could be more convenient for an athlete to take to training and then consume immediately after exercise is completed. However, with thoughtful planning it is possible for an athlete to obtain all the nutrients they require through regular foods. For example, high-quality protein in eggs or chicken leftover from the previous evening's dinner could be brought on a sandwich in a cooler bag with an ice block to keep cool until after training.

SPORTS SUPPLEMENTS

Sports supplements are different from sports foods because they typically contain unusual amounts of nutrients or other components of foods that would not normally be obtained through food alone. There are many sports supplements that are marketed as being able to enhance exercise performance, but the scientific evidence to support the proposed benefits is not convincing for several supplements. Nevertheless, the way in which many sports supplements are marketed makes them very attractive to athletes and exercising individuals. In fact, many athletes hold strong beliefs about the positive effects of certain supplements. This may be due to a genuine benefit, or it may be due to a placebo or belief effect. The **placebo effect** occurs when an individual experiences or perceives a benefit from a supplement due to the belief that it will be beneficial rather than as a result of any direct physiological effect. Many scientists discount placebo effects as not being real, and these effects are often tightly controlled for in experiments evaluating the effectiveness of a sports supplement. However, there have also been well-controlled studies investigating the placebo effect using supplements such as caffeine that are known to enhance performance. These studies have shown that exercise performance is enhanced when participants are told they are receiving the supplement despite actually being given an inactive substance (Beedie & Foad 2009). Interestingly, although the placebo effect enhances performance, the magnitude of this effect is usually slightly less than the amount of performance improvement observed from the actual supplement. These studies have clearly shown that some placebo effects are likely to occur with sports supplements. Interestingly, this may have some implications for ethical practice in sports nutrition (Halson & Martin 2013). It might not be considered ethical to deliberately deceive an athlete by advising them to consume a supplement that does not cause any performance-enhancing physiological effects. However, most athletes want to perform at their best regardless of how that is achieved and are more than willing to consume sports supplements, even if the benefits are only due to a placebo effect. This area is complex, but the placebo effect should be taken into consideration when providing advice about sports supplements and also when monitoring the effects of sports supplements.

Despite many sports supplements lacking scientific evidence to support their marketing claims, a number of sports supplements have been shown to be effective at enhancing performance under certain conditions. The Australian Institute of Sport has developed a classification system that ranks sports supplements into groups based on scientific evidence and other practical considerations that determine whether a product is safe, legal and effective at improving sports performance. There are four categories of sports supplements in this system:

Placebo effect
When an individual experiences or perceives a benefit from a supplement due to the belief that it will be beneficial rather than any direct physiological effect.

1. **Group A Supplements**—there is sufficient scientific evidence to recommend these supplements in specific situations using evidence-based protocols.
2. **Group B Supplements**—research is promising regarding the benefits of these supplements, but it is inconclusive to date and these supplements should only be used if they are part of a research project or when it is possible to monitor how athletes respond.
3. **Group C Supplements**—there is very little scientific evidence that these supplements are beneficial and supplements in this category are generally not recommended.
4. **Group D Supplements**—these supplements are either banned or are at high risk of contamination with substances that could lead to a positive drug test and are definitely not recommended for athletes.

This framework provides a useful guide for athletes, coaches and sports nutrition practitioners when deciding on which supplements to include in their overall sports nutrition program. The list of supplements in each category changes over time as new evidence emerges about each of the different supplements. We will focus on the Group A supplements in this chapter. A range of sports foods and medical supplements are currently included in Group A, in addition to the following sports supplements:

- caffeine
- creatine
- nitrates
- bicarbonate
- beta-alanine.

Caffeine is one of the most widely used pharmacologically active substances in the world and has been shown to improve performance in a variety of exercise tasks. Caffeine is present in many commonly consumed foods and in beverages such as coffee, tea, chocolate- and cola-flavoured beverages. The physiological effects of caffeine occur due to its similarity to the **adenosine** molecule. Among its many actions, adenosine causes a decrease in alertness and arousal when it binds to receptors on the surface of cells in the brain. Caffeine also binds to these receptors and blocks the effects of adenosine. Therefore, caffeine can increase alertness and arousal and subsequently reduces the perception of effort during exercise. The reduced perception of effort during exercise can enhance performance by delaying fatigue and allowing an athlete to exercise at a higher intensity for longer periods of time.

Adenosine
A chemical that naturally occurs in humans and which causes a decrease in alertness and arousal when it binds to receptors on the surface of cells in the brain.

Interestingly, the dose of caffeine required to achieve optimal improvements in exercise performance is relatively small. Doses of approximately 3 mg/kg body mass appear to be most effective, with no additional benefit occurring with higher doses (Desbrow et al. 2012). This dose is equivalent to approximately 600 millilitres of a standard energy drink or two cups of coffee and is actually quite similar to the usual daily consumption of caffeine for many adults. Consumption of caffeine at these relatively low doses is unlikely to result in any negative side-effects in most people, which is perhaps one reason why caffeine use in sport has not been restricted since 2004. Caffeine has been shown to improve performance when consumed in tablet form, coffee or in energy drinks (Quinlivan et al. 2015). However, the amount of caffeine in coffee can vary significantly. In fact, some Australian studies have shown that there is a tenfold difference in the caffeine content of coffee purchased at different retail outlets (Desbrow et al. 2007). Using energy drinks as a source of caffeine can also have limitations for athletes. Some athletes experience uncomfortable gastrointestinal symptoms when energy drinks are consumed before exercise. Therefore, it is recommended that caffeine be consumed in tablet form when used as a sports supplement in order to be certain of the exact dose ingested and to reduce any unwanted gastrointestinal side-effects.

Caffeine is most effective when consumed approximately one hour before exercise, although many studies have shown caffeine enhances performance when it is given to participants at a variety of different times before and/or during the exercise task. It has even been shown that very small amounts of caffeine consumed in cola beverages can enhance performance in the concluding stages of an endurance exercise task. The benefit to performance in this instance actually occurred despite very little change in the caffeine concentration in the blood. In fact, the amount of caffeine appearing in the blood does not seem to be related to the performance benefit. Nevertheless, the studies that have directly compared different times of ingestion suggest that approximately one hour before exercise is optimal, but there may well be variations to this for different individuals.

Contrary to popular belief, caffeine consumption does not cause dehydration during exercise. Even though caffeine acts as a mild diuretic by causing small increases in urine volume, these effects are negated by exercise, possibly due to the changes in hormones and cardiovascular function during exercise (Zhang et al. 2015). In fact, caffeine has actually been shown to cause similar performance benefits when consumed before exercise performed in hot conditions compared with more neutral environmental conditions.

Regular consumption of caffeine can cause the body's cells to adapt and generate more adenosine receptors. This has the potential to make regular caffeine consumers less able to experience the performance enhancements associated with caffeine supplementation. However, studies have shown that individuals who normally consume large amounts of caffeine in their diet still receive similar benefits when consuming caffeine before exercise compared with athletes who do not consume much caffeine on a regular basis. It also does not appear that there is any benefit gained from abstaining from caffeine for a few days before using a caffeine supplement. It is important to note that, while we are confident that caffeine supplementation is effective at improving exercise performance, there are a limited number of studies that have thoroughly investigated the factors that might moderate the ergogenic effects of caffeine and more research in this area is certainly warranted.

Creatine has been used by athletes as an **ergogenic aid** for several decades. Supplementation with creatine monohydrate increases the creatine pool in muscles which allows for more rapid ATP regeneration during repeated bouts of high-intensity exercise (see Chapter 2). This mechanism may enable a higher training intensity and improved adaptation to training, particularly resistance training which involves repeated, high-force muscle contractions. Creatine supplementation also appears to positively influence anabolic processes in muscles, which results in an increase in lean muscle mass after supplementation. Many studies have shown that creatine supplementation during a period of resistance training enhances gains in muscle strength and lean body mass. Typical creatine supplementation protocols involve a short loading phase, lasting 5–7 days, during which 20 g/day of creatine monohydrate is consumed in four daily intakes of 5 grams each, evenly spaced throughout the day. This is then followed by a maintenance phase in which 3–5 g/day is consumed. The maintenance phase typically lasts for the duration of the training cycle in which improvements in maximal muscle strength and lean body mass are the primary goals.

Ergogenic aid
Any substance or aid that improves physical performance.

Dietary nitrate is becoming increasingly popular as a sports supplement due to its capacity to enhance endurance exercise performance (McMahon et al. 2017). Many green leafy vegetables and beetroot are examples of foods with a high nitrate content. The nitrate content of foods can vary significantly due to growing conditions and loss of nitrate during cooking and preparation, which makes it difficult to predict how much dietary nitrate is being consumed through different foods. There are now many sports foods and beverages available that are made with concentrated beetroot juice and contain a known amount of nitrate. Once ingested, dietary nitrate can be converted to nitrite by bacteria in the mouth. Circulating nitrite is then converted into nitric oxide in blood and other tissues. Enhancing nitric oxide availability may improve muscle function and consequently exercise performance. Nitrate supplementation appears to specifically enhance the efficiency of oxygen use during exercise, which allows individuals to perform greater work for the same energy cost (Jones 2014). This results in an improved capacity to exercise at a fixed intensity for a longer duration before exhaustion occurs. Daily intake of 400–500 milligrams of nitrate for approximately one week appears to be most effective at enhancing performance; however, benefits have also been shown after a single dose consumed 2–3 hours before exercise. Interestingly, the benefits of dietary nitrate supplementation are less evident in highly trained athletes, particularly when exercise performance is measured via a time-trial test rather than time to exhaustion tests. This suggests that recreational exercisers are likely to experience improved exercise performance after nitrate supplementation. However, elite athletes may wish to monitor their individual response to nitrate supplementation to determine if this is likely to be an effective nutrition strategy that contributes to their performance goals.

Performance in short-duration, high-intensity exercise can be improved after the ingestion of sodium bicarbonate (Peart et al. 2012). Increasing bicarbonate in the blood enhances the capacity to buffer acid produced by the muscle during exercise (see Chapter 2). This has the potential to delay fatigue during high-intensity exercise. Although there is a clear mechanistic rationale for bicarbonate to enhance performance, not all studies show a performance benefit. This may be due to side-effects associated with gastrointestinal discomfort offsetting the benefit of an improved buffer capacity. As with nitrate supplementation, the benefits of bicarbonate ingestion appear to be less evident in highly trained individuals, possibly due to the already high buffer capacity developed through training in this population. Doses of 200–400 mg/kg body mass consumed 60–90 minutes before exercise appear to be optimal, but it is recommended that athletes trial this on several occasions during training to ensure that no adverse gastrointestinal side-effects are likely to occur in competition.

Beta-alanine is a component of the dipeptide carnosine, which plays a role in buffering acid produced in the muscle during high-intensity exercise (see Chapter 1). This has the potential to delay fatigue and enhance performance, particularly in events lasting approximately 1–4 minutes. Beta-alanine supplementation over several weeks has been shown to result in increased muscle carnosine and improved performance in short-duration (1–4 minutes), high-intensity exercise. A daily dose of 6.4 grams is used in most studies and it appears that at least four weeks of beta-alanine supplementation is required to elevate muscle carnosine concentration. However, further increases in muscle carnosine concentration are observed after ten weeks of supplementation. The daily dose is usually consumed on 3–4 occasions spread throughout the day in order to reduce the acute side-effects associated with consumption of large doses of beta-alanine. Side-effects can include tingling, flushing and a prickly sensation on the skin which peaks around 30–60 minutes after the ingestion of beta-alanine.

Protocol
The official procedure or set of rules or methods that need to be followed.

The **protocol** for beta-alanine supplementation is much more difficult for athletes to adhere to than protocols for other supplements, as it involves several daily doses taken for several weeks. Therefore, beta-alanine supplementation is only recommended for highly motivated athletes who are able to commit to a relatively long supplementation regime.

Supplements such as caffeine, creatine, nitrate, sodium bicarbonate and beta-alanine have all been shown to enhance exercise performance in many different studies. Most studies compare the effects of a single supplement against a placebo under relatively well-controlled conditions. However, many athletes looking for a competitive edge will consume multiple supplements at the same time in order to derive as much benefit as possible. Unfortunately, the beneficial effects of taking multiple different supplements may not be additive. Findings of studies investigating combinations of supplements are somewhat inconsistent, with some showing additive effects and others showing that performance gains from multiple supplements are no greater than those from a single supplement. Research into the effects of consuming multiple supplements is relatively scant at present due to the difficulty of conducting studies involving multiple interventions. While further research is required, it is also likely that different athletes will have somewhat different responses to each supplement. It is therefore important for athletes to monitor and evaluate their own individual responses to supplements to most effectively use sports supplements to enhance their performance.

Research into sports supplements continues to evolve and there are many new supplements that have shown promising results, but there is not enough scientific evidence to date to provide clear recommendations on the benefit of these supplements. Examples of these supplements include pickle juice (any sort containing salt and vinegar) to reduce muscle cramps; tart cherry juice to enhance recovery; citrulline, carnitine and quercetin for enhanced endurance performance; curcumin for reducing inflammation and enhancing recovery; glutamine for enhancing immune function; and gelatin for enhancing tissue repair and injury prevention. All of these supplements have the potential to provide significant benefit, but the evidence is insufficient at the moment to be confident that most athletes will respond positively when these supplements are consumed.

SUMMARY AND KEY MESSAGES

Thoughtfully selected foods and overall dietary patterns can enhance an athlete's performance. Small additional benefits are possible through the intake of sports foods and sports supplements. The mechanism of action of sports supplements is complex and the benefits of most supplements are usually specific to a certain type of exercise or sport activity. Supplements such as caffeine, creatine, bicarbonate, nitrate and beta-alanine have the strongest scientific evidence supporting their benefits in sport.

Key messages
- Most of the benefits of nutrition for an athlete are the result of thoughtfully selected foods and overall dietary patterns.
- Sports foods are specially formulated products in which nutrients are packaged in convenient forms for athletes and exercising individuals to help them achieve specific nutritional or performance goals.
- Sports supplements are different from sports foods because they typically contain unusual amounts of nutrients or other components of foods that would not normally be obtained through food alone.
- Sports supplements that have good evidence for enhancing performance include caffeine, creatine, bicarbonate, nitrate and beta-alanine.
- There is also emerging evidence for the benefits of pickle juice, tart cherry juice, citrulline, carnitine, quercetin, curcumin, glutamine and gelatin.
- Given individual variation in how athletes respond to different supplements, it is important that athletes monitor and evaluate their own individual responses to supplements in order to receive the greatest benefit.

REFERENCES

Beedie, C.J. & Foad, A.J., 2009, 'The placebo effect in sports performance: A brief review', *Sports Medicine*, vol. 39, no. 4, pp. 313–29.

Desbrow, B., Biddulph, C., Devlin, B. et al., 2012, 'The effects of different doses of caffeine on endurance cycling time trial performance', *Journal of Sports Science*, vol. 30, no. 2, pp. 115–20.

Desbrow, B., Hughes, R., Leveritt, M. et al., 2007, 'An examination of consumer exposure to caffeine from retail coffee outlets', *Food & Chemical Toxicology*, vol. 45, no. 9, pp. 1588–92.

Halson, S.L. & Martin, D.T., 2013, 'Lying to win—Placebos and sport science', *International Journal of Sports Physiology & Performance*, vol. 8, no. 6, pp. 597–9.

Jones, A.M., 2014, 'Influence of dietary nitrate on the physiological determinants of exercise performance: a critical review', *Applied Physiology & Nutritional Metabolism*, vol. 39, no. 9, pp. 1019–28.

McMahon, N.F., Leveritt, M.D. & Pavey, T.G., 2017, 'The effect of dietary nitrate supplementation on endurance exercise performance in healthy adults: A systematic review and meta-analysis', *Sports Medicine*, vol. 47, no. 4, pp. 735–56.

Peart, D.J., Siegler, J.C. & Vince, R.V., 2012, 'Practical recommendations for coaches and athletes: A meta-analysis of sodium bicarbonate use for athletic performance', *Journal of Strength & Conditioning Research*, vol. 26, no. 7, pp. 1975–83.

Quinlivan, A., Irwin, C., Grant, G.D. et al., 2015, 'The effects of Red Bull energy drink compared with caffeine on cycling time-trial performance', *Internatinal Journal of Sports Physiology & Performance*, vol. 10, no. 7, pp. 897–901.

Zhang, Y., Coca, A., Casa, D.J., et al., 2015, 'Caffeine and diuresis during rest and exercise: A meta-analysis', *Journal of Science and Medicine in Sport*, vol. 18, no. 5, pp. 569–74.

CHAPTER

13

Changing body composition and anthropometry

Patria Hume

Body composition changes with growth and maturation, and due to influences such as diet and exercise. Anthropometry is the comparative study of sizes and proportions of the human body. This chapter provides an overview of body composition, anthropometric methods used to assess body composition, and how body composition can be modified through diet and exercise.

LEARNING OUTCOMES

Upon completion of this chapter you will be able to:
- provide a definition of body composition
- outline techniques used to assess body composition
- describe how body composition can be modified.

WHAT IS BODY COMPOSITION?

Body composition is a term that is commonly used when referring to the amount of fat relative to muscle you have in your body. However, this technically is **total body fat** and **fat-free mass** (FFM), which includes muscle, water and bone. Body composition is, therefore, the relative proportions of fat, protein, water and mineral components in the body. Almost 99 per cent of the human body mass is composed of six elements: oxygen, carbon, nitrogen, hydrogen (and smaller quantities of their stable **isotopes**), calcium and phosphorus.

Isotope
Atoms that have the same number of protons and electrons but a different number of neutrons.

Body density
The compactness of a body, defined as the mass divide by its volume.

Body composition varies among individuals due to differences in **body density** and degree of obesity. Bone is more dense than muscle, which is more dense than fat. If there is relative loss of bone density (osteoporosis) or decrease in muscle mass (with reduced training), fat mass may be overestimated when using densitometry techniques to calculate the ratio of fat mass to fat-free mass. Densitometry techniques include underwater (hydrostatic) weighing and air displacement plethysmography (Bod Pod®).

TECHNIQUES USED TO ASSESS BODY COMPOSITION

Extracellular water
Water that is outside the cells, including the water between the cells and the plasma.

Visceral adipose tissue
The adipose tissue within the abdominal cavity, which is wrapped around the organs.

Subcutaneous adipose tissue
Adipose tissue directly under the skin.

Intermuscular adipose tissue
Adipose tissue located within the skeletal muscle.

Ectopic fat depots
Excess adipose tissue in locations not usually associated with adipose tissue storage, such as in the liver or around the heart.

Anthropometry is the comparative study of sizes and proportions of the human body. We most commonly use surface anthropometry techniques to assess body composition.

However, there are a variety of body composition (physique assessment) techniques that can be selected. Assessment of body composition may be conducted using **non-imaging** (surface anthropometry, air displacement plesthmyography, three-dimensional body scanning, doubly-labelled water, bioelectrical impedance, new innovations), and **imaging** techniques (dual energy X-ray absorptiometry, ultrasound, computed tomography and magnetic resonance imaging). See the recently published guidelines for more information on how to use selected physique assessment methods and report data to athletes and coaches (Hume et al. 2017).

Combinations of techniques allow measurement of fat, fat-free mass, bone mineral content, total body water, **extracellular** water, total adipose tissue and its subdepots (**visceral**, **subcutaneous** and **intermuscular**), skeletal muscle, select organs, and **ectopic fat depots** (Lee & Gallagher 2008). Clinicians and scientists can quantify a number of body components and can track changes in physique with the aim of determining efficacy of training, nutrition and clinical interventions.

Selection of techniques to assess body composition is dependent upon factors including the validity, reliability, cost, safety, time for data collection and analysis, skill required for the practitioner and accessibility of the technology. It is important to consider:

- why you measure body composition using the techniques and technologies
- precision and accuracy, validity, practicality, and sensitivity to monitor changes in body composition using the technique
- advantages and disadvantages of the technique
- the equipment/hardware, calibration, software, skills required, training and accreditation for techniques
- client presentation and preparation protocols for the techniques.

Athlete presentation for measurement is important, as hydration levels will affect the results. Factors such as time of day, prior food or fluid intake, exercise, body temperature, hydration status and gastrointestinal tract contents should be standardised wherever possible prior to any physique assessment. Given the **diurnal** variation in body mass, fasted early morning assessments following bladder and possibly bowel evacuation are the most reliable where practical.

Diurnal
The 24-hour period or daily cycle, such as being active during the day and resting at night.

Surface anthropometry assessment

The International Society for the Advancement of Kinanthropometry (ISAK) provides international standards for surface anthropometry assessment, using basic measures of skinfolds, girths, lengths and breadths. A restricted profile includes two basic measures (body mass, height), eight skinfolds (triceps, biceps, subscapular, iliac crest, supraspinale, abdominal, front thigh, calf), five girths (upper arm relaxed, upper arm tensed, waist, hips, calf) and two breadths (elbow, knee). A full profile includes all the restricted profile measures plus additional measures, resulting in a total of four basic measures, eight skinfolds, 13 girths, eight lengths and nine breadths.

The advantages of ISAK surface anthropometry methods are that assessments take approximately ten minutes for a restricted profile and up to 30 minutes for a full profile, and the equipment is readily available and easily calibrated. The methods are valid and reliable if ISAK training is undertaken to ensure correct use of anatomical bony landmarks (Hume & Marfell-Jones 2008) and correct use of calipers. The disadvantage of the ISAK surface anthropometry technique is that skinfold calipers compress the adipose (fat) tissue, resulting in variation in measurements. To help reduce the effects of skinfold compressibility, a complete set of skinfold measurements is obtained before repeating the measurements.

Air displacement plethysmography (Bod Pod®)

Air displacement plethysmography is used to measure body volume and calculate estimates of body density. The Bod Pod® (COSMED USA Inc., Concord, CA) device consists of a measurement pod of two isolated chambers to measure body volume, a calibratable set of scales and a computer attached to each measurement device. The Bod Pod® is easy to use and non-invasive. Completion of the test including accurate body mass, multiple measures of body volume, and either measurement or estimation of lung gas volume, takes approximately ten minutes from stepping on the scales to stepping out of the Bod Pod®.

During measurement the client sits quietly in the measurement chamber, breathing normally and minimising movement. The chamber has a magnetically locking door with a clear window. Within the measurement pod, the technology allows estimation of lung volume. Two measurements of body volume are undertaken, with a third required if the first two measures are not within 150 millilitres. Once body volume has been calculated the software provides body-fat percentage and absolute values of fat mass and fat-free mass. The Bod Pod® will underestimate fat mass compared to other physique assessment techniques if there are poor standardisation practices in athlete presentation.

Bioelectrical impedance analysis (BIA)

Bioelectrical impedance analysis (BIA) allows measurement of total body water, which is used to estimate fat-free body mass and, by difference with body mass, body fat. BIA assessment devices are readily available and assessment is quick compared to other methods. A client appointment of 15 minutes is needed for body mass and standing stature measurement, electrode placement and then one minute of data collection. The technique is client-friendly as it is non-invasive and there is low health risk. The procedure is simple and there is good portability of the equipment. BIA is relatively low cost compared to other methods of body composition analysis. However, precision and validity is low.

Sensitivity to monitor change of physique is low given that variation in client presentation for testing can affect the results (for example, levels of hydration) (Kerr et al. 2017). The techniques to collect the data are simple; however, interpretation of the data is impeded given that the formulas used by the equipment to calculate body-fat/fat-free mass are not readily available and instead only a final figure/figures are displayed. Client preparation for measurement is important given the effect of hydration on results. Training of the technician is needed to ensure correct preparation of the skin and reliable placement of electrodes on the ankle and the wrist. Regional body assessment is possible but is invalid.

Deuterium dilution–doubly-labelled water technique

The doubly-labelled water technique (commonly known as deuterium dilution) is used to measure body water and total energy expenditure. The technique requires the client to consume a stable isotope water (known as doubly-labelled water) and then provide urine samples for several days after the initial ingestion. The technique is a non-invasive way of measuring the rate of carbon dioxide production in clients over a period of seven to 14 days. The most sensitive means of measuring the isotopes of deuterium and oxygen-18 in the samples is by isotope ratio mass spectroscopy. Due to the technical nature, cost and lack of availability of the equipment, the use of the technique is uncommon. The reliability of the technique is high. Regional body assessment is not possible; instead, total body water, fat-free mass and fat mass are calculated. The time commitment for clients is approximately six hours given the repeat samples required.

Ultrasound

The ultrasound technique for measurement of subcutaneous adipose tissue and embedded fibrous structures employs image capture from any standard-brightness mode ultrasound machine, followed by an image-analysis procedure. The technique avoids compression of the tissues and movement that occurs when using skinfold calipers. As with skinfolds, the ultrasound technique only samples the subcutaneous adipose tissue and does not measure the fat stored in deeper depots. It is an accurate and reliable technique for measurement of subcutaneous adipose tissue provided the practitioner has had certified training in the data collection and use of the analysis software

All participants must be marked prior to measurement. Measurements are taken from eight standard measurement sites: upper abdomen, lower abdomen, erector spinae, distal triceps, brachioradialis, lateral thigh, front thigh, medial calf. The operator places the centre of the ultrasound probe over the marked site to capture an ultrasound image.

Magnetic resonance imaging (MRI) and computed tomography (CT)

Magnetic resonance imaging and computed tomography are imaging techniques that provide highly accurate measures of body composition at the tissue-organ level. Computed tomography works through measuring the attenuation of X-rays through body tissues, whereas magnetic resonance imaging uses a strong magnetic field to align positively charged protons in the body's tissues which are then digitised to provide an image. Magnetic resonance imaging is a safer method than computed tomography as it does not expose participants to radiation. Due to high cost and low availability, these techniques are generally only used for clients as part of a medical assessment or for research purposes. Both techniques are considered reference methods for body composition assessment due to their high precision and validity.

Dual energy X-ray absorptiometry (DXA)

Dual energy X-ray absorptiometry (DXA) is regarded as the current gold standard for determining body-fat percentage and lean mass. The DXA machine emits sources of X-ray energies which pass through the body, enabling determination of bone mineral content, lean mass and fat mass for the whole body and for regional areas. Given the use of X-rays (exposure to radiation), the International Society for Clinical Densitometry has established clinical practice guidelines relating to the collection and analysis of DXA data. Standardisation of how athletes present for scanning is important. Ideally it should be done in the morning and they should be well hydrated (urine specific gravity (USG) measurements may be taken), glycogen replete (not having exercised heavily the day before), overnight-fasted and in minimal clothing (such as singlet and underwear). They should be correctly positioned on the scanning bed, being centrally aligned in a standard position using custom-made positioning aids (foam blocks). Following the scan, images should be reviewed so that the automatic segmentation of body regional areas of the scan can be checked and adjusted manually if required. Body composition assessment using such a protocol will ensure a high level of precision, while still being practical for clients. An assessment can usually be completed within ten minutes.

Three-dimensional body scanning

Three-dimensional body scanning is used to determine surface anthropometry characteristics such as body volume, segment lengths and girths. Three-dimensional scanning systems use laser, light or infra-red technologies to acquire shape and software to allow manual or automatically extracted measures. Body posture during scanning is important to ensure accurate measures can be made from the images. The images vary depending on the configuration, resolution and accuracy of the scanner. Training is required to ensure successful use of three-dimensional scanning hardware and software. The hardware for full body scanning is expensive, so the technique is not commonly available yet. Three-dimensional body scanning protocols (Stewart & Hume 2014) are available at the J.E. Lindsay Carter Kinanthropometry Archive <https://www.aut.ac.nz/study/study-options/sport-and-recreation/research/j.e.-lindsay-carter-clinic-for-kinanthropometry>.

Three-dimensional body scanning systems integrated with other imaging modalities to create multifaceted digital human profiles, and artificial intelligence techniques such as deep learning and artificial neural networks, are set to revolutionise the physique assessment landscape over the coming decade. Using computer vision techniques, it is now possible to register an individual's DXA-derived body composition with the mesh exported by the same individual's three-dimensional body scan. Technological and computing innovations are rapidly transforming the tools we employ for measuring, recording, collating and interpreting body dimension and composition assessments.

HOW BODY COMPOSITION CAN BE MODIFIED

Body composition changes with growth and maturation, and due to influences such as diet and exercise. Body characteristics such as stature (height), skeletal lengths and breadths are not adaptable except during the growth periods, but body mass, lean mass and fat mass are more modifiable and can be manipulated. The influence of a person's genetic profile impacts on their presenting body shape (**morphology**), as well as their responsiveness to interventions that aim to change body composition and shape (Ivey et al. 2000) and the associated physique capacity (Kouri et al. 1995).

Morphology
The body shape.

Morphological prediction
The prediction of the adult body shape from a growing child or adolescent.

Morphological prototype
The best body shape and distribution of soft tissue to maximise performance in a given sport.

Anticipating adult physique in a growing child (**morphological prediction**) has implications for athlete talent identification and development for sports performance (Hume & Stewart 2012). During growth, segment breadths are most useful for prediction of adult dimensions because they remain stable in relation to stature throughout adolescence. Changes in soft tissue for maximum functional effectiveness (**morphological prototype**) respond to training. Alignment of morphology to performance, and recognition of the wide individual variability in maturation rate, helps avoid biasing athlete selection or overlooking individuals with athletic potential.

Body composition information can be used to monitor the effectiveness of physique manipulation via exercise or nutrition (Cole et al. 2005) interventions. Physique assessment allows identification of clients who require additional support to restore or maintain physique status (for example, at-risk clients who have lost or gained weight rapidly). Monitoring the progress of clients in meeting their physique goals (such as strength and conditioning goals to increase muscle mass) provides motivation to continue in the intervention.

Dietary approaches to change body composition

Gaining weight

When an athlete is interested in weight gain, in most cases muscle gain is desired. For muscle gain to occur, two key things need to be present: excess energy intake to provide energy for anabolism, and a good training program to activate the muscle tissue and encourage growth and development.

From a dietary perspective, an excess of 2000–4000 kJ/day is usually required to generate consistent muscle gain. This is best achieved by eating regular meals and snacks that are high in energy and nutrients. It is realistic to expect muscle gain of 2–4 kilograms per month; however, rates of muscle gain vary between individuals and genetics can play a considerable role. Consistency, in terms of both diet and training program, is key for successful muscle gain. Excessive energy intake without appropriate training will result in fat gain instead of muscle gain.

As an example, the following foods combinations can provide an additional 2000 kJ:
- full-fat fruit yoghurt (200 g) plus 25 almonds plus medium banana OR
- half a large avocado spread on two slices of toast and an apple.

Eating enough food to obtain the additional energy can be challenging for some athletes, so simple meal and snack ideas can make a big difference. In recent times, the popularity of 'shakes' and smoothies has been helpful for athletes trying to gain weight, as some find it easy to throw ingredients in the blender, mix and drink versus eating.

Working with individual athletes to put together a realistic eating plan is very important; if a plan is not followed consistently, results are likely to be slow. Additionally, prioritising real foods over weight-gain supplements is highly recommended, as the nutrient density of wholesome real foods is likely to outweigh commercial protein powder-based products.

Losing weight

Generally, when weight loss is desired it is 'fat' loss people think about; while fat is the most common form of weight athletes may want to lose, there are circumstances—such as in weight category sports—where athletes may not be concerned about what weight type they lose as long as they weigh in below the cut-off (see Chapter 17).

Nutrition professionals generally recommend that weight is lost slowly, aiming for about 500 grams weight loss per week. This can be achieved through a 2000 kJ/day energy restriction—that is, reducing energy intake by 2000 kJ every day below total requirements. This should be planned based on current dietary intake and on what the individual's body composition has been over the last 2–3 months, as well as any planned changes in training. If training is to remain consistent and weight has been stable, then reducing the athlete's usual diet by 2000 kJ per day can often be effective. This can be done by reducing portion sizes at each meal time or by cutting out unnecessary items and discretionary foods.

The best approach will vary from athlete to athlete, and hence should be planned in a collaborative way. However, if weight has not been stable over the last 2–3 months (either increasing or decreasing) and/or training is about to change considerably, then more care will need to be taken to determine a suitable total dietary intake to enable healthy weight loss to occur.

ISSUES TO CONSIDER FOR BODY COMPOSITION ASSESSMENT

Data interpretation

Physique assessment provides valuable information; however, taken in isolation physique assessment can easily be misinterpreted or misused. Additional information, such as dietary intake and training load, and input from exercise and health professionals, is required to fully interpret findings and make recommendations.

Physique and sport

Profiling of athletes at all levels of participation in sport can help determine potential suitability for sport and effectiveness of interventions such as diet and training. As scientists and clinicians, we ask what physique characteristics are important for athletes in the sports we work with to help improve performance (Keogh et al. 2009) or reduce injury risk; what should we measure and monitor? Athletes, and their coaches, often ask how the athletes' physique compares to elite athletes in their sport. Accessing normative data for athletes at all levels of participation from development to elite can be difficult. Consideration of population trends for physique characteristics in normative databases is needed. Where possible, current research data should be gained to enable comparisons of physique characteristics for athletes of similar age, gender, ethnicity and sports participation level.

Large-scale surveys of world-class athletes have been conducted at Olympic Games (Kerr et al. 2007) and world championship events for over 60 years. These projects have provided data for identifying unique physique characteristics for selected sports that aim to optimise power, leverage or have a high metabolic demand. Physique characteristics play an important role in the self-selection of individuals for competitive sport. However, as a large number of factors are involved in the physical make-up of a champion sportsman or sportswoman, there is not necessarily one perfect body shape for a particular sport or event within that sport. Anthropometric tools have been used in profiling athletes' trajectory to optimising the trainable parameters at the times that matter most. This is important for weight category sports, where athletes may be at risk of employing unsafe weight control practices in order to 'make weight'. Rowing and powerlifting are two sports that require body mass to meet weight class categories for competition. Gymnastics is a sport that has pressure for leanness due to aesthetic reasons (see Chapter 17). We need to understand what physique characteristics are important for athletes to help improve performance or reduce injury risk.

Body image

The concept of body image includes how we perceive, think, feel and, ultimately, behave due to our own conception of our physical image. Body-image dissatisfaction is when there is a difference between our perceived body image and our desired body image. The prevalence of **body-image disorders** in athletic populations remains worryingly high. The assessment of body image in people may progress with the use of modern three-dimensional scanning technology together with volumetric assessment. The novel iPad SomatoMac application may be useful for estimates of body-image dissatisfaction and distortion, especially in athletes (Macfarlane et al. 2016). The SomatoMac application uses male and female **somatotype** photographs that allow more comprehensive estimates of body-image dissatisfaction than existing figural silhouettes and pictorial scales.

Body-image disorder
A mental disorder in which an individual continually focuses on one or more perceived flaws in appearance that are minor or not observable to others.

Somatotype
Classification of the human physical shape according to the body build or shape.

TRAINING OF PHYSIQUE ASSESSMENT PROVIDERS

Training, accreditation and quality-assurance schemes ensure appropriate levels of professionalism and safety for the public who utilise physique assessment programs. There are only two international training and certification programs for surface anthropometry and ultrasound techniques. Manufacturers' training on equipment is provided for three-dimensional scanning, Bod Pod®, bioelectrical impedance analysis, dual energy X-ray absorptiometry, magnetic resonance imaging and computed tomography. Ethical considerations in assessing anthropometry profiles for clients are important. Practitioners need to maintain professional objectivity and integrity and respect the client during physique assessment. Client safety and wellbeing are paramount in assessments, and practitioners must ensure the client understands all procedures and that consent is gained to conduct the physique assessment.

SUMMARY AND KEY MESSAGES

After reading this chapter, you should understand what body composition is, understand the importance of the validity and reliability of methods used to assess body composition, and be familiar with how body composition can be modified. You will have identified anthropometric methods that can help you to monitor your ability to achieve goals of modifying body composition.

Key messages

- Body composition is the relative proportions of fat, protein, water and mineral components in the body.
- Anthropometry is the comparative study of sizes and proportions of the human body.
- There are valid and reliable techniques used to assess body composition; however, practitioner training is required and client presentation for assessment can affect results.
- Body composition can be modified via growth and development, diet and exercise.
- Athletes aiming to gain muscle mass need to make sure they consistently eat appropriate foods containing the required amount of additional energy (excess of 2000–4000 kJ/day) and exercise appropriately.
- Athletes aiming to lose fat mass need to make sure they consistently have an energy deficit of 2000 kJ/day.
- Physique assessment provides an objective measure of body composition status in relation to physical performance, health status and diet.

REFERENCES

Cole, C.R., Salvaterra, G.F., Davis, J.E.J et al., 2005, 'Evaluation of dietary practices of national collegiate athletic association division I football players', *Journal of Strength and Conditioning Research*, vol. 19, no. 3, pp. 490–4.

Hume, P. & Marfell-Jones, M., 2008, 'The importance of accurate site location for skinfold measurement', *Journal of Sports Science*, vol. 26, no. 12, pp. 1333–40.

Hume, P.A., Kerr, D. & Ackland, T. (eds), 2017, *Best Practice Protocols for Physique Assessment in Sport*, Singapore: Springer Nature Singapore.

Hume, P.A. & Stewart, A.D., 2012, 'Body composition change', in Stewart, A.D. & Sutton, L. (eds), *Body Composition in Sport, Exercise and Health*, London, UK: Taylor and Francis, pp. 147–165.

Ivey, F.M., Roth, S.M., Ferrell, R.E. et al., 2000, 'Effects of age, gender, and myostatin genotype on the hypertrophic response to heavy resistance strength training', *Journal of Gerontology*, vol. 55, no. 11, pp. M641–8.

Keogh, J.W.L., Hume, P.A., Mellow, P. et al., 2009, 'Can absolute and proportional anthropometric characteristics distinguish stronger and weaker powerlifters?', *Journal of Strength and Conditioning Research*, vol. 23, no. 8, pp. 2256–65.

Kerr, A., Slater, G. & Byrne, N., 2017, 'Impact of food and fluid intake on technical and biological measurement error in body composition assessment methods in athletes', *British Journal of Nutrition*, vol. 117, no. 4, pp. 591–601.

Kerr, D.A., Ross, W.D., Norton, K.P. et al., 2007, 'Olympic lightweight and open-class rowers possess distinctive physical and proportionality characteristics', *Journal of Sports Sciences*, vol. 25, no. 1, pp. 43–5.

Kouri, E.M., Pope, H.G., Katz, D.L. et al., 1995, 'Fat-free mass index in users and nonusers of anabolic-androgenic steroids', *Clinical Journal of Sports Medicine*, vol. 5, no. 4, pp. 223–8.

Lee, S.Y. & Gallagher, D., 2008, 'Assessment methods in human body composition', *Current Opinion in Clinical Nutrition and Metabolic Care*, vol. 11, no. 11, pp. 566–72.

Macfarlane, D.J., Lee, A., Hume, P. et al., 2016, 'Development and reliability of a novel iPad-based application to rapidly assess body image: 3776 Board# 215', *Medicine & Science in Sports & Exercise*, vol. 48, no. 6, p. 1056.

Stewart, A.D. & Hume, P.A., 2014, *Bideltoid Breadth Measurement* [Online], J.E. Lindsay Carter Kinanthropometry Archive 3D Scanning Protocols, available at: www.sprinz.aut.ac.nz/clinics/j.e.-lindsay-carter-kinanthropometry-clinic/archive.

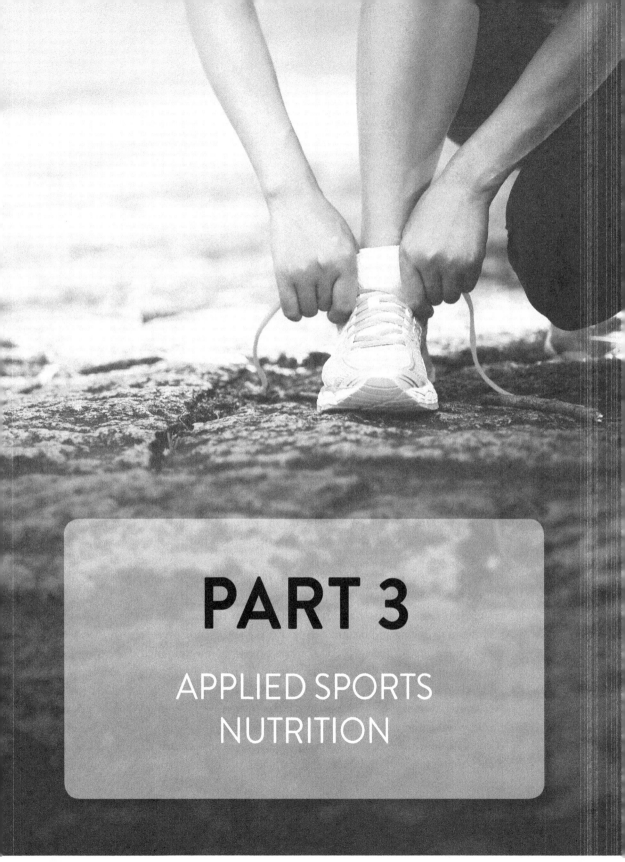

PART 3

APPLIED SPORTS NUTRITION

CHAPTER 14

Endurance sports

Gregory Cox

Endurance sport encompasses a variety of activities (running, swimming, cycling, paddling), sometimes in combination (adventure racing, triathlon) across a range of distances and intensities (5-kilometre ocean swim, 10-kilometre run, ironman triathlon or multi-day stage cycling race). Other activities, while not considered endurance sports by definition as the actual competition only lasts 3–6 minutes (for example, sprint canoe, rowing, middle-distance running), routinely incorporate endurance training sessions. We now acknowledge that endurance sport athletes have unique requirements to maximise favourable responses to training, assist recovery, maintain health and wellbeing and facilitate daily training and competition performance. Given the requirements to manage body composition while meeting high daily energy and nutrient demands, purposeful dietary planning is required for endurance athletes.

Understanding the sport culture, the individual athletes' food preferences and beliefs, the dynamics of weekly training, the environmental conditions in which they train and race, and the logistics for nutrition support for racing will define the effectiveness of nutrition support to endurance sport athletes. This chapter will explore daily training needs of endurance sport athletes and outline various nutrition considerations for endurance competition.

LEARNING OUTCOMES

Upon completion of this chapter you will be able to:

- understand the nutrition challenges faced by endurance athletes in daily training
- describe daily carbohydrate requirements for endurance athletes and identify important considerations when managing individual athletes
- assess an athlete's daily food and fluid intake and identify key areas to modify to optimise daily training performance, recovery and the favoured metabolic adaptations to training
- identify important considerations for racing and the need to customise nutrition support across the wide variety of endurance events
- manipulate fluid intake advice according to an athlete's likely requirements.

NUTRITION PRINCIPLES FOR DAILY TRAINING

Endurance athletes (recreational and elite) commit considerable effort, time and finances to training and racing. Yet few invest in the services of experienced qualified sports nutrition professionals to assist them in individualising their daily food and fluid intakes or in developing a race nutrition plan. Rather, endurance athletes rely heavily on information from other athletes, online forums, sport-specific magazines, supplement company websites and coaches. A common mistake for recreational endurance athletes is to model their daily and/or race nutrition choices on an elite athlete. Social media is commonly used by endurance athletes to inform the broader community about their food and fluid preferences. Daily training, physiology and annual race calendars vary considerably between athletes, and ultimately dictate daily nutritional needs and race-day nutrition tactics. Given the delicate balance involved in maintaining health and wellbeing while optimising daily training performance and recovery, expert nutrition advice should be sought by endurance athletes.

Elite and recreational endurance athletes alike are time-poor. Elite endurance athletes can train up to five sessions daily while juggling sponsor commitments, travel and performance support appointments. Recreational endurance athletes, while not training at the same level, are required to balance lifestyle commitments such as work, study and family in between daily workouts. Careful planning of daily meals and snacks that provide nutritious options aligned to the training goals while offering convenience and taste is a high priority for endurance athletes. Further, consideration of the annual training plan is required, as the emphasis changes throughout the year (see Chapter 9).

Matching daily energy needs

Dietary surveys of endurance athletes commonly report dietary intakes that fall below recommendations for energy (kilojoules), carbohydrate and various vitamins and minerals. This mismatch of daily energy intake with the daily energy requirements for training is likely due to a combination of issues. Firstly, there is no strong biological drive to match energy intake to activity-induced energy expenditure. Hunger is often suppressed in endurance athletes following intense training, particularly in activities such as running which can cause gastrointestinal discomfort and upset. Secondly, given the importance of maintaining a light and lean physique to optimise endurance performance, many endurance athletes adopt an overly restrictive approach with their food and fluid choices in an attempt to minimise body-fat levels. Finally, athletes may not be sufficiently organised to ensure appropriate foods and fluids are available on heavy training days, creating a practical barrier to meeting their daily energy needs. Interestingly, when athletes are well supported and organised—such as athletes contesting the Tour de France—research has demonstrated that they are able to match energy intake with daily energy expenditure even on the most strenuous of cycling stages (Saris et al. 1989).

Given daily fluctuations in training, endurance athletes should be educated so that they possess the necessary food knowledge and skills to customise daily food and fluid intakes in order to manipulate daily energy, and subsequently nutrient, intakes. Athletes need to be well organised to include additional extras in the way of training food and fluids, between-meal snacks and/or main meal extras on heavy training days to increase their daily energy intake. When additional foods and fluids are included throughout the day should be determined by the primary goal of individual training sessions, the time for recovery between training and food and fluid tolerance, as well as logistics. Conversely, on rest days or lighter training days when daily energy requirements are reduced, food and fluids intake should be adjusted accordingly.

Endurance athletes, male and female, are at increased risk of suffering from low energy availability. This is not surprising, given the high daily training loads common to many endurance training programs coupled with an emphasis on maintaining lean physiques. Low energy availability occurs with a reduction in energy intake and/ or an increased exercise load, leading to the disruption of hormonal and metabolic systems. Low energy availability is central to **RED-S** (relative energy deficiency in sport), which affects numerous aspects of health and performance, including metabolic rate, menstrual function, bone health, immunity, protein synthesis, cardiovascular and psychological health.

Disordered eating is common in cases of low energy availability; however, mismanaged attempts to quickly reduce body mass or fat mass or acute increases in daily training

RED-S
Relative energy deficiency in sport, a syndrome of impaired physiological function caused by relative energy deficiency.

Disordered eating
Eating behaviours that are not healthy or normal, including restrained eating, binge eating, fasting, heavy exercise, using excessive laxatives or purging.

loads may result in low energy availability. Performance support staff and coaches should communicate regularly to discuss the health and wellbeing of the athletes in their care. Communication around the annual plan and weekly training load is central and allows the sports nutrition professional to adjust messaging around daily fuel requirements. The inclusion of assessment tools such as resting energy expenditure, dietary intake, hormone profiling, body composition and bone health are useful tools in managing endurance athletes to better understand their health and wellbeing.

Carbohydrate intake guidelines for daily training

For endurance athletes training strenuously, daily carbohydrate demands can exceed the body's capacity to store carbohydrate. Thus, the availability of carbohydrate as fuel to support training performance and assist recovery is crucial. During intense sustained or intermittent exercise typical of endurance events or high-intensity endurance training sessions, carbohydrate is the primary fuel to support exercise performance. Carbohydrate intake should be modified in response to fluctuations in daily training load. Further, the intake of additional carbohydrate should be strategically coordinated around training to optimise training performance, facilitate recovery and enhance the adaptation to training.

The International Olympic Committee on Nutrition for Sport updated its carbohydrate intake guidelines in 2010—see Table 14.1 for an abridged version. This update provided the impetus for sports nutrition professionals to interrogate the guidelines, understand daily training patterns and subsequently customise carbohydrate intake recommendations for individual athletes on a daily basis. No longer are carbohydrate guidelines provided generically to athletes based on body size or type of sport. In assessing daily carbohydrate needs when managing endurance athletes, you should consider:

- daily training intensity, frequency and duration
- body weight and composition of the athlete
- body composition adjustments, whether it be weight loss or additional requirements associated with growth
- subjective feedback from the athlete relating to training performance and recovery
- gender
- training state and training age
- changes in the training environment, such as altitude and heat.

Box 14.1 provides a meal plan example for an elite female triathlete. The meal plan highlights the importance of considering the broader nutritional goals of the athlete when planning daily carbohydrate intake. Specific attention should be given to

Table 14.1. Daily carbohydrate intake recommendations for endurance athletes

Situation		Carbohydrate targets	Comments on type and timing of carbohydrate intake
DAILY CARBOHYDRATE NEEDS TO SUPPORT TRAINING AND RECOVERY—these general recommendations should be fine-tuned with individual consideration of total energy needs, body composition, daily training loads and feedback from training performance.			Timing of carbohydrate intake around training should support the primary goal for each session. Convenience, athlete tolerance, individual preferences and logistics are important considerations. Nutrient-rich carbohydrate food/fluids assist the athlete to meet overall nutrition goals and should be prioritised. Timely intake of a carbohydrate-containing food/fluid immediately after training should align with overall nutrition goals and consider timing of next training session and scheduled meal.
Light	Low intensity or skill-based activities	3–5 g/kg/d	
Moderate	Moderate exercise program (i.e. ~1 hr per day)	5–7 g/kg/d	
High	Endurance program (e.g. 1–3 hr/d moderate- to high-intensity exercise)	6–10 g/kg/d	
Very high	Extreme commitment (e.g. >4–5 hr/d moderate- to high-intensity exercise)	8–12 g/kg/d	
ACUTE FUELLING STRATEGIES—these guidelines promote high carbohydrate availability to promote optimal performance in endurance competition or key training sessions. Event demands and body composition should be considered when interpreting these guidelines.			
General fuelling up	Endurance events <90 min	5–10 g/kg/d	Athletes may choose compact carbohydrate-rich sources that are low in fibre/residue and easily consumed to ensure that fuel targets are met while avoiding issues relating to gastrointestinal discomfort.
Carbohydrate loading	Endurance events >90 min	36–48 h of 8–12 g/kg/d	
Pre-event fuelling	Before exercise (>60 min)	1–4 g/kg consumed 1–4 hr before exercise	Timing, amount and type of carbohydrate food and drinks should be chosen to suit the practical needs of the event and individual preferences/experiences of the athlete. Choices high in fat/protein/fibre may need to be avoided to reduce risk of gastrointestinal issues. Low glycaemic index choices may provide a more sustained source of fuel for situations where carbohydrate cannot be consumed during exercise, although being familiar with these foods items is important. Liquid carbohydrate-containing options provide a convenient option, particularly for athletes unable to tolerate foods due to 'pre-race nerves'.

Source: Modified from Burke et al. 2011.

Box 14.1: Example meal plan for an elite female triathlete

Pre-training snack (6.30am)	Slice of toast with honey Coffee with milk
Training (7.00am)	12 km Tempo run ~60minutes. Components of performance running for the last 15–20 minutes
Breakfast (8.15am)	Mixed wholegrain cereal with milk, high-protein yoghurt with mixed berries and almonds Grain toast with poached egg, spinach, mushrooms and tomato
Training (10.30am)	Swim set – 75–90 minutes Total swim 4.5 km, with quality main set of 1500 km
Immediately post-training prior to physiotherapy appointment	Liquid meal supplement (provides ~20 g protein and ~40 g carbohydrate) Banana
Lunch out with friends (1.30pm)	Toasted chicken, avocado and salad wrap Fruit salad with yoghurt Skinny flat white coffee
Afternoon snack	2 x Rice cakes with spread Fluid top-up
Afternoon training (4.30pm)	Cycle – 1 h 15 minutes criterium cycle race (40 minutes quality) with 4 km run off the bike at race pace Carbohydrate gel, water and sports drink (300–400 ml) during criterium cycle
Post-training drink while at ice-bath (6.15pm)	Flavoured milk (250 ml) Water Nut and dried fruit mix
Dinner (7.30pm)	Lean beef and vegetable stir-fry (assorted vegetables included) Brown rice Piece of fruit ± yoghurt
Supper	Glass of milk

Source: Gregory Cox.

the timing of carbohydrate intake and use of different carbohydrate foods and fluid to coordinate carbohydrate intake around training to support daily performance and recovery.

The meal plan in Box 14.1 is based on an elite female triathlete. Elite triathletes train 2–5 times daily using a mix of low-intensity aerobic and high-intensity repeat-effort work. Elite triathletes need to be well organised to meet daily energy, carbohydrate and nutrient needs to maintain training performance, health and well-being. Timing appropriate snacks around training and including nutritious foods at meals that provide antioxidants in addition to carbohydrate, protein and healthy fats will assist training performance and recovery.

How aggressive refuelling strategies are employed after exercise should reflect the glycogen likely to have been used in the session, the timing of the next session, the next meal time and the broader nutrition goals of the athlete. Hence, the approach taken to refuelling strategies should be periodised throughout the week, or even the training year, depending on the key training goals. A well thought-out timetable will allow preparation before, and recovery after, key training sessions and competition. It may not matter that lower intensity sessions are undertaken without full refuelling—in fact, there may actually be some advantages to this (see Box 14.2).

Box 14.2: How much glycogen do endurance athletes use?

An intense high-quality endurance cycling session consisting of 8 × 5-minute maximal efforts will deplete muscle glycogen stores by about 50 per cent (Stepto et al. 2001). A sports nutrition professional should be familiar with the specific carbohydrate requirements of the athletes they manage when providing advice regarding strategies for carbohydrate intake around daily training and racing.

In the 1–2 hours after hard exercise, the muscle is primed to absorb and store carbohydrate—this is referred to as the **window of opportunity**. While early feeding promotes refuelling at the high end of the storage range, muscle will continue to take up carbohydrate in response to food consumed at meals throughout the day. It is worth taking advantage of this window when recovery time is short and refuelling needs are particularly important (for example,

Window of opportunity
In sports nutrition and training this refers to the 1–2 hours after hard exercise in which the muscle is primed to absorb and store carbohydrate.

after a Friday morning run with the next session scheduled on Sunday morning). The overall carbohydrate intake, not the timing of carbohydrate intake, will be the driving force behind how much muscle glycogen is restored during recovery periods that extend over 24–28 hours.

Training with low carbohydrate availability

In recent times, much has been written about purposely training and/or sleeping with low muscle glycogen stores to accelerate favourable adaptations that occur in response to aerobic exercise. Training when fasted, withholding carbohydrate during extended sessions, limiting carbohydrate during recovery between training sessions, and sleeping with low muscle glycogen stores have all been investigated to determine the likely benefits of 'training low'. Whether to strategically incorporate training low techniques into the weekly training schedule should be discussed with the athlete support team as there are several performance and health implications to consider.

Protein to promote recovery and gains in lean body mass

While much of the research focus on endurance athletes has centred on carbohydrate, protein plays a particularly important role for endurance athletes. While protein requirements for endurance athletes are increased, they are typically met as the athlete increases their daily energy intake. However, strategic timing of protein-containing foods and/or fluids immediately after training and/or during extended training sessions can assist in maintaining or increasing lean body mass as well as enhancing favourable metabolic responses to endurance exercise. Sports nutrition professionals should be purposeful in their planning by including protein-containing foods and fluids immediately following targeted endurance training sessions (see Box 14.1).

Iron is an important micronutrient for endurance athletes

Endurance athletes are prone to having low iron status caused by inadequate dietary intake in combination with increased iron losses (for instance, through **gastrointestinal bleeding**, sweating and **haemolysis**), increased iron needs (for instance, when training at altitude) and reduced iron absorption (which occurs during the post-exercise window, particularly when exercise is undertaken with low glycogen stores). Regardless of the stage of iron depletion, all types of iron deficiency should be carefully managed. A planned assessment schedule for iron status should be considered within

Gastrointestinal bleeding
Bleeding that occurs from any part of the gastrointestinal tract, but typically from the small intestine, large intestine, rectum or anus. Gastrointestinal bleeding is not a disease, but is a symptom of many diseases. For athletes, bleeding may occur due to sloughing of intestinal lining as a result of the continual jarring that occurs when running on hard surfaces.

Haemolysis
The rupture of red blood cells.

the annual training, competition and travel plans of endurance athletes. Athletes will benefit from education that highlights dietary sources of iron as well as ways to improve iron absorption (Table 14.2). The use of iron supplements may be necessary at specific times for certain athletes and should be managed by the sports medicine physician and sports dietitian.

Table 14.2. Components in food that affect bioavailability of iron

Iron enhancers	Iron inhibitors
Vitamin C-rich foods (ascorbic acid) • salad, lightly cooked green vegetables, some fruits and citrus fruit juices or vitamin C-fortified fruit juices	Phytates • found in cereal grains, wheat bran, legumes, nuts, peanut butter, seeds, bran, soy products, soy protein and spinach
Some fermented foods • miso, some types of soy sauce	Polyphenolic compounds • strong tea and coffee, herb tea, cocoa, red wine, some spices, e.g. oregano
Meat enhancer factor • found in beef, liver, lamb, chicken and fish	Calcium inhibits both haem and non-haem iron absorption as iron and calcium co-compete for absorption across the gut (milk, cheese)
Alcohol and some organic acids • very low-pH foods containing citric acid, tartaric acid, e.g. citrus fruit	Peptides from partially digested plant proteins • soy protein isolates, soy products
Vitamin A and beta-carotene • liver, animal fats, carrots, sweet potato	

RACE-DAY NUTRITION STRATEGIES

Optimal performance during competition is achieved by targeting the factors that would otherwise cause fatigue or a reduction in work output and/or skill. Nutritional factors that can cause fatigue include depletion of glycogen stores, low blood glucose levels (**hypoglycaemia**), dehydration, low blood sodium levels (**hyponatraemia**), and gastrointestinal upset. Eating strategies in preparation for the race and during the race should be implemented to avoid or reduce the impact of these problems.

Hypoglycaemia
Low blood glucose levels.

Hyponatraemia
Low blood sodium levels.

Bonking
An athletic term describing a sudden and overwhelming feeling of running out of energy, often also termed 'hitting the wall' during endurance events.

Carbohydrate loading for endurance racing
Carbohydrate is stored within the muscle as glycogen. Carbohydrate loading, if done appropriately, increases muscle glycogen stores—thereby delaying the point of fatigue, commonly referred to as '**bonking**' in endurance circles. Carbohydrate

loading emerged in the late 1960s, when Scandinavian researchers found that 3–4 days of carbohydrate deprivation, followed by three days of high carbohydrate eating resulted in a supercompensation of muscle glycogen and a subsequent improvement in endurance exercise capacity (Bergstrom et al. 1967). This method was later refined, when Sherman et al. (1981) found that muscle glycogen stores increased to similar levels without the three days of depletion prior to 3–4 days of high carbohydrate eating and rest.

Despite a greater reliance on muscle glycogen when pre-exercise concentrations are elevated with carbohydrate loading prior to exercise, carbohydrate loading is generally associated with enhanced performance when exercise duration exceeds 90 minutes. In shorter duration endurance events (for example, 10-kilometre road runs, a 40-kilometre cycling time-trial or a 2–3-kilometre open water swim), suitable fuel stores in the muscle are achieved by a combination of tapered exercise or rest, plus adequate carbohydrate intake (5–10 g per kg body mass) over the 24–36 hours before the event. For many athletes, this dietary prescription is already achieved in the everyday training diet, so no extra effort or planning is required. However, for some athletes (often women or athletes on a weight-reduction diet) increasing total dietary energy and carbohydrate above their normal intake may be needed to achieve these fuelling-up goals.

For longer duration events, such as marathon, 70.3 or ironman triathlon, achieving a high carbohydrate intake (8–12 g per kg body mass) for 24–72 hours before an event will require athletes to modify their typical daily food and fluid intake. It is unlikely that an athlete's typical carbohydrate intake will fall within this range to supercompensate muscle glycogen stores. A well-structured and considered carbohydrate loading plan will ensure an athlete increases their carbohydrate intake while avoiding gastrointestinal issues. Box 14.3 provides some common practice considerations for sports nutrition professionals.

Pre-race meal

A carbohydrate-rich meal or snack scheduled 1–4 hours before a race has a role in fine-tuning competition preparation by topping-up muscle glycogen stores and restoring liver glycogen stores (following an overnight fast). Including fluid (~400–600 mL) with the pre-exercise meal will maximise fluid retention and ensure the athlete is well-hydrated, especially where a fluid deficit is likely to occur during the event. The pre-race meal should be carbohydrate-focused, relatively low in fat and contain moderate amounts of protein. Above all, the pre-race meal should be familiar to the athlete to achieve gut comfort throughout the event, preventing the athlete from either becoming hungry or suffering gastrointestinal disturbance or upset. Liquid meal alternatives that contain carbohydrate and protein provide an excellent option for athletes who cannot tolerate solid foods immediately before race start. Given the variety of endurance

Box 14.3: Carbohydrate loading practice considerations

- Athletes should be provided with adequate information regarding the carbohydrate content of foods. Many athletes have limited understanding of the carbohydrate content of everyday foods and fluids or formulated supplementary sports foods such as carbohydrate gels, sports drinks and energy bars. Providing a carbohydrate ready reckoner will assist the athlete in achieving required carbohydrate intakes (see the suggestions in Box 14.4).
- Low-fibre foods should be included within a carbohydrate loading plan to help maintain a normal fibre intake for the athlete.
- When devising a carbohydrate loading plan, it is important to understand the athlete's likely exercise routine for the final 2–3 days before competition. Additional training should be considered in dietary planning to ensure adequate energy is available to allow additional carbohydrate consumed to be available for glycogen storage rather than used to meet energy needs.
- When formulating a carbohydrate loading plan, it is important to consider the likely glycogen storage capacity of the athlete when determining the subsequent amount of carbohydrate to be consumed. For well-trained elite athletes with a long training history and low body-fat stores, higher amounts of carbohydrate within the guidelines should be considered. For recreationally engaged endurance athletes and those with higher body-fat levels, carbohydrate intake goals should be modified to the lower end of suggested intake range.
- If formulating a carbohydrate loading meal plan that includes discretionary foods such as confectionery, soft drink and sports drink, it is worthwhile including a disclaimer such as: *The food suggestions and volumes specified in the carbohydrate loading meal plan are specific to carbohydrate loading and should not be misinterpreted to reflect everyday healthy eating habits or strategies. Many of the above suggestions are contrary to everyday healthy eating guidelines and are specific to pre-race endurance competition nutrition requirements.*

races, scheduling of events, food availability and environmental conditions, athletes are best advised to plan and subsequently rehearse their pre-race meal. Fine-tuning may require input from a skilled sports nutrition professional to avoid gastrointestinal upset and optimise the readiness to compete. Box 14.4 provides some examples of carbohydrate-rich pre-race meals.

Important considerations for carbohydrate intake during racing

Reported race-day carbohydrate intake rates vary considerably between athletes undertaking endurance exercise. This is not surprising, as some events or disciplines within a

---

Box 14.4: Examples of pre-race meals

Early morning race start. Choices need to be simple and easy to prepare and consumed 1½–2 hours before race start. Water should be included and varied according to anticipated fluid requirements, environmental conditions, other fluids contained within the meal and the athlete's thirst level.
- Cooked oats + low-fat milk with honey, + banana + glass of fruit juice
- ¾–1½ cups of cereal + low-fat milk + slice of toast with savoury spread + milk coffee
- Toasted muffin/s or crumpet/s or bread + jam or honey + banana with 400–600 mL of sports drink + ½–1 sports bar
- 1–2 pancakes with syrup + liquid meal replacement
- 400–600 mL of sports drink + sports bar
- Fruit smoothie (banana, low-fat milk, yoghurt and honey) or fruit smoothie

Late race start. A normal schedule of meals should be consumed before the pre-race meal. Timing of pre-race meal can be varied to suit athlete preference (1–3 hours pre-race). Water should be included and varied according to anticipated fluid requirements, environmental conditions, other fluids contained within the meal and the athlete's thirst level.
- Roll(s) or sandwich(es) + 400–600 mL of sports drink
- Spaghetti with tomato or low-fat sauce + glass of fruit juice
- ½–1 cup of creamed rice + 2 slices of toast with savoury spread and 400–600 mL of sports drink

multidiscipline event provide better access to and tolerance of the intake of food and fluids. For example, Kimber et al. (2002) found that 73 per cent of the total energy consumed during an ironman triathlon was consumed during the cycle leg of the race. One interesting finding from this study was that overall finishing time was inversely related to carbohydrate intake during the run for male competitors. Pfeiffer et al. (2012), also found that high rates of carbohydrate intake were usually observed in faster athletes; however, high rates of carbohydrate intake are associated with increased rates of gastrointestinal upset, such as nausea and flatulence. While there are obvious benefits to exercise performance of providing carbohydrate during endurance sports (Stellingwerff & Cox 2014), it is important that carbohydrate intake suggestions are well tolerated by the athlete. Many athletes do not consume carbohydrate routinely during training (Burke et al. 2003), which may partly explain why they suffer gastro-intestinal upset and discomfort when they compete and ingest carbohydrate-containing fluids and foods.

Researchers at the Australian Institute of Sport were the first to demonstrate that athletes are able to increase their use of ingested carbohydrate during a simulated race if they routinely consume carbohydrate during daily training for four weeks (Cox et al. 2010). It appears that athletes can train their gut to increase absorption and subsequent delivery of the ingested carbohydrate to the working muscle. The practical significance of this research highlights the importance of 'training the way you race'. In preparation for endurance racing, athletes should rehearse their race carbohydrate intake strategies in race-like training sessions that mimic the demands of competition.

The amount, timing, type, frequency of intake and form of carbohydrate should be considered when advising endurance athletes in relation to carbohydrate intake during training and racing (Table 14.3). In brief, in high-intensity endurance sports lasting less than 45 minutes, there appears to be little benefit to consuming carbohydrate during exercise. While the athlete should start exercise with normalised muscle glycogen stores, there is little to gain by consuming carbohydrate in these brief endurance events or training sessions. However, consuming small amounts of carbohydrate—even rinsing the mouth with carbohydrate—provides a performance advantage in endurance exercise lasting 45–75 minutes (Rollo & Williams 2011). Consuming carbohydrate in these events provides a central stimulus, altering the perception of effort and allowing for greater work outputs. The frequency of exposure, not the amount of carbohydrate consumed, is central to planning carbohydrate intake strategies for these events.

As the duration of the endurance event extends beyond 90 minutes, providing carbohydrate during exercise will provide an alternate fuel for the exercising muscle while maintaining high rates of carbohydrate oxidation. Furthermore, carbohy-drate intake will assist in maintaining blood glucose levels within normal ranges.

Table 14.3. Carbohydrate intake recommendations for endurance athletes during exercise

	Situation	Carbohydrate targets	Comments on type and timing of carbohydrate intake
During brief exercise	<45 minutes (e.g. 10 km track event)	Not needed	
During sustained high-intensity training sessions or races	45–75 minutes (e.g. half marathon, road cycling time-trial)	Small amounts including mouth rinse	Carbohydrate-containing drinks, including sports drinks and carbohydrate gels, provide practical options for athletes undertaking high-intensity endurance sports.
During endurance events or extended training sessions	1–2.5 hours (e.g. marathon)	30–60 g/h	Most endurance events require athletes to refuel/rehydrate while they are actually racing. The availability of foods and fluids varies according to the race. Race organisers may provide selected foods and fluids from feed/aid stations on the course, whereas some athletes may carry their own supplies. A range of everyday foods/fluids and specialised sports supplements, including sports drinks and gels, provides convenient, well-tolerated options. Athletes should practice in training to find a refuelling plan that suits their individual goals, including hydration needs and gut comfort.
During ultra-endurance exercise	>2.5–3 hours (e.g. ultramarathons, ironman triathlons, cycling stage races)	Up to 90 g/h	As above. Higher intakes of carbohydrate are associated with better performance. Specifically designed sports foods and fluids providing multiple transportable carbohydrates (glucose:fructose mixtures) will achieve high rates of oxidation of carbohydrate consumed during exercise. Including a variety of tastes and textures during longer or multi-day endurance races is important to avoid 'flavour fatigue'.

Source: Adapted from Burke et al. 2011.

For extended-duration endurance events there is a dose-response benefit to consuming carbohydrate (Smith et al. 2013). The maximal amount tolerated and available for oxidation will be increased by consuming multiple transportable carbohydrates (glucose and fructose), as they are absorbed across the gut on different transporters.

Further, as previously mentioned, rehearsing race-day carbohydrate intakes, particularly high rates of carbohydrate, will improve tolerance.

There is a myriad of sports foods, fluids and everyday food items that can be incorporated into a race-day plan for an endurance athlete. The combination of everyday food items and specialised sports foods should be based on the ease of intake and the athlete's food and fluid preferences. Box 14.5 provides various suggestions for race-day food and fluid intakes.

Box 14.5: Carbohydrate food and fluid suggestions for endurance racing

High-intensity endurance events 45–75 minutes
- Small quantities (exposures) of carbohydrate.
- Mouth rinse or frequent intake of carbohydrate-containing drinks (e.g. sports drink) if practical and tolerated + water as tolerated.

High-intensity endurance events 90–150 minutes
- Carbohydrate intake target of 30–60 g of carbohydrate per hour.
- Water should be consumed to alleviate thirst in addition to fluids listed to top-up fluid intake.

Hourly suggestions
- 200–300 mL of sports drink ± sports gel (25–30 g CHO per gel) OR
- ~200–300 mL of cola soft drink ± sports gel (25–30 g CHO per gel) OR
- 400–600 mL of sports drink OR
- 1–2 x sports gel (25–30 g CHO per gel).

Endurance events >2½–3 hours
- Carbohydrate intake target is up to 90 g of carbohydrate per hour.
- For ultra-endurance races a variety of tastes (sweet and savoury) should be included to avoid flavour fatigue.
- The amount of carbohydrate consumed should reflect the nature of the event and specific requirements of the athlete.
- The combination of solid vs liquid forms of carbohydrate should be modified to reflect the intensity of exercise and the duration of the event.

- Intake of carbohydrate-containing fluids should be managed to control hourly carbohydrate intake.
- Water should be consumed to alleviate thirst in addition to fluids listed to top-up fluid intake.

Hourly carbohydrate suggestions for 40–60 g/h

- 300–400 mL of sports drink + 1 x sport gel (25–30 g CHO per gel) OR
- 2 x sport gels (25–30 g CHO per gel) OR
- 400–600 mL of sports drink + banana OR
- 600 mL of sports drink + nut muesli bar OR
- 400–500 mL of cola drink

Hourly carbohydrate suggestions for 70–90 g/h

- 600 mL of sports drink + 2 x sport gels (25–30 g CHO per gel) OR
- 500–600 mL of sports drink + sandwich (savoury or sweet spread) OR
- 200 mL of sports gel concentrate—8 x sports gels (~25 g CHO per gel) added to a 600 mL drink bottle topped up with water to 600 mL OR
- 600 mL of cola drink + ½ sports bar (40 g CHO per bar) OR
- 250 mL of liquid meal supplement + cereal bar or granola bar OR
- 400–600 mL of sweetened iced tea + 40 g of dried fruit and nut mix + ½–1 sandwich (savoury spread) OR
- 300–500 mL of sports drink + 60 g chocolate bar + 20 g packet of crisps OR
- 40 g of confectionery or sports confectionery + 2 pikelets and jam + fun-size chocolate bar.

Source: Gregory Cox.

Fluid intake considerations for endurance athletes

In many endurance sports, sweat losses are considerable, resulting in significant loss of fluid and dehydration. This is magnified in hot, humid environments and in sports where there are practical barriers to drinking (for example, mountain bike racing and marathon running). Earlier laboratory studies consistently reported that the stress associated with exercise increased in response to the level of fluid deficit. However, there is some controversy regarding the effect of dehydration on endurance exercise performance, particularly in field settings (Goulet 2012). The point at which the effects become apparent depend on the individual—their level of training and fitness, their starting hydration status and their acclimation—and the environment (effects are greater in the heat or at altitude).

Race and/or training fluid intake advice should be individualised to ensure athletes use available opportunities to drink fluids at a rate that prevents thirst and keeps their accumulating fluid deficit below two per cent of body mass. Figure 14.1 provides an insight into the complex nature of providing individualised fluid intake advice. For instance, an elite male triathlete racing at high speeds in a hot Olympic-distance triathlon should create opportunities to maximise fluid intake and take visual cues from other athletes as a reminder to drink as sweat losses will be high and opportunities to drink limited. Further, the speed of racing will impact on tolerance and gut comfort when ingesting fluids. In contrast, a recreational female runner who runs/walks a marathon in cool weather can expect lower sweat rates, while having ample opportunity to slow or stop at aid stations. For this athlete, controlling her opportunities, rather than drinking as much as tolerated, should underpin her fluid intake advice to minimise the risk of over-drinking. While not common, overzealous fluid intake combined with low sweat

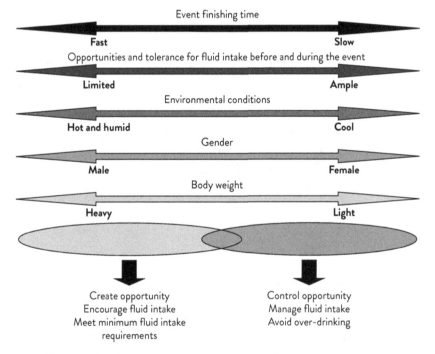

Figure 14.1. Fluid intake advice

Source: Adapted from Burke & Cox 2010.

losses may lead to the potentially fatal condition of hyponatraemia (low blood sodium concentration, often known as water intoxication). The development of a race fluid intake plan can be assisted by undertaking fluid balance assessments during race-like training sessions in similar environmental conditions so that the athlete can gauge their typical sweat rates in comparison to their opportunity/ability to rehydrate.

The most suitable drink choices and delivery methods will depend on the sport and the need to address other nutritional goals. Fluids need to be palatable (temperature, taste) and available to encourage intake. Other characteristics to consider include the beverage temperature, which can be manipulated both to improve palatability in the specific environment and to contribute to body temperature regulation; cold fluids and ice slushies can reduce core temperature in hot conditions, while warm fluids may increase body temperature in cold environments. Many endurance events offer a range of fluids, most commonly, water, sports drink, cola soft drinks and, in extended races, warm broths or soups. Sports drinks are formulated to meet a range of needs and simultaneously provide fluid, electrolytes and carbohydrate. Cola soft drinks provide additional carbohydrate and small amounts of caffeine which, when included later in exercise, may provide a performance benefit (Cox et al. 2002). Above all, athletes should be familiar with the sports drink on offer at the endurance event and/or plan to provide their preferred choice.

SUMMARY AND KEY MESSAGES

After reading this chapter, you should be familiar with the training and competition demands of endurance athletes. You should understand the carbohydrate requirements associated with different event durations and intensities, and be able to tailor a nutrition plan based on these requirements with consideration of the individual athlete and environmental conditions.

Key messages

- In planning daily energy and carbohydrate intakes, it is critical to understand the daily training schedule and purpose of training sessions to optimise training performance, facilitate recovery and promote favourable adaptations to training.
- Well-selected protein-containing foods and fluids during recovery post-exercise will optimise recovery and promote gains in lean body mass.
- Endurance athletes commonly suffer from low iron status and, as such, should be carefully monitored and managed.
- Carbohydrate loading offers particular advantage to endurance athletes competing in events longer than 90 minutes. Dietary strategies should be employed to achieve high carbohydrate intakes while avoiding high intakes of fibre.

- The pre-race meal should be carbohydrate-focused and customised to suit the athlete and race schedule. Above all, food and fluids should be familiar to the athlete.
- Carbohydrate intake for racing should be scaled according to the duration and intensity of the event. For athletes consuming high rates of carbohydrate, race-day nutrition plans should be rehearsed to minimise the risk of gastrointestinal discomfort during the race.
- Race-day carbohydrate and fluid intakes should be adjusted to suit individual athlete preferences. Given the variety of endurance events, sports nutrition professionals should become familiar with the practical challenges faced by athletes in meeting their race-day nutrition goals.

REFERENCES

Bergstrom, J., Hermansen, L., Hultman, E. et al., 1967, 'Diet, muscle glycogen and physical performance', *Acta Physiologica Scandinavia*, vol. 71, pp. 140–50.

Burke, L.M. & Cox, G.R., 2010, *The Complete Guide to Food for Sports Performance. Peak Nutrition for Your Sport*, Crows Nest, NSW: Allen & Unwin.

Burke, L.M., Hawley, J.A., Wong, S.H. et al., 2011, 'Carbohydrates for training and competition', *Journal of Sports Science*, vol. 29, pp. S17–27.

Burke, L.M., Slater, G., Broad, E.M. et al., 2003, 'Eating patterns and meal frequency of elite Australian athletes', *International Journal of Sport Nutrition & Exercise Metabolism*, vol. 13, no. 4, pp. 521–38.

Cox, G.R., Clark, S.A., Cox, A.J. et al., 2010, 'Daily training with high carbohydrate availability increases exogenous carbohydrate oxidation during endurance cycling', *Journal of Applied Physiology*, vol. 109, no. 1, pp. 126–34.

Cox, G. R., Desbrow, B., Montgomery, P. G. et al., 2002, 'Effect of different protocols of caffeine intake on metabolism and endurance performance', *Journal of Applied Physiology*, vol. 93, no. 3, pp. 990–9.

Goulet, E.D., 2012, 'Dehydration and endurance performance in competitive athletes', *Nutrition Reviews*, vol. 70, suppl. 2, pp. S132–6.

Kimber, N.E., Ross, J.J., Mason, S.L. et al., 2002, 'Energy balance during an ironman triathlon in male and female triathletes', *International Journal of Sport Nutrition & Exercise Metabolism*, vol. 12, no. 1, pp. 47–62.

Pfeiffer, B., Stellingwerff, T., Hodgson, A.B. et al., 2012, 'Nutritional intake and gastrointestinal problems during competitive endurance events', *Medicine & Science in Sports & Exercise*, vol. 44, no. 2, pp. 344–51.

Rollo, I. & Williams, C., 2011, 'Effect of mouth-rinsing carbohydrate solutions on endurance performance', *Sports Medicine*, vol. 41, no. 6, pp. 449–61.

Saris, W.H., Van Erp-Baart, M.A., Brouns, F. et al., 1989, 'Study on food intake and energy expenditure during extreme sustained exercise: The Tour de France', *International Journal of Sports Medicine*, vol. 10, suppl. 1, pp. S26–31.

Sherman, W.M., Costill, D.L., Fink, W.J. et al., 1981, 'Effect of exercise-diet manipulation on muscle glycogen and its subsequent utilization during performance', *International Journal of Sports Medicine*, vol. 2, suppl. 2, pp. 114–8.

Smith, J.W., Pascoe, D.D., Passe, D.H. et al., 2013, 'Curvilinear dose-response relationship of carbohydrate (0–120 g.h(−1)) and performance', *Medicine & Science in Sports & Exercise*, vol. 45, no. 2, pp. 336–41.

Stellingwerff, T. & Cox, G.R., 2014, 'Systematic review: Carbohydrate supplementation on exercise performance or capacity of varying durations', *Applied, Physiology, Nutrition and Metabolism*, vol. 39, no. 9, pp. 998–1011.

Stepto, N.K., Martin, D.T., Fallon, K.E. et al., 2001, 'Metabolic demands of intense aerobic interval training in competitive cyclists', *Medicine & Science in Sports & Exercise*, vol. 33, no. 2, pp. 303–10.

CHAPTER

15

Strength and power athletes

Gary Slater and Lachlan Mitchell

The ability to generate explosive muscle power and strength is critical to success in crossfit, Olympic weightlifting and powerlifting, throwing events including javelin, discus, shot put and hammer, and 100- and 200-metre sprints in track and field. The athletes competing in these events will typically incorporate some form of resistance exercise into their overall training program, as well as diverse sport-specific training. Given the disparity between the sport-specific training programs of strength and power athletes and their subsequent metabolic implications, this chapter will focus on the nutritional implications of resistance training among strength and power athletes. The sport of bodybuilding will also be addressed given the focus on resistance exercise in overall training program prescription.

LEARNING OUTCOMES

Upon completion of this chapter you will be able to:
* understand the training nutrition needs of strength and power athletes, including macronutrient needs over the day

- identify appropriate nutrition strategies to facilitate recovery
- appreciate the issues regarding supplement use in this population
- understand the competition demands of strength and power athletes and translate that into specific nutrition guidance
- appreciate the importance of physique traits among this athlete population and how to manipulate these through dietary interventions.

TRAINING PROGRAMS

Athletics competitors participating in throwing events typically undertake periodised training programs (Chapter 9) that aim to develop maximum strength and power of the major muscle groups. Training involves a range of modalities including **plyometric exercises**, sprinting, power lifts, Olympic lifts and weighted throwing drills to complement technical throwing training. Periodisation of resistance training typically involves a transition from high-volume, high-force, low-velocity movements requiring less coordination characteristic of traditional powerlifting to more **explosive**, lower-force, low-repetition training using Olympic lifts in preparation for competition. The focus on explosive Olympic lifts over more traditional strength-based lifting results in more favourable power and strength gains, derived primarily from neural rather than skeletal muscle **hypertrophy** adaptations. Consequently, this style of training enhances traits important to athletic development and is common among other explosive athletics disciplines like sprinting and jumping events, as well as increasingly being incorporated into the training practices of powerlifters.

Plyometric exercises
Exercises in which muscles exert maximum force in short intervals of time, with the goal of increasing power—for example, jump training.

Explosive
Requiring a maximum or near maximum power output from the athlete in a short amount of time.

Hypertrophy
An increase in skeletal muscle size through growth in size of its cells.

Unlike other sports that use resistance exercise to complement sport-specific training, crossfit, powerlifting, Olympic lifting and bodybuilding use resistance training as a primary mode of training. While Olympic and powerlifting athletes are primarily concerned with enhancing power and strength respectively, bodybuilding training primarily aims to induce skeletal muscle hypertrophy. Consequently, the training programs of bodybuilders are unique, typically of greater volume than those of other athletes, using higher repetition ranges with multiple sets per muscle group and little rest between sets.

TRAINING NUTRITION

Nutrition plays an important role in three aspects of training for strength and power athletes: (1) fuelling of sport-specific and strength training, (2) recovery from this training and (3) the promotion of training adaptations, including skeletal muscle hypertrophy. Resistance exercise requires a high rate of energy supply, derived from both the phosphagen energy systems and glycogenolysis (see Chapter 2) (Lambert & Flynn 2002; Tesch et al. 1986), with the contribution of each dependent upon the relative power output, the work-to-rest ratio and muscle blood flow (Tesch et al. 1986). The source of fatigue during resistance exercise is likely multifactorial, including neuromuscular and peripheral metabolic factors such as decline in intramuscular pH (MacDougall et al. 1999), the latter somewhat dependent on the intensity and volume of training undertaken as well as the time point within a resistance training session. Metabolic fatigue during the earlier part of a workout may be due at least partly to reductions in phosphagen energy system stores and mild acidosis, while subsequent fatigue may result more from acidosis and impaired energy production from glycogenolysis (MacDougall et al. 1999).

Acidosis

A process causing increased acidity in the blood and other body tissue.

Given the extreme muscularity of these individuals and the association between muscle mass and total energy expenditure, it is not surprising that these athletes have generous energy intakes (Slater & Phillips 2011). However, when expressed relative to body mass the energy intakes of strength and power athletes are generally unremarkable relative to those reported for athletes in other sports but lower than current strength athlete guidelines of ~185–210 kJ/kgBM/day (Manore et al. 2000). This likely reflects the fact that taller and/or more muscular individuals have lower resting and total energy requirements relative to body mass. Given this, consideration may need to be given to the allometric scaling of traditional sports nutrition guidelines for macronutrients among larger athletes, reflective of their lower relative energy requirements. Consideration should also be given to distribution of nutrient intake (Thomas et al. 2016), with limited information available on daily distribution of energy and nutrient intake, making it difficult to infer compliance with guidelines relating to key periods of nutrient intake, including before, during and after exercise.

Allometric scaling

Basing an individual's basal metabolic rate (BMR) and hence requirements on their body mass.

Carbohydrate

A single resistance training session can result in reductions in muscle glycogen stores of as much as 40 per cent (Tesch et al. 1986; MacDougall et al. 1999), with the amount of depletion depending on the duration, intensity and overall work accomplished during the session. Higher repetition, moderate load training characteristic of programming prescribed to promote skeletal muscle hypertrophy results in the greatest reductions in muscle glycogen stores. Reductions in muscle glycogen stores has been associated with performance impairment and, therefore, lower training capacity, although this effect is not always evident and may be dependent on the method used to induce a state of glycogen depletion. Nonetheless, it is possible that impaired training or competition performance could occur in any session or event that relied on rapid and repeated glycogen breakdown.

Given that resistance training is merely one component of the overall training program of sprint and throwing event athletes, and that the skeletal muscle damage that accompanies resistance training impairs muscle glycogen resynthesis, it would seem pertinent to encourage strength trained athletes to maintain a moderate carbohydrate intake. Guidelines proposing an intake within the range of 6 g/kg BM/day for male strength athletes (Lambert & Flynn 2002), and possibly less for females (Volek et al. 2006), have been advocated. Lifters and throwers typically report carbohydrate intakes of 3–5 g/kg BM/day, while bodybuilders maintain daily intakes equivalent to 4–7 g/kg BM/day, independent of gender (Slater & Phillips 2011). While this may appear low relative to endurance athletes, conclusive evidence of benefit from maintaining a habitual high carbohydrate intake among strength athletes remains to be confirmed. Given the lower relative energy expenditure of larger athletes and their requirements for other nutrients, plus the impact of adjusting carbohydrate on total energy intake, recommendations for carbohydrate intake at strategic times, including before, during and after exercise, may be more applicable to the strength athlete, ensuring carbohydrate availability is optimised at critical time points. Thus, we would consider a range of daily carbohydrate intakes of 4–7 g/kg BM as reasonable for these athletes, depending on their phase of training and daily training loads.

Protein

Strength-trained athletes have advocated high-protein diets for many years. While debate continues on the need for additional protein among resistance-trained individuals, general guidelines now recommend athletes undertaking strength training ingest approximately twice the current recommendations for protein of their sedentary counterparts, or as much as 1.2–2.0 g protein/kg BM/day (Phillips & Van Loon 2011). Given the relatively wide distribution of protein in the meal plan and increased energy intake of athletes, it should not be surprising to learn that the majority of strength-trained athletes easily achieve these increased protein needs (Slater & Phillips 2011). Exceeding the upper range of protein intake guidelines offers no further benefit as excess protein is broken down and excreted. Furthermore, there is evidence that an intense period of resistance training reduces protein turnover and improves net protein retention, thus reducing relative dietary protein requirements of experienced resistance-trained athletes.

Simply contrasting an athlete's current daily protein intake against guidelines does not indicate whether dietary intake has been optimised to promote gains in muscle mass or enhance repair of damaged tissues. Rather, consideration should be given to other dietary factors, including total energy intake, the daily distribution of protein intake (especially as it relates to training), and the source of dietary protein (Morton et al. 2015). While there is very little information available on the eating patterns of strength athletes, available literature suggests the majority of daily protein intake is ingested at main meals from an even mix of animal- and plant-based sources, with a skewed pattern of intake towards the evening meal, indicating a significant proportion of athletes fail to achieve optimal protein intake at breakfast and lunch. Thus, rather than focusing on total daily intake, athletes are encouraged to focus more on optimising protein quality and distribution throughout the day. Given muscle protein synthesis becomes less efficient in response to persistently high levels of amino acids in the blood, it has been suggested 4–5 evenly spaced feedings of ~20 g (0.25 g/kg BM) high biological value protein should be recommended for strength athletes (Phillips & Van Loon 2011).

Fat

The dietary fat intake of strength and power athletes is generally greater than that recommended for healthy individuals and is often derived from sources rich in saturated fat, presumably from an emphasis on animal foods in the pursuit of a higher protein intake. While it is unclear what the impacts of such dietary practices are on athletes' blood lipid profiles, it may explain in part the lower dietary carbohydrate intakes reported among strength and power athletes. Given that replacing fat with **isoenergetic** amounts of carbohydrate has a favourable effect on protein balance, it is tempting to recommend a reduction in dietary fat intake, especially for those individuals exceeding current guidelines. However, consideration must be given to the practical implications of substituting a high energy-density macronutrient with a lower energy macronutrient and the impact this may have on energy balance, especially among strength and power athletes with very high energy needs. Conversely, there may be situations in which a higher intake of foods rich in unsaturated fats may be advocated for strength and power athletes struggling to achieve energy needs because of an emphasis on the selection of lower energy-density foods in the meal plan.

Isoenergetic
Containing the same number of calories/kilojoules.

Pre-exercise and during exercise

Athletes are encouraged to pay particular attention to dietary intake in the hours before exercise, on the assumption that pre-exercise nutritional strategies can influence exercise performance. While this is a widely accepted practice prior to endurance exercise to enhance work capacity, evidence is also emerging for a beneficial role of carbohydrate consumed immediately prior to strength training. For example, Lambert at al. (1991) reported that supplemental carbohydrate ingestion prior to and during resistance exercise (1 g/kg before, 0.5 g/kg during) increased total work capacity, a response which has been replicated elsewhere. However, not all studies have shown a benefit from consuming carbohydrate prior to exercise; we propose that the **ergogenic** potential for carbohydrate ingestion is most likely to be observed when undertaking longer-duration, high-volume resistance training. At present, a specific recommendation for an optimum rate or timing of carbohydrate ingestion for strength and power athletes before and during any given training session cannot be determined. Given the lower relative energy expenditure of resistance exercise to endurance exercise, the lower range of existing exercise carbohydrate intake guidance for endurance athletes (for instance, 1 g/kg before and 0.5 g/kg carbohydrate during exercise) may be a reasonable proxy until more specific resistance training research is undertaken. As with all athletes, strength and power athletes should be encouraged to initiate training in a **euhydrated** state given that even moderate **hypohydration** can impair resistance-training work capacity.

Ergogenic
Enhancing physical performance.

Euhydrated
Normal state of body water content.

Hypohydration
Dehydration of the body.

Recently, there has been interest in combining carbohydrate and essential amino acids both before and during resistance exercise, presumably to increase substrate availability and thus exercise performance, to promote a more anabolic (muscle-building) hormonal environment, to stimulate muscle protein synthesis and to reduce muscle damage and soreness. Initial research found that greater muscle protein synthesis occurred when nutritional support was provided before rather than after resistance exercise, but this has not been replicated elsewhere. Consequently, current guidelines recommend that protein be consumed after exercise because this is when there is maximal stimulation of muscle protein synthesis.

Recovery

Given that resistance training typically forms only one component of an athlete's training schedule, recovery strategies proven to enhance restoration of muscle glycogen stores, such as eating carbohydrate after exercise, should be routinely implemented following resistance training. General sports nutrition guidelines advocate carbohydrate should be consumed at a rate of 1.0–1.2 g/kg BM immediately after exercise. However, this has no influence on muscle protein metabolism. In contrast, consuming protein after exercise results in an exacerbated elevation in muscle protein synthesis at the same time as a minor suppression in muscle protein breakdown, resulting in a positive net protein balance. The ingestion of approximately 20 grams (0.25 g/kg BM) of high biological-value protein after resistance exercise appears to be sufficient to maximally stimulate muscle protein synthesis, with higher doses recommended following resistance-training sessions engaging the whole body and among elderly or injured athletes. So, eating both carbohydrate and protein immediately after resistance training results in more favourable recovery outcomes, including restoration of muscle glycogen stores and muscle protein metabolism, than consuming either nutrient alone. Eating protein after exercise also reduces the amount of carbohydrate required in the acute recovery period, with an energy-matched intake of 0.8 g/kg BM/hour carbohydrate plus 0.4 g/kg BM/hour protein resulting in similar muscle glycogen resynthesis over five hours compared to 1.2 g/kg BM/hour carbohydrate alone following intermittent exercise, with a similar response evident following resistance exercise. Preliminary evidence also suggests that consuming both carbohydrate and protein after exercise may reduce muscle damage often seen in strength-trained athletes; whether such a change has a functional benefit is unclear.

Supplementation practices

Supplement use is reported to be higher among athletes than their sedentary counterparts, with particularly high rates of supplement use among weightlifters and bodybuilders. The high prevalence of supplement use among bodybuilders, Olympic weightlifters, track and field athletes, and those who frequent commercial fitness centres is not unexpected, given the range of products targeted at this market. While multivitamin and mineral supplements are very popular among all athletes, other products such as protein powders and specific amino acid supplements, caffeine and creatine monohydrate are also frequently used by strength-trained athletes.

Recognising the nutritional value of food sources of protein and essential amino acids, creatine monohydrate appears to be the only supplement that has been reported to enhance skeletal muscle hypertrophy and functional capacity in response to resistance training. However, liquid meal supplements rich in carbohydrate and protein may be valuable in the post-exercise period to boost total energy and specific nutrient intake at a time when the appetite is often suppressed. There is also evidence that caffeine enhances muscular strength. While other dietary supplements such as individual amino acids and their metabolites have been advocated for use among bodybuilders, research supporting their ergogenic potential is limited, and thus cannot currently be recommended based on available preliminary literature.

Strength-trained athletes continue to seek supplement information from readily accessible sources, including websites, social media, magazines, fellow athletes and coaches.

The accuracy of such information may vary (see the Introduction for more details), leaving the athlete vulnerable to inappropriate and/or ineffective supplementation protocols and an increased risk of inadvertent doping. The presence of muscle dysmorphia, a body dysmorphic disorder characterised by a pre-occupation with a sense of inadequate muscularity common among bodybuilders, may also influence supplementation practices and lead to **anabolic steroid** use.

Anabolic steroids
Drugs which help the repair and build of muscle tissues, derived from the male hormone testosterone.

COMPETITION

Competition demands of strength sports are typically characterised by explosive single efforts where athletes are given a designated number of opportunities to produce a maximal performance, with significant recovery between each effort. This recovery time means that muscle energy reserves are unlikely to be challenged, even in the face of challenging environmental conditions of competitions like the summer Olympic Games. Consequently, nutrition priorities should focus on more general goals like optimising gastrointestinal tract comfort and preventing weight gain during the competition taper.

Olympic weightlifting, powerlifting and bodybuilding are unique among strength and power sports in that competition is undertaken via weight categories or, on occasion in bodybuilding, by height class. As such, these athletes are likely to engage in acute weight-loss practices common to other weight category sports including short-term restriction of food and fluids, resulting in a state of glycogen depletion and hypohydration. While performance is typically compromised in sports requiring a significant contribution from aerobic and/or anaerobic energy metabolism (Chapter 2), activities demanding high power output and absolute strength are less likely to be influenced by acute weight loss. Furthermore, the weigh-in is typically undertaken two hours prior to the commencement of weightlifting competition, affording athletes an opportunity to recover, at least partially, from any acute weight-loss strategies undertaken prior to the weigh-in. The body mass management guidelines for Olympic combat sport athletes (Reale et al. 2017) would also appear applicable for Olympic weightlifters.

Given the association between lower body-fat levels and competitive success, bodybuilders typically adjust their training and diet several months out from competition in an attempt to decrease body fat while maintaining or increasing muscle mass. While a compromise in muscle mass has been observed when attempting to achieve the extremely low body-fat levels desired for competition, this is not always the case. The performance implications of any skeletal muscle loss are unknown given the subjective nature of bodybuilding competition. Among female bodybuilders such dietary restrictions are often associated with compromised micronutrient intake and menstrual dysfunction, presumably because energy availability falls below the threshold of ~125 kJ/kg fat-free mass/day required to maintain normal endocrine (hormonal) regulation of the menstrual cycle (refer to Chapter 18 for more information).

If muscle protein breakdown is experienced by an Olympic weightlifter or power-lifter as they attempt to 'make weight' for competition, a compromise in force-generating capacity, and thus weightlifting performance, is at least theoretically possible. More details on weight category sports and weight-making can be found in Chapter 17.

PHYSIQUE

Within the lifting events, physique traits influence performance in several ways. While the expression of strength has a significant **neural** component, lifting performance is closely associated with skeletal muscle mass. Excluding the open weight category, weightlifters also tend to have low body-fat levels, enhancing development of strength per unit of body mass. Successful weightlifters also have a higher sitting height-to-stature ratio with shorter limbs, creating a biomechanical advantage. An association between physique traits and competitive success in the Olympic throwing events has been recognised for some time, with successful athletes heavier and taller than their counterparts and growing in size at a rate well in excess of general population trends. In contrast to other strength sports, bodybuilding is unique in that competitive success is judged purely on the basis of the size, symmetry and definition of musculature. Not surprisingly, bodybuilders are the most muscular of all the strength athletes. Successful bodybuilders have lower body fat, yet are taller and heavier with wider skeletal proportions, and are much broader across the shoulders than the hips.

Neural
Relating to a nerve or the nervous system.

While it is reasonable to presume that the nutritional focus of strength and power athletes remains on skeletal muscle hypertrophy throughout the year, in reality this is rarely the case, except perhaps during the 'off-season' for bodybuilders or specified times of the annual **macrocycle** of other strength and power athletes. Furthermore, significant changes in body mass among bodybuilders, Olympic weightlifters and powerlifters will likely influence the weight category they compete in and those they compete against. Thus, the intention to promote skeletal muscle hypertro-phy must be given serious consideration by athletes and their coaches before being implemented.

Macrocycle
Refers to the overall training period, usually representing a year.

SUMMARY AND KEY MESSAGES

After reading this chapter, you should have a broad understanding of the important role nutrition plays for athletes competing in sports where the expression of explosive power and strength are critical to competitive success. While total energy intake of strength and power athletes tends to be greater than endurance-focused athletes, intake relative to body mass is often unremarkable, with less known about distribution of nutrient intake over the day. Strength and power athletes will benefit from a greater focus on the strategic timing of nutrient intake before, during and after exercise to assist them in optimising resistance-training work capacity, recovery and body composition. Strength and power athletes create unique challenges for the nutrition service provider given their reliance on readily-accessible sources of information, susceptibility to sports supplement marketing, potentially distorted body image and challenges associated with achieving a specified weight category in some sports plus the general void of scientific investigation in recent years relating specifically to this unique group of athletes.

Key messages
- Strength and power athletes tend to consume more total energy, but less energy relative to their body mass, than endurance-focused athletes.
- Strategic timing of nutrient intake before, during and after exercise will help to optimise training work capacity, recovery and body composition.
- Strength and power athletes are recommended to consume daily carbohydrate intakes of 4–7 g/kg body mass, and daily protein intakes between 1.0 and 1.2 g/kg body mass in the form of 4–5 evenly spaced feedings of ~20 grams (0.25 g/kg body mass) high biological-value protein.
- Athletes should consume carbohydrate at a rate of 1 g/kg before and 0.5 g/kg during training, and focus their protein intake after training during maximal stimulation of muscle protein synthesis.
- Recovery should include consumption of 20 grams of protein (0.25 g/kg body mass) to stimulate muscle protein synthesis, and 0.8 g/kg BM/hour carbohydrate plus 0.4 g/kg BM/hour protein to promote glycogen repletion.
- Athletes' dietary practices may be influenced by inaccurate nutrition information, sports supplement marketing and distorted body image.

REFERENCES

Lambert, C.P. & Flynn, M.G., 2002, 'Fatigue during high-intensity intermittent exercise: Application to bodybuilding', *Sports Medicine*, vol. 32, no. 8, pp. 511–22.

Lambert, C.P., Flynn, M.G., Boone, J.B.J. et al., 1991, 'Effects of carbohydrate feeding on multiple-bout resistance exercise', *Journal of Strength and Conditioning Research*, vol. 5, no. 4, pp. 192–7.

MacDougall, J.D., Ray, S., Sale, D.G. et al., 1999, 'Muscle substrate utilization and lactate production during weightlifting', *Canadian Journal of Applied Physiology-Revue Canadienne De Physiologie Appliquee*, vol. 24, no. 3, pp. 209–15.

Manore, M.M., Barr, S.I. & Butterfield, G.E., 2000, 'Joint Position Statement: Nutrition and Athletic performance. American College of Sports Medicine, American Dietetic Association, and Dietitians of Canada', *Medicine & Science in Sports & Exercise*, vol. 32, no. 12, pp. 2130–45.

Morton, R.W., McGlory, C. & Phillips, S.M., 2015, 'Nutritional interventions to augment resistance training-induced skeletal muscle hypertrophy', *Frontiers in Physiology*, vol. 6, pp. 245.

Phillips, S.M. & Van Loon, L.J., 2011, 'Dietary protein for athletes: From requirements to optimum adaptation', *Journal of Sports Science*, vol. 29, suppl. 1, pp. S29–38.

Reale, R., Slater, G. & Burke, L.M., 2017, 'Individualised dietary strategies for Olympic combat sports: Acute weight loss, recovery and competition nutrition', *European Journal of Sport Science*, vol. 17, no. 6, pp. 727–40.

Slater, G. & Phillips, S.M., 2011, 'Nutrition guidelines for strength sports: Sprinting, weightlifting, throwing events, and bodybuilding', *Journal of Sports Science*, vol. 29, suppl. 1, pp. S67–7.

Tesch, P.A., Colliander, E.B. & Kaiser, P., 1986, 'Muscle metabolism during intense, heavy-resistance exercise', *European Journal of Applied Physiology & Occupational Physiology*, vol. 55, no. 4, pp. 362–6.

Thomas, D.T., Erdman, K.A. & Burke, L.M., 2016, 'Position of the Academy of Nutrition and Dietetics, Dietitians of Canada, and the American College of Sports Medicine: Nutrition and Athletic Performance', *Journal of the Academy of Nutrition & Dietetics*, vol. 116, no. 3, pp. 501–28.

Volek, J.S., Forsythe, C.E. & Kraemer, W.J., 2006, 'Nutritional aspects of women strength athletes', *British Journal of Sports Medicine*, vol. 40, no. 9, pp. 742–8.

CHAPTER 16

Team sport athletes

Stephen J. Keenan and Brooke Devlin

Team sports are popular at a variety of levels, ranging from amateur social competitions for health and fitness to Olympic, national and international elite competitions. The physical demands of team sports are multifaceted and, as such, a thorough understanding of the physiological demands, duration and intensity of each team sport is required in order to ensure appropriate nutrition strategies are in place. Furthermore, team sports present unique challenges with regards to nutrition. In the first section, this chapter will discuss why it is important to consider the differences between team sport athletes and individual athletes, and the importance of individualised nutrition advice in a team setting. The second section will focus on how the structure and characteristics of competition and the demands of travel influence and impact on nutrition strategies and practices. Finally, the chapter will conclude with discussion of food service provision for team sport athletes, why this is important and some of the issues nutrition professionals need to consider when catering to large groups.

LEARNING OUTCOMES

Upon completion of this chapter you will:
- have an understanding of the differences between team sport athletes and individual athletes and the importance of pack mentality in team sports

- understand the importance of individualised nutrition advice and why blanket style nutrition recommendations are not advised
- recognise the challenges nutrition professionals need to overcome when working with team sport athletes
- understand that each sport presents unique nutritional challenges related to the game and competition structure
- develop an understanding of food service provision and catering for team sport athletes.

WHAT IS DIFFERENT ABOUT TEAM SPORT ATHLETES?

Popular team sports for men and women in Australia, New Zealand and the Asia-Pacific region include basketball, netball, cricket, volleyball, rugby league, rugby union, hockey, soccer (football) and Australian football. These sports differ in their competitive seasons, game lengths, skill requirements and movement patterns performed during play. Additionally, the time of year each sport is played differs, with some being summer sports (such as cricket) and others winter sports (such as Australian football). All these factors need to be taken into consideration when preparing nutrition recommendations. Additionally, a thorough understanding of the physiological demands of the sport is required to ensure appropriate nutrition strategies are in place and fuel requirements are met.

As with individual athletes, the nutritional requirements of team sport athletes depend on the physiological demands, predominant energy systems, duration, frequency and intensity of the sport. Within a team sport, there are a number of different positions that athletes can play (such as offensive or defensive). The position an athlete plays also influences their nutritional requirements. For example, in a sport such as soccer, the nutrition requirements of the goal keeper will be very different to a position such as a mid-fielder due to differences in the distance, frequency and intensity of running movements.

Unlike many individual sports and events, in team sports athletes are often required to repeat regular short, high-intensity efforts interspersed with longer periods of rest and low- to moderate-intensity efforts, such as jogging and walking. Therefore, team sports are typically both anaerobic and aerobic (Chapter 2) in nature and, consequently, athletes are required to develop not only speed, agility, muscular strength and power but also endurance (Bradley et al. 2013). Furthermore, technical and tactical elements are incorporated into the games, with the specific skill required dependent on the game and position played.

While sports nutrition principles and practices will be similar between individual athletes and team sport athletes, there are additional factors and issues that are important to consider regarding nutrition practices of team sport athletes. These issues are discussed throughout this chapter.

Pack mentality

Depending on the sport, the number of athletes in a team can vary from five up to groups as large as 50. Regardless of the size of the team, group dynamics can have a major influence on nutrition practices of athletes.

Pack mentality

For team sport athletes, a pack mentality occurs when individual athletes within the team act in a similar manner to others in the group.

In team sport, it is common for there to be a '**pack mentality**' that influences athletes' behaviours, including their nutrition practices. In the case of nutritional intake, if there are some athletes within the team who follow suboptimal practices or have extreme dietary behaviour, this can influence the overall nutrition practices of the whole team.

While pack mentality may be seen to negatively influence nutritional intake in some cases, it is important to consider using the team environment and pack mentality to assist in improving the nutrition practices of the athletes and making positive changes to the nutritional intake of the team. As with any team environment, there will be natural tendencies for some individuals to be leaders and have stronger personalities. Working with leaders in a team environment who follow optimal nutrition practices is an effective strategy to influence the nutrition practices of athletes in a team and improve the culture. As an example, alcohol intake following a game is quite common due to the social nature of team sports. However, when a key team member limits their alcohol consumption, it can positively influence the overall alcohol intake of the team. To improve and influence nutritional intake of athletes in team sports it is vital to consider the team environment, culture and natural tendency for a pack mentality to occur.

Blanket approaches to nutrition advice

High-level competitive team sports have a large team of coaching and support staff, such as sports scientists, working with athletes. There are a range of factors that influence the performance of an athlete, and coaching and support staff work to improve these factors, including fitness, strength and game tactics. Despite its ability to influence performance, nutrition is not always a priority among coaching and support staff due to budget constraints and competing pressures.

In these high-pressure and simultaneously time- and resource-poor environments, it is common for blanket nutrition advice to be provided to a team of athletes. Blanket nutrition advice can be described as nutrition advice that is the same for all the athletes, regardless of their individual differences. Furthermore, the way in which this advice is delivered is also the same for all athletes. It groups all athletes together (under one blanket), and assumes the information and nutrition advice they need is the same. This is problematic, as it is well established that individual athletes within a team are unique and will respond differently to nutrition interventions and advice. For example, caffeine has been found to improve athletic performance (Burke 2008), but not all athletes respond to caffeine in the same way. The performance benefit of caffeine is substantial for some athletes, insignificant for others. Athletes will also vary in their tolerance of caffeine-containing beverages and supplements. Therefore, athletes require specific, individually tailored, **personalised nutrition advice** that takes into consideration a range of individual health, social and sport-specific factors.

Personalised nutrition advice
Specific and individualised advice for each athlete based on their own personal situation including playing position, body composition, culture, taste preferences and past experiences.

GROUP NUTRITION EDUCATION AND NUTRITION KNOWLEDGE

As outlined, it is important that athletes are provided individual nutrition advice as far as possible within the context of the team setting. However, it is common for team sport athletes to receive group nutrition education. Group nutrition education sessions are advantageous as a time- and cost-effective method to educate and influence nutritional practices. They can also assist in building a positive team environment and culture. However, education provided in a group setting often employs 'blanket' nutrition advice and does not cater for the differing needs of individual athletes. Athletes will also have different learning styles, and these should be taken into consideration when planning group nutrition education sessions.

Group nutrition education sessions are used to improve nutrition knowledge, and sometimes also food and cooking skills, with the aim of positively influencing nutrition practices. In team sports, group nutrition education sessions and cooking classes are commonly used to educate a number of athletes at one time. Evaluation of such sessions is important to identify their effectiveness in improving nutrition knowledge, food skills and dietary practices, to identify areas for improvement and to advocate for increased nutrition services.

FOOD AND FLUID PROVISION FOR TEAM SPORTS

The implementation of nutrition strategies in team sports is often subject to rules and regulations that restrict opportunities for intake of food and fluids. While sports such as basketball or Australian football include numerous breaks in play that allow delivery of food or fluids to players, opportunities in other codes, such as soccer (football), are much more limited. Often substitutions, treatment of injured players and half-time breaks are the only times players can access food and fluid, and to do this they may need to dash to the sidelines. This can pose challenges when trying to replace large fluid losses or provide large quantities of carbohydrate; providing these in large **boluses** at half-time breaks may lead to gastro-intestinal disturbance. Studies that have informed fluid and carbohydrate intake guidelines have often used protocols that involve providing small amounts periodically, which is impractical in team sports. Therefore, nutrition support needs to be customised to both the sport and the individual.

Bolus
A portion, with respect to food, that is swallowed at one time.

Competition structure and access to food/fluid during the game

The structure of competition varies between sports and can create difficulties when trying to optimise fluid and food ingestion. Depending on the intensity and duration of the event, and the environment in which it is played, a greater emphasis may need to be placed on ensuring athletes take every opportunity to rehydrate or ingest carbo-hydrates. Cricket, for example, may be played in extreme heat, with some formats of the game lasting 6–7 hours per day for five days. Although originally developed in temperate English weather, it is now also played in the harsh Australian summer, the severe heat of Dubai and the extreme humidity in India, with temperatures occasion-ally reaching over 40°C. While those in the outfield may have access to drinks on the boundary line, batsmen—who are generally also wearing heavy pads, gloves and a helmet—may have much more limited access to fluids, with drinks breaks generally scheduled only once per hour (though they break for meals over the course of the day). In Australia, soccer is also played in the summer, with drinks generally only available at the break between 45-minute halves or if there is an extended stoppage in play. In circumstances such as these, it is important to think strategically about providing athletes with optimal nourishment. In cricket, for example, if there is a break in play for injury, to change the ball or if the batsman calls for a new bat or gloves, a drinks runner should be sent out to the players at the same time if possible. In soccer, placing drink bottles around the ground, allowing players to access fluids quickly during stop-pages or substitutions, will allow them to maintain a better hydration status. For events lasting 90 minutes or more, it is important to provide fluids such as sports drinks that contain carbohydrate and electrolytes, with added flavours to promote greater intake (see Chapter 11 for more information on hydration).

Although it is important to ensure that opportunities are created for athletes to ingest food and fluid during play where possible, the importance of designated breaks should not be ignored. Sports drinks, along with any food or supplements such as fruit, gels or lollies, should be presented in a way that allows easy access for the athletes. Often the athletes will have treatment or presentations from the coaching staff during their designated breaks, and eating and drinking may slip their mind. Setting up their food and drinks on a table just inside the door to the change rooms may help ensure they grab something on the way in and way out, reducing the risk of missing an opportunity to refuel. For those who have more individualised refuelling strategies, placing the appropriate amount of food and drink in, or in front of, their locker may allow them to adhere to this more easily. While structured breaks such as half-time allow greater opportunity for food and fluid intake, it should also be stressed that trying to achieve recommended intakes needs to be balanced with gastrointestinal comfort, and force-feeding athletes may actually lead to poorer performance.

Catering for the team

Catering for athletes in the team environment may occur on many different levels, from individual to team-wide provision of food, both of which provide unique challenges. Training and competition schedules, personal preferences and body composition goals can all influence the type and amount of food provided. Addressing all of these concerns at once can be difficult, and while ideally clubs could utilise in-house catering staff to accommodate each player's different requirements (as is the case in some larger organisations around the world), smaller clubs may need to bring in outside catering to ensure adherence to budget.

On-site, team-wide catering offers a cost-efficient method of providing nutritious food to athletes. This can be particularly important when the training schedule runs over normal meal times. It is not uncommon for players to complete two training sessions each day, especially over the pre-season period, and this may involve long days with limited opportunities to seek food.

Providing a meal can help ensure that players refuel to train and compete at the intensity required; however, it is not as simple as providing sufficient carbohydrate, protein and fat. In one team, not only are there differing taste preferences, there are also different nutrition priorities. The first player in the lunch line may be trying to add muscle mass, while the second is looking to reduce body fat, the third is recovering from injury and the fourth has just managed to get his body composition where it needs to be, and is trying to maintain that. On top of this, each player is a different size and may have a different training load. How do you then cater for each player with one generic meal? To allow each individual to customise their meal, education and presentation of food is critical; these are discussed below.

Education

As discussed earlier, while group education may be cost-effective, individual nutrition knowledge is important to help athletes make appropriate food choices, especially when faced with buffet-style catering. Each player should be aware of their own goals, and how nutrition contributes to them, to enable them to make appropriate food choices. Putting up posters or noticeboards in the food-provision area may help create an environment that reinforces this education. Having the team dietitian and/or other nutrition support staff present occasionally during food service will allow the players to confirm their food choices.

Presentation

Presentation of the food is critical to allow players to customise their own meals. Mixed-meal dishes such as stir-fries and casseroles may not be ideal, as players may have differing protein, carbohydrate and fat requirements. Separating the protein, carbohydrate and, potentially, the fat (although most meals provided are likely to have low to moderate fat content), allows the athlete to pick and choose ingredients and portion sizes to suit their needs. For example, instead of a stew, it may be more appropriate to offer roast meat, separate starchy and non-starchy vegetables and a jug of gravy or sauce. Some options, such as burgers, may not need separation, as the athlete can pull them apart to consume what they require. Options such as pasta may not allow easy separation of components but are often very popular among teams, especially in the lead-up to competition. In such circumstances, it may be worthwhile offering multiple options, so that players with lower loads who may be periodising carbohydrate intake (see Chapter 9) are still able to achieve this.

Catering for the individual within the team

Ideally, players will gain the skills necessary to prepare appropriate food matching their nutrition goals. Occasionally, however, due to lack of time, motivation or available facilities, this will not occur. In this case, it may be worthwhile exploring catering options for the individual. There are many food service companies that provide meals appropriate for the athlete, and are often able to customise meal plans.

Post-game meals

Post-game meals pose some unique challenges. Not only are there many athletes who subscribe to the idea that they can 'eat whatever they want' post-game due to their workloads (potentially undoing a great deal of good work if they are trying to improve their body composition), some will have large appetites while others will have none at all. Providing foods that meet their nutritional needs for recovery in several different forms can help work around these issues, as long as the athlete is well-educated on what they should be putting into their bodies. Liquids such as flavoured milks, providing around 20 grams of protein and 60 grams of carbohydrate per 600 millilitres, are a popular post-match recovery option for those with smaller appetites, while fruit, sandwiches, wraps, protein shakes or bars, muesli bars and hot meals such as pasta and rice dishes all provide nutritious recovery options. While all of these can be great choices, logistics often precludes offering all of them at once, meaning there are always likely to be some athletes who miss out on their preferred option. A good compromise can be organising a smaller range of more portable foods (such as milks, fruit, sandwiches, shakes and bars) in the change rooms post-match with a subsequent meal at a nearby restaurant, depending on the timing of the match.

TRAVEL

Teams that travel for competition or training need to consider a number of factors relating to nutrition. These vary depending on whether the travel is domestic or international in nature, with domestic travel posing fewer challenges than international travel. When travelling anywhere via air, consideration should be given to food and fluid provision; this is discussed in Chapter 21.

When travelling to a country where the types of foods consumed are significantly different from those in the athletes' home country, efforts should be made to educate players on appropriate food choices. Topics to cover may include avoiding food from areas that have a high risk of food contamination, such as street stalls, and ensuring athletes drink bottled water in areas that do not have safe tap water. Where possible, it is ideal to contact the accommodation or restaurants in which the team will be eating before they travel. Organising a menu of suitable, familiar foods will help reduce the risk of gastrointestinal issues, or players not eating. Again, having a stockpile of suitable snacks for players will also help them achieve their nutritional goals.

SUMMARY AND KEY MESSAGES

Although 'pack mentality' is common among teams of athletes, it needs to be recognised that each individual athlete is likely to have different goals, taste preferences, learning styles and motivations. Each of these needs to be taken into consideration, along with the intricacies of each sport, including training schedules and competition structures when providing food for teams or advising athletes on what to consume. Education is key to empowering individual athletes to make appropriate food choices, and while a blanket approach to nutritional advice may seem tempting, a customised approach is likely to be much more effective. Once each individual is sufficiently educated, it is important to ensure that their food environment is conducive to making good choices. Pre-planning by the nutrition and catering staff will help make the good choice the easy choice.

Key messages

- The different game factors (game length, skill requirements, position played, movement, game breaks and season played) must all be considered when formulating nutrition advice for individuals in team sports.
- 'Pack mentality' can be used in a positive way to influence nutrition intake of team sport athletes.
- Ideally, blanket nutrition recommendations need to be avoided and individualised nutrition advice provided in a team sport setting.
- Providing appropriate food and fluid during competition can be complicated by game structure.
- Thinking strategically will ensure athletes have a maximum number of opportunities to refuel.
- Team-wide catering is a valuable tool, but individuals need to be properly educated to make the right choices.
- When travelling, differences in culture and hygiene standards need to be considered.

REFERENCES AND FURTHER READING

Bishop, D. & Girard, O., 2013, 'Determinants of team-sport performance: Implications for altitude training by team-sport athletes', *British Journal of Sports Medicine*, vol. 47, suppl. 1, pp. S17–21.

Bradley, P.S., Carling, C., Diaz, A.G. et al., 2013, 'Match performance and physical capacity of players in the top three competitive standards of English professional soccer', *Human Movement Science*, vol. 32, no. 4, pp. 808–21.

Burke, L.M., 2008, 'Caffeine and sports performance', *Applied Physiology, Nutrition, and Metabolism*, vol. 33, no. 6, pp. 1319–34.

Cortese, R.D.M., Veiros, M.B., Feldman, C. et al., 2016, 'Food safety and hygiene practices of vendors during the chain of street food production in Florianopolis, Brazil: A cross-sectional study', *Food Control*, vol. 62, pp. 178–86.

Liu, Z., Zhang, G. & Zhang, X., 2014, 'Urban street foods in Shijiazhuang city, China: Current status, safety practices and risk mitigating strategies', *Food Control*, vol. 41, pp. 212–18.

Reilly, T., Waterhouse, J., Burke, L.M. et al., 2009, 'Nutrition for travel', *Journal of Sports Sciences*, vol. 25, suppl. 1, pp. S125–34.

Weight category and aesthetic sport athletes

Regina Belski

Weight category and aesthetic sport athletes have some additional nutrition considerations that are not strictly linked to performance. For weight category sports, which include sports like boxing and lightweight rowing, athletes are required to be under a certain weight. If an athlete is over the cut-off during the weigh-in, they cannot compete. This can lead to suboptimal practices to 'make weight', including severe fluid and food restriction, use of laxatives and diuretics, and extreme use of saunas. Timing of weigh-ins also varies from sport to sport and even among competitions, with some being immediately before an event and others several days beforehand, so it is vital to understand the rules and processes of the sport and competition in which the athlete is competing.

For aesthetic sports, which include sports like gymnastics, ballet and diving, there is a strong focus on appearance as part of the way performance is assessed. Problems relating to nutrition can result, as this focus on aesthetics can lead to problems with body image and suboptimal dietary practices to try to control body size or shape.

This chapter discusses the common challenges faced when working with weight category and aesthetic sport athletes and provides some practical strategies on how best to support these athlete groups.

LEARNING OUTCOMES

Upon completion of this chapter you will:

* understand the additional challenges faced by athletes competing in weight category sports
* understand the additional challenges faced by athletes competing in aesthetic sports
* be able to propose two different approaches to managing weight-making behaviours of athletes.

WEIGHT CATEGORY SPORTS

Weight category sports are those sports where athletes are required to compete in weight categories or classes—for example, boxing, lightweight rowing and judo—and sports such as horseracing, where jockeys are weighed prior to every race.

Weight categories were introduced to these sports as it is widely believed that additional weight, and accompanying increases in strength if that weight is derived from muscle mass, puts athletes at a competitive advantage. To create a fair competition, a maximum weight limit is set. Some examples of weight categories used in Australia and New Zealand can be seen in Table 17.1.

For example, a lightweight rower in great health and achieving personal bests may still have a problem if they weigh in 500 grams over their cut-off, as this means that—regardless of how talented and prepared they are—they cannot compete.

For professional jockeys there is even more pressure, with failure to meet the weight cut-off for a given race potentially leading to fines and suspensions as well as loss of income. While riding weights in Australia range from the set minimum of 53 kilograms (which includes the saddle and riding equipment, but not the whip and cap) up to approximately 61 kilograms, most jockeys strive to be the minimum weight as this increases the number of races they are suitable for/able to race in (based on horse handicapping). For this reason, it is not unusual for **weight-making** behaviours to occur in these sports.

Weight-making
Any behaviour used to quickly lose weight regardless of what that 'weight' is (water, fat, muscle) before a competition weigh-in.

COMMON WEIGHT-MAKING PRACTICES

While making weight may not always lead to problems, extreme weight-making behaviours are problematic. Such weight-making practices include extensive use of saunas to dehydrate the body, use of diuretics, excessive exercise, running dressed in heavy, non-breathable clothing to promote sweating, not eating or drinking, and the use and abuse of diet pills, purging and other such practices (Crighton et al. 2015). Unfortunately, these more extreme weight-making behaviours have both short-term and long-term health effects and have contributed to the death of athletes in some cases.

Table 17.1. Weight categories for selected sports (Australia and New Zealand)

Sport	Sex	Weight
Lightweight rowing	Men	≤72.5 kg (team average weight ≤70 kg)
	Women	≤59 kg (team average weight ≤ 57 kg)
Judo	Men	>100 kg >90 kg and up to and including 100 kg >81 kg and up to and including 90 kg >73 kg and up to and including 81 kg >66 kg and up to and including 73 kg >60 kg and up to and including 66 kg ≤60 kg Open, with no weight restriction.
	Women	>78 kg >70 kg and up to and including 78 kg >63 kg and up to and including 70 kg >57 kg and up to and including 63 kg >52 kg and up to and including 57 kg >48 kg and up to and including 52 kg ≤48 kg Open, with no weight restriction.
Boxing (amateur, youth and elite divisions)	Men	>91 kg >81 kg and up to and including 91 kg >75 kg and up to and including 81 kg >69 kg and up to and including 75 kg >64 kg and up to and including 69 kg >60 kg and up to and including 64 kg >56 kg and up to and including 60 kg >52 kg and up to and including 56 kg >49 kg and up to and including 52 kg >46 kg and up to and including 49 kg
	Women	>81 kg >75 kg and up to and including 81 kg >69 kg and up to and including 75 kg >64 kg and up to and including 69 kg >60 kg and up to and including 64 kg >57 kg and up to and including 60 kg >54 kg and up to and including 57 kg >51 kg and up to and including 54 kg >48 kg and up to and including 51 kg >45 kg and up to and including 48 kg

Source: International Rowing Federation <http://www.worldrowing.com/>; International Judo Federation <https://www.ijf.org/>; The International Boxing Association <https://www.aiba.org/>.

It is not unusual to see athletes trying to lose two–five kilograms in the days leading up to competition. It is not surprising to see athletes resort to extreme measures, such as cutting/shaving their hair, trimming fingernails and even inducing vomiting or nosebleeds in situations where they are a few grams over the cut-off at weigh-ins.

The potential negative health effects of extreme weight-making include:

- dehydration leading to significant plasma volume loss and increasing risk of heat illness
- drop in metabolic rate with repeated weight-making practices utilising fasting as a result of muscle loss
- impaired cognitive functioning, including increased fatigue, confusion and mood changes
- lean tissue loss
- impaired bone synthesis during periods of severe energy restriction, which may make athletes more susceptible to injury and have a long-term impact on bone health.

MANAGING WEIGHT-MAKING

When working with athletes in weight category sports, there are two main avenues that can be taken to address weight-making: (1) support the athlete to achieve a 'regular' weight that fits their weight category, thereby removing the need to make weight; or, if this is not possible, (2) support the athlete to 'make weight' in a safe way.

While the first option is obviously desirable from a health perspective, it is not realistic for most athletes, as many prefer to compete at a weight that is far from ideal for their actual body type and shape. Considering that athletes in most weight category sports require significant lean body mass, which increases their overall weight, there arises a conflict between building muscle and being able to compete. It is unfortunately common for coaches to encourage athletes to compete in a lighter weight division than that to which they are naturally best suited, as they are seen as having an advantage over naturally smaller/lighter athletes. While this may be true from a physical strength perspective, an athlete who is severely dehydrated and has not properly eaten is not in a position to perform at their best.

Weigh-in times in different sports, and even between different levels of competition, vary. Some sports/competitions have athletes weigh in the day before competition, allowing refuelling and rehydration if required, but others have weigh-ins immediately before competition or even, in some cases, before every bout/match, making rehydration challenging for those who have utilised dehydration techniques to make weight. As discussed in Chapter 11 (Hydration) this has a significant impact on performance.

Let's take a closer look at each of the approaches athletes may choose to take.

Regular weight = competition weight approach

This is considered the more sensible and healthy approach, as it eliminates the need to 'make weight' and undertake risky diet and/or dehydration behaviours. The approach involves selection of the most appropriate weight category (within five per cent of natural weight if possible) for an athlete based on the weight they are able to attain and maintain while eating appropriately, training well and performing at a high level. This will involve losing weight for some athletes and gaining weight for others. While this may sound easy and obvious, it is an approach athletes and coaches are often not comfortable with, mostly because once athletes find a place in their 'category' the notion of moving into another category is almost as daunting as changing sports, with changes in the competition and the competitors. It may also be challenging for athletes who do not actually know what their 'normal' non-dieting weight is; this is particularly true for younger athletes who started in a weight category in their late teens and remained in the same category into their twenties despite significant growth in height. These cases can require time to identify the best option—and time is not something that is always easy to find for competitive athletes. Where possible, nutrition professionals can encourage athletes to use the off-season to find a more 'natural' weight. Anthropometric assessment (see Chapter 13 for more details) by a trained professional should be used to help athletes assess the most appropriate weight category in which they should compete.

Where an athlete naturally sits just above a weight class it may not be clear which weight category is best. One option is to encourage the athlete to work on gaining additional muscle mass to gain further strength and get their weight up, closer to the top of the weight category, or alternatively support them to make weight for the lower category in a safe and healthy way in the lead-up to competition.

Safer weight-making practices

From a health perspective it would be best if athletes did not have to make weight at all; however, this is unfortunately unlikely to be the case where sports remain categorised by weight class. Therefore, it is important to help athletes to make weight in the safest way possible, without compromising short- or long-term health.

This means that athletes need to be encouraged to allow enough time before competition to lose the extra weight. They should avoid dehydration practices or, if they must use them, have adequate time to rehydrate before competition. It should be made clear to athletes that any weight-making strategies are short-term measures—for example, if significant energy or fluid restriction is taking place, that it is only for a clearly defined period of time, after which a healthy way of eating and drinking returns. It is easy for athletes to fall into a very restrictive way of eating or disordered eating involving bingeing, purging or utilising laxatives and/or diuretics as part of their usual routine, compromising their wellbeing and performance. Appropriate strategies for managing weight in weight category athletes are outlined in Box 17.1.

It is important that athletes have an opportunity to consider their options and discuss them with their support team when making a decision about the best approach for them. Advice needs to be aligned with the rules of the sport, timing of weigh-ins and the physiological needs of the athlete. It is strongly recommended that any athlete participating in a weight category sport should seek the advice of a qualified sports dietitian to individualise their weight management plan.

Box 17.1: Examples of advice for weight category athletes

Well ahead of competition:
- Develop a long-term plan for weight on- and off-season.
- If necessary, consume an appropriate energy restricted diet aiming for a maximum of 500 grams of weight loss per week (see Chapter 13 for more details on changing body composition).

Shortly before competition/weigh-in:
- Avoid high-salt foods that may lead to water retention (for example, processed foods such as deli meat, canned soups/foods, frozen meals, potato chips, soy sauce, pickles, fast food).
- Aim for a low-residue, low-fibre diet (for example, consume white bread instead of wholegrain, peel fruit and vegetables before cooking/eating, avoid food made with seeds and nuts).
- Consume appropriate amounts of fluid, making sure that fluid loss does not exceed two per cent loss of body weight and is replaced before competition.

Refuelling strategies (if fluid and/or energy restriction was used to make weight):
- Where possible, allow enough time to rehydrate (2–4 days).
- Consume 150 per cent of the fluid loss (for instance, drink 1.5 litres of fluid for each kilogram of weight lost).
- Utilise drinks containing electrolytes and carbohydrate to maximise hydration (see Chapter 11 for more details on optimising rehydration).
- Consume carbohydrates to maximise glycogen stores.

AESTHETIC SPORTS

Aesthetic sports are those sports where there is a strong focus on appearance as part of the way performance is assessed. These include dance, gymnastics, aerobics, figure skating, cheerleading, ballet and diving. In many of these aesthetic sports, how an athlete looks while performing will be a component of how their performance is evaluated. Execution of particular technical movements is important, but so is the grace and beauty of that movement. This is where problems relating to nutrition can arise, as this focus on aesthetics can lead to problems with body image and suboptimal dietary practices to try to control body size or shape. Most commonly this manifests as **disordered eating** and energy restriction (de Bruin et al. 2007). Another factor that is not particularly helpful is that athletes often get involved in these sports at a young age, and their bodies continue to grow, develop and change shape as they age. However, for many athletes these changes can be seen as undesirable; for example, the development of larger breasts and wider hips is not considered desirable for a ballerina. These pressures make teenage girls in aesthetic sports particularly vulnerable to restrictive or disordered eating. More details of disordered eating and the challenges of working with young athletes can be found in Chapter 18.

Disordered eating
A variety of abnormal eating behaviours that, by themselves, do not warrant diagnosis of an eating disorder but are usually not optimal for health and performance.

Nutrition recommendations for athletes in aesthetic sports need to be particularly mindful of how dietary changes could impact on the physical appearance of the individual athlete. While muscle gain is desirable in many sports, for aesthetic athletes a muscle distribution that is considered to be less physically attractive can lead to lower competition scores.

It is important to acknowledge the stereotypical body shapes and physiques found in many aesthetic sports, but also to remind athletes that they are individuals and not everyone is exactly the same. Where possible, it is wise to have some examples of high-performing athletes in their sport with different body shapes from the standard. In gymnastics, a very good example is the difference in physique between two top 2008 Beijing Olympic gymnasts, Nastia Liukin and Shawn Johnson (both from the USA team). These two gymnasts have vastly different body shapes; they won both gold and silver medals in the same events, demonstrating that different body shapes can still lead to great outcomes. Simple visual examples can have a significant effect on young, impressionable athletes, and help to encourage even aesthetic sport athletes to focus on optimising their performance more than worrying about the exact size and shape of their bodies. In situations where body-image concerns are present, it is wise to consider the involvement of a sports psychologist to support the athlete.

SUMMARY AND KEY MESSAGES

After reading this chapter, you should understand that athletes who compete in weight category sports are under extreme pressures to achieve a specific weight to avoid exclusion from competition. Weight-making is a common practice among athletes in weight category sports and can lead to both short- and long-term negative health outcomes; therefore, athletes need professional guidance and support to either attain and compete at a weight that is easily sustainable for the athlete or to support them to make weight in a safer manner.

Aesthetic sport athletes are under an additional spotlight in relation to their physical appearance, as how they look when performing is a component of how their performance is evaluated. These athletes are more likely to develop concerns regarding their body image and should be supported to adopt healthy eating practices in line with personalised goals.

Key messages

- Athletes in weight category sports are prone to undertake risky weight-making behaviours.
- Weight category sport athletes should be supported to minimise the need to make weight, or do so in a safer manner.
- Aesthetic sport athletes are at higher risk of disordered body image and, hence, disordered eating.
- Aesthetic sport athletes should be supported to focus on their personal goals and performance, rather than on body size or shape.

REFERENCES

Crighton, B., Close, G.L. & Morton, J.P., 2016, 'Alarming weight cutting behaviours in mixed martial arts: A cause for concern and a call for action', *British Journal of Sports Medicine*, vol. 50, no. 8, pp. 446–7, doi: 10.1136/bjsports-2015-094732.

de Bruin, A.K., Oudejans, R.R. & Bakker, F.C., 2007, 'Dieting and body image in aesthetic sports: A comparison of Dutch female gymnasts and non-aesthetic sport participants', *Psychology of Sport and Exercise*, vol. 8, no. 4, pp. 507–20.

CHAPTER

18

Young athletes

Helen O'Connor and Bronwen Lundy

Engagement in physical activity has a range of important physical, social and mental health benefits for young people. Sports participation can be at a range of levels, from active recreational engagement through to elite, internationally representative competition. Young prepubertal athletes can often be engaged in more than one sport, even at a relatively high level. However, as they progress into adolescence and reach national or internationally representative levels, sports participation becomes increasingly specialised, typically focusing on only one sport.

Nutrition is important for young athletes, to support overall growth and development as well as optimal sports performance. Engagement in sport has the potential to motivate improved dietary practices to support performance improvement. In developed countries, and increasingly in developing countries, young athletes experience an obesogenic environment and the literature suggests that athletes—even those at elite or professional levels—consume diets that are not consistent with public health or sports nutrition guidelines (although there is evidence that the dietary intakes of young athletes are superior to their non-athletic counterparts). Typical (Croll et al. 2006) food habits in childhood and adolescence—which include a preference for fast foods, inadequate vegetable intake and high intakes of nutrient-poor discretionary foods and sugar-sweetened beverages—are also reported in young athletes (Parnell et al. 2016).

There is a need for nutrition education which includes skills in shopping and cooking throughout these developmental years. As young athletes may spend much of their spare time training, they often have less time to participate in or observe food preparation skills in the home.

Young athletes have special nutrition needs. They can also be at an increased risk of inadequate or inappropriate dietary intake or supplement use. These risks may result from the additional demands of serious training on their capacity to consume a diet that has sufficient energy and macro- and micronutrients. Additionally, pressure to attain a specific weight or body composition can encourage restrictive eating practices or use of inappropriate dietary supplements or ergogenic aids, contributing to this risk. Clearly, childhood and adolescence is an important life stage for growth and development, as well as an opportunity to establish healthy eating habits, a positive relationship with food and a robust body image.

LEARNING OUTCOMES

Upon completion of this chapter you will be able to:
- identify special nutritional requirements and considerations for young athletes
- understand the challenges of ensuring young athletes consume sufficient energy and nutrients to sustain growth as well as optimise training adaptations and sports performance
- outline the risks associated with energy restriction, including relative energy deficiency in sport (RED-S), and the associated negative physical, mental health and body-image consequences
- understand differences in thermoregulation between young and adult athletes and how this may impact hydration strategies and the risk of exertional heat illness
- understand how dietary supplements are attractive to young athletes but also the potential risks associated with their use at the early phase of their development and sports career.

THE ROLE OF NUTRITION IN SUPPORTING GROWTH AND DEVELOPMENT OF YOUNG ATHLETES

During childhood, growth and development is relatively steady and occurs at a similar rate in boys and girls. The physical strength and exercise capacity of prepubertal boys and girls is generally similar at this age stage and, although they often compete separately, many recreational sports permit girls and boys to compete together. During puberty, the rate of growth increases until peak height velocity is reached. This more rapid rate of growth is often referred to as the pubertal growth spurt, although it is important to recognise that the onset and growth rate during this 'spurt' varies widely.

Girls generally commence their growth spurt and reach peak height velocity two years earlier (~12 years) than boys.

High-level engagement in sport can sometimes make it more difficult for young athletes to consume sufficient energy to meet the demands of training, especially during the pubertal growth spurt when there are additional energy demands for growth. Inadequate energy intake can result in delayed growth and, sometimes, increased fatigue, poor recovery and a range of more serious consequences if this is chronic. Although increased physical activity usually increases appetite to a level that helps the young athlete match their energy needs, young athletes will still need specific guidance to help plan their dietary intake around training demands. This can also sometimes be the case when there is a relatively rapid increase in the duration or intensity of training, which can occur when a young athlete is identified for a talented athlete program or if they move up to a new training level.

There are a number of practical factors that can also make it more difficult for young athletes to consume sufficient energy. The demands of busy training schedules, either before or after school, can reduce the time available for food preparation and consumption. Some young athletes avoid food and/or fluid close to, or even during, training sessions due to issues with gastrointestinal discomfort or the fear of experiencing a 'stitch'. These issues are more common in sports that involve running, jumping or tumbling, as opposed to swimming and cycling where the torso experiences less impact. Young athletes usually need to consume additional food and fluids during school hours to meet their higher energy demands; preparing and carrying the additional food, or purchasing or accessing this at school, presents another challenge. Higher intakes can sometimes also result in comments from other, less active peers about the volume of food consumed, which can make some young athletes feel self-conscious. Fussy eating is a further factor challenging the attainment of sufficient energy intake, and addressing this merely by increasing the volume of a limited range of foods can make the diet extremely monotonous and unappetising. Younger athletes need support and encouragement to widen the range of foods consumed, which is valuable for positive longer-term health and performance outcomes.

SPECIAL NUTRIENT REQUIREMENTS OF YOUNG ATHLETES

Protein

Children and adolescents need additional protein (compared to adults) to support growth (for example, the Australian recommended dietary intake for protein is 0.75 and 0.84 g/kg BM/day for adult women and men respectively, versus 0.77–0.91 and 0.91–0.99 g/kg BM/day for girls and boys respectively [NHMRC 2006]).

Adult athletes need additional protein to assist in the growth and/or maintenance of lean body mass. Although few studies have been performed with young athletes, there is some evidence for an increased protein requirement (1.35–1.6 g/kg BM/ day), especially in adolescents with high musculature or undergoing heavy training (Aerenhouts et al. 2011). As young athletes in developed countries typically consume around 1.2–1.6 g/kg BM/day of protein, it is anticipated that almost all would obtain sufficient protein from food and not require supplemental protein (Desbrow & Leveritt 2015).

Adequate energy intake is critical to the maintenance of positive nitrogen balance in athletes. In practice, inadequate energy is more often a factor limiting muscle gain than inadequate protein; however, younger athletes on restrictive diets may be at risk of both inadequate energy and protein intake. Although the research on protein requirements in athletes focuses on adult athletes, it seems likely that younger athletes would benefit from strategies used by adults to optimise development and maintenance of muscle, including distribution of protein over the day and protein intake around the time of training (see Chapter 9).

Carbohydrate

As with protein requirements, there is limited research on how the carbohydrate requirements of young athletes differ from those of adults. Early muscle biopsy studies found that young athletes have greater oxidative enzyme concentration and aerobic capacity, and less adaptation to anaerobic enzyme capacity (Erickson & Saltin 1974). They have been reported to rely more on oxidative (aerobic) metabolism during exercise (Taylor et al. 1997). Other studies have shown no difference in adaptation compared to adults (Haralambie 1982). Taken together, there is little evidence to support major differences in carbohydrate adaptation or fuel utilisation between younger and adult athletes.

Athletes should focus on planning carbohydrate intake around exercise duration and intensity (see Chapter 9 for recommended intake ranges). Young athletes typically have lower training volumes than adults, although this depends on both the sport and the individual athlete. It is usually the case for endurance and team sports, where training loads are built gradually until training loads are similar to those of adults in late adolescence. For this reason, carbohydrate loading is not necessary for young athletes until they undertake longer-duration endurance events in late adolescence.

Micronutrients at risk in young athletes

Young athletes commonly have low levels of calcium and iron (Desbrow & Leveritt 2015), especially female athletes after menarche when menstrual loss increases iron requirements. Iron loss may also be greater in athletes participating in endurance sports (see Chapter 14). Iron intake is usually lower in athletes restricting energy intake and sometimes in those who are vegetarian or eat less animal protein (see Chapter 5).

Calcium is another key nutrient, given the increased requirement during childhood and adolescence to support bone development. Inadequate calcium intake is often reported during childhood and adolescence in the general population and is also commonly reported in studies of young athletes. The risk of inadequate intake is increased in those who avoid or restrict dairy products.

Vitamin D is another nutrient which may be lower in athletes who train longer hours indoors or in latitudes where there is less sunlight and foods are not fortified with vitamin D. Sunscreen use, while important to prevent sun damage, does limit synthesis of vitamin D from the skin, so sun exposure without burning, where possible, is a valuable strategy to support adequate vitamin D levels. Athletes with darker skin and those who wear full-length clothing will produce less vitamin D from sun exposure and may be more reliant on obtaining vitamin D from dietary sources.

It is important to recognise that use of supplements to treat an existing nutrient deficiency may be warranted. This should be undertaken after a medical diagnosis and in conjunction with professional support from a sports dietitian to assist the athlete to improve dietary intake and prevent future deficiency through a balanced intake of whole foods.

THERMOREGULATION AND HYDRATION IN YOUNG ATHLETES

We used to believe that children were less able to regulate their body temperature than adults, but we now know that this is not the case. Children's greater surface area-to-mass ratio is actually an advantage for heat loss in most circumstances, except when environmental temperature is greater than skin temperature (>3°C) (Rowland 2008). In practice, younger athletes do not usually train or compete at the same work rates as adults; rather, they exercise at loads commensurate with their age and body size, which protects them from excessive heat storage (Rowland 2008). Children also have higher skin blood flow during exercise, and this promotes increased convective heat loss. Children do sweat less than adults but this actually helps to reduce the risk of hypohydration. Relative to their body mass, prepubertal athletes have been shown to have better evaporative cooling than young adults. The smaller, more diffuse sweat drops produced in prepubertal children promote better evaporation than larger sweat drops in adults, which tend to join together and drip rather than evaporate from the body. The lower body mass in children essentially means they need to produce less sweat than adults to maintain heat balance for the same change in core temperature (Rowland 2008).

In 2011, the American Academy of Pediatrics released a policy statement (American Academy of Pediatrics et al. 2011) concluding that young athletes do not have less effective thermoregulatory ability, insufficient cardiovascular capacity or lower physical exertion tolerance compared with adults during exercise in the heat, as long as adequate hydration is maintained. Aside from inadequate hydration, the primary determinants of reduced performance and exertional heat-illness risk in youth during sports in hot environments include undue physical exertion, insufficient recovery between repeated bouts of exercise and closely scheduled same-day training sessions or competition rounds. Inappropriate clothing, uniforms and protective equipment also plays a role in excessive heat retention. In practice, serious heat illness in young athletes is infrequently reported in the medical literature, suggesting that such events are rare (Rowland 2008). In practice, many of the strategies for hydration and competition refuelling used for adults are appropriate to young athletes. Although the volumes of fluid required are less for young athletes, they should still aim to reduce net fluid loss to <2 per cent of body weight (see also Chapter 11).

RISKS AND CHALLENGES ASSOCIATED WITH OPTIMISING PHYSIQUE ATTRIBUTES IN YOUNG ATHLETES

Physique is an important attribute for success in many sports. Characteristics such as larger stature and arm span are important for shooting and reach in sports such as basketball, swimming and tennis, while in gymnastics, diving and figure skating a shorter, compact frame facilitates the ease of aerial rotation. Other physique characteristics important to many sports include increased muscularity and lower levels of body fat. Although these can be modified by diet and training, they are also under genetic control and so there are limits to the capacity for change. Natural physique attributes are often early influencers of sport selection. Boys who are muscular and tall for their age may be attracted to sports such as rugby union rather than gymnastics.

The timing of the onset of puberty may also influence sport success. In contact football sports such as rugby, there is concern that early pubertal development provides an unfair advantage for talent identification over athletes of the same age who are relatively prepubertal but similarly or more talented than their earlier-developing counterparts. The reverse is also true in some women's sports, where the desired body shape and size is closer to the prepubertal physique. Normal changes that occur during puberty, including an increase in both muscularity and, predominantly in females, acquisition of body fat, may result in some talented athletes developing a physique that is less desirable for their sport (Cobley et al. 2009).

RESTRICTIVE EATING, DIETING, DISORDERED EATING AND ENERGY DEFICIENCY IN YOUNG ATHLETES

Risks of restrictive eating and dieting

Young athletes in sports where leanness is highly desirable (such as gymnastics, ballet, diving or figure skating) or where they need to make weight to compete (as in lightweight rowing, boxing and martial arts) are at an increased risk of restrictive eating, which can have negative short- and long-term consequences. In the short term, they may consume inadequate energy to train effectively, recover, adapt and improve performance. Growth may also be compromised. Inadequate carbohydrate intake may result in glycogen depletion, and this can increase fatigue and reduce training capacity and the potential for optimal metabolic adaptation. Inadequate protein intake may compromise growth and lean mass development. When overall food intake is reduced, there is also an increased risk of deficiency of key micronutrients.

Disordered eating and eating disorders

In the longer term, short-term dieting may develop into disordered eating. This can happen gradually and without the awareness of the young athlete, coach or parent. The disordered eating patterns can eventually progress to an eating disorder such as anorexia or bulimia nervosa. Although prevention should always be the primary aim, when disordered eating behaviours develop, early intervention is essential and is associated with significantly better longer-term outcomes. Although disordered eating can be difficult to identify in its early stages, athlete, coach and parent education can assist with earlier recognition of the problem (Jeacocke & Beals 2015).

Young athletes should not be encouraged to reduce weight or body fat without serious consideration of the potential negative effects. Weight management in young athletes requires the clinical expertise and professional support from a sports dietitian. Critical comments about weight or body composition often initiate inappropriate dieting, and this increases the risk of adverse outcomes in young athletes who are vulnerable to misinformation and may seek to rectify their weight 'problems' with 'fad' diets or non-evidence-based approaches. Once disordered eating practices develop they are difficult to reverse and intensive clinical intervention from a psychologist/psychiatrist and a dietitian is required. Medication, family therapy and, sometimes, hospitalisation may be needed. The development of an eating disorder can seriously jeopardise the future sports prospects of the athlete and lead to poorer longer-term physical and mental health. Making the decision about whether a young athlete with disordered eating should continue participating in sport can be challenging. Guidelines for sport exclusion and return to play have been developed on a score-based system and can help coaches and practitioners make objective decisions (De Souza et al. 2014).

RELATIVE ENERGY DEFICIENCY IN SPORT

There has been awareness for some time that young athletes, most often females, may experience health issues related to insufficient energy intake to fuel their training and maintain other essential body functions such as growth, repair of tissues such as bone and normal reproductive function. This issue was initially described as the 'Female Athlete Triad', which acknowledged the cluster of symptoms observed, including low bone-mineral density, low energy availability, eating disorder or disordered eating and menstrual dysfunction (Drinkwater et al. 2005). Energy availability (EA) is a relatively new concept that describes the energy remaining to maintain essential body functions after accounting for expenditure for exercise training (Loucks 2003).

EA is defined by the following equation:

$$EA\ (kJ/kg\ FFM) = (energy\ intake - energy\ cost\ of\ exercise)\ /\ fat\text{-}free\ mass$$

Low energy availability (LEA) may occur accidentally through a misunderstanding of the energy needs for sport, as a result of dietary restraint or as the consequence of disordered eating (Mountjoy et al. 2014). LEA is considered to occur when EA drops below a threshold of 125 kJ/kg FFM.

Awareness and improved understanding of the impact of LEA has continued to evolve and it is now clear that the consequences go beyond menstrual dysfunction and decreased bone health (Mountjoy et al. 2014). Evidence of negative consequences is also evident in male athletes, although this is less well characterised than in females. The term 'relative energy deficiency in sport' (RED-S) (Mountjoy et al. 2014) expands and reconceptualises the 'Female Athlete Triad' issues, acknowledging that both male and female athletes may be affected and that LEA may affect multiple body systems, including gastrointestinal, immunological, cardiovascular and endocrine function. In young athletes, growth and the attainment of optimal peak bone mass may also be affected (Box 18.1).

Identifying RED-S in young individual athletes and teams

Identification and assessment of LEA in field settings is difficult due to challenges in accurately measuring energy intake and exercise energy expenditure (Melin & Lundy 2015). Even when accurate measurements can be obtained, these assessments represent only a single point in time and cannot identify whether the reported energy availability is representative of the usual diet or is a short-term change. Measurement of resting metabolic rate can be a useful screening tool as it is often suppressed in LEA. Relevant indicators in the athlete's clinical history may also help to identify RED-S (Box 18.2). A helpful screening tool, the LEAF-Q (Low Energy Availability in Females questionnaire) is freely available, non-threatening and quick to complete (Melin et al. 2014).

Box 18.1: Consequences of RED-S

- Metabolic
- Endocrine
- Bone health
- Menstrual function
- Immunological
- Gastrointestinal
- Cardiovascular
- Psychological
- Growth and development
- Haematological

Source: Adapted from Mountjoy et al. 2014.

Box 18.2: Questions to consider if RED-S is suspected

1. Does the athlete have a history of frequent illness or injury?
2. For females, do they have a normal menstrual cycle?
3. Has body composition been a focus of their training or personally?
4. Do they have normal bone health?
5. Subjectively, what is their diet plan like?
6. Do they have a strong focus on healthy eating?
7. Do they adequately fuel training sessions?

For teams or squads of young female athletes, this may be helpful to identify those who require further medical and or nutrition support and follow up. The development of a similar tool for male athletes would be welcomed.

SPORTS SUPPLEMENT USE IN YOUNG ATHLETES

Young adolescent athletes in sports where larger mass and muscularity are important may be attracted to use supplements to support lean mass gain. While cautious use of supplements, particularly balanced products such as liquid meals (for example, Sustagen™) can assist young athletes in meeting energy needs more easily, heavy use of single nutrient supplements, such as protein powders and amino acids, may displace healthy foods and potentially increase the risk of ingestion of substances prohibited for use in sport. Even if the athlete is not yet undergoing drug testing, some of these substances (for example, stimulants and anabolic steroids) are detrimental to health. Stimulant abuse can result in a wide range of negative health consequences, including addiction/dependence, headaches, gastrointestinal upset and interrupted sleep patterns. Anabolic steroids can result in increased aggression, liver or heart damage along with a range of other serious effects.

These substances may be contaminants in the product and not disclosed on the label. There is also evidence that early use of supplements for lean mass gain may later influence inclination to use substances prohibited by sports drug agencies. For these reasons, a 'food first' approach is recommended for athletes younger than 18, with supplement use limited to sports foods (carbohydrate-electrolyte drinks, gels, sports bars and liquid meals) rather than ergogenic aids (Barkoukis et al. 2015). Young athletes have so much development potential from training, and the use of ergogenic aids at this stage introduces additional risk; performance assistance is best incorporated after optimising young athletes' preparation through a well-designed eating plan, effective training, psychological strategies and technical development. Supplements are often viewed as the 'magic bullet' and can contribute to a 'win at all costs' mentality. The risks of supplement use often remain poorly understood at this developmental stage (Desbrow & Leveritt 2015).

SUMMARY AND KEY MESSAGES

Young athletes have special nutrition needs to support growth and development as well as training. These mostly revolve around the need for additional energy and for key nutrients such as protein, carbohydrate, iron and calcium. The additional needs for protein and carbohydrate are generally consistent with adult athletes per kilogram of body weight, although more research is required. Strategies such as carbohydrate loading are not needed until late adolescence, as the durations and distances of endurance events are shorter for young athletes. At this stage, developing athletes are often conscious of body image and can be vulnerable to restrictive eating, energy and nutrient deficiency. Support to maintain a positive body image and a healthy diet is crucial to optimal physical and mental health. Where warning signs of RED-S or disordered eating emerge, early professional intervention supports more positive longer-term outcomes. Despite earlier concerns, younger athletes are not at a greater risk of exertional heat illness than adults. Finally, young athletes are often attracted to dietary supplements and ergogenic aids. At this age, a 'food first' approach is recommended with an overarching philosophy of encouraging healthy eating and physical, mental and technical development over the use of supplements (unless there is a deficiency), particularly ergogenic aids.

Key messages

- Young athletes have special nutrition needs. There is an increased requirement for energy, especially during adolescence, to support the accelerated rate in growth and development, in addition to the needs of training.

- Young athletes may undertake restrictive eating to reduce weight or body fat and this can result in insufficient energy consumption. This not only increases fatigue and compromises training adaptations and performance but also places the young athlete at increased risk of relative energy deficiency in sport (RED-S).

- RED-S compromises reproductive, immune and cardiac function as well as bone health, with some of these negative outcomes irreversible.

- Young athletes on restrictive diets are at risk for micronutrient deficiency, as requirements for nutrients such as iron and calcium are increased during growth and development.

- Eating disorders, and restrictive eating that progresses to disordered eating, pose a serious risk to both physical and mental health. Disordered eating can be triggered by negative comments about weight or shape or the recommendation to lose weight or fat without support from a qualified health professional. Young athletes are at a vulnerable stage of life and a positive body image must be nurtured.

- Limited research in young athletes indicates that macronutrient requirements per kilogram of body weight are similar to those for adult athletes, although, as they usually train and compete for shorter durations, carbohydrate intake should be periodised to training loads and strategies such as glycogen loading are not needed until late adolescence.

- Although young athletes had initially been reported to thermoregulate less effectively than adults, recent research indicates they are not at significantly greater risk of exertional heat stress when compared to adults. Many of the strategies used for hydration and competition fuelling can also be applied in principle to young athletes.

- Ergogenic aids, while popular at this stage, should generally be avoided and a 'food first' approach encouraged. A key strategy for sports nutrition at this phase of development is to ensure the athlete develops knowledge, skills and increasing independence in selecting a healthy diet.

REFERENCES

Aerenhouts, D., Deriemaeker, P., Hebbelinck, M. et al., 2011, 'Energy and macronutrient intake in adolescent sprint athletes: A follow-up study', *Journal of Sports Science*, vol. 29, no.1, pp. 73–82.

American Academy of Pediatrics, Council on Sports Medicine Fitness, Council on School Health et al., 2011, 'Policy statement: Climatic heat stress and exercising children and adolescents', *Pediatrics*, vol. 128, no. 3, pp. e741–7.

Barkoukis, V., Lazuras, L., Lucidi, F. et al., 2015, 'Nutritional supplement and doping use in sport: Possible underlying social cognitive processes', *Scandavian Journal of Medical Science in Sports*, vol. 25, no. 6, pp. e582–8.

Cobley, S., Baker, J., Wattie, N. et al., 2009, 'Annual age-grouping and athlete development: A meta-analytical review of relative age effects in sport', *Sports Medicine*, vol. 39, no. 3, pp. 235–56.

Croll, J.K., Neumark-Sztainer, D., Story, M. et al., 2006, 'Adolescents involved in weight-related and power team sports have better eating patterns and nutrient intakes than non-sport-involved adolescents', *Journal of American Dietetic Association*, vol. 106, no. 5, pp. 709–17.

De Souza, M.J., Nattiv, A., Joy, E. et al., 2014, 'Female Athlete Triad Coalition Consensus Statement on Treatment and Return to Play of the Female Athlete Triad: 1st International Conference held in San Francisco, California, May 2012 and 2nd International Conference held in Indianapolis, Indiana, May 2013', *British Journal of Sports Medicine*, vol. 48, no. 4, p. 289.

Desbrow, B. & Leveritt, M., 2015, 'Nutritional issues for young athletes: Children and adolescents', in Burke, L.M. & Deakin, V. (eds), *Clinical Sports Nutrition*, 5th edn, North Ryde, NSW: McGraw-Hill Education, pp. 592–618.

Drinkwater, B.L., Loucks, A.B., Sherman, R.T. et al., 2005, 'Position Stand on the female athlete triad', in Sangenis, P. (ed.), *IOC Medical Commission Working Group Women in Sport*, International Olympic Committee, Lausanne, Switzerland, pp. 2–46.

Erickson, B.O. & Saltin, B., 1974, 'Muscle metabolism in boys aged 11–16 years', *Acta Pediatrica Belgica*, vol. 28, pp. 257–65.

Haralambie, G., 1982, 'Enzyme activities in skeletal muscle of 13–15 years old adolescents', *Bulletin Europeen de Physiopathologie Respiratoire*, vol. 18, no. 1. pp. 65–74.

Jeacocke, N. & Beals, K.A., 2015, 'Eating disorders and disordered eating in athletes', in Burke, L.M. & Deakin, V. (eds), *Clinical Sports Nutrition*, 5th edn, North Ryde, NSW: McGraw-Hill Education, pp. 213–232.

Loucks, A.B., 2003, 'Introduction to menstrual disturbances in athletes', *Medicine & Science in Sports & Exercise*, vol. 35, pp. 1551–2.

Melin, A. & Lundy, B., 2015, 'Measuring energy availability', in Burke, L.M. & Deakin, V. (eds), *Clinical Sports Nutrition*, 5th edn, North Ryde, NSW: McGraw-Hill Education, pp. 146–157.

Melin, A., Tornberg, A.B., Skouby, S. et al., 2014, 'The LEAF questionnaire: A screening tool for the identification of female athletes at risk for the female athlete triad', *British Journal of Sports Medicine*, vol. 48, no. 7, pp. 540–5.

Mountjoy, M., Sundgot-Borgen, J., Burke, L. et al., 2014, 'The IOC consensus statement: Beyond the female athlete triad—Relative energy deficiency in sport (RED-S)', *British Journal of Sports Medicine*, vol. 48, no. 7, pp. 491–7.

National Health and Medical Research Council (NHMRC), 2006, *Nutrient reference values for Australia and New Zealand including recommended dietary intakes*, Canberra, ACT: Commonwealth of Australia, pp. 27–8, retrieved from <https://nhmrc.gov.au/sites/default/files/images/nutrient-refererence-dietary-intakes.pdf>.

Parnell, J.A., Wiens, K.P. & Erdman, K.A., 2016, 'Dietary intakes and supplement use in pre-adolescent and adolescent Canadian athletes', *Nutrients*, vol. 8, no. 9, pp. 526.

Rowland, T., 2008, 'Thermoregulation during exercise in the heat in children: Old concepts revisited', *Journal of Applied Physiology*, vol. 105, no. 2, pp. 718–24.

Taylor D.J., Kemp G.J., Thompson C.H. & Radda G.K., 1997, 'Ageing: Effects on oxidative function of skeletal muscle *in vivo*', in Gellerich, F.N. & Zierz, S. (eds), *Detection of Mitochondrial Diseases. Developments in Molecular and Cellular Biochemistry*, vol. 21, Boston, MA: Springer.

CHAPTER 19

Masters athletes

Janelle Gifford and Helen O'Connor

The incidence of chronic conditions such as obesity, Type 2 diabetes, cardiovascular disease (CVD) and musculoskeletal disorders increases with age, placing added pressure on health and societal systems for their management and treatment. Adopting or maintaining a healthy lifestyle with attention to good nutrition and physical activity reduces the risk of developing these conditions and may be effective in their management. Older people who participate in competition or systematic training can be defined as masters (older, veteran, senior, mature) athletes. They may have been active all their lives, or have become active to improve their health or treat one or more lifestyle-related conditions (Gifford et al. 2015). As with younger athletes, the nutritional needs of masters athletes vary according to the type, duration and intensity of activity, but there are changes in the underlying physiological processes with ageing and any health conditions that may be present add complexity to determining needs. Physical activity also has positive effects on the physiology of ageing, which may have beneficial outcomes. Each masters athlete is, therefore, unique in their physiological profile and requirements. This chapter provides an overview of nutrition requirements in ageing and selected chronic health conditions in older athletes and addresses the use of supplements in this group.

LEARNING OUTCOMES

Upon completion of this chapter you will be able to:

- define the term 'masters athlete'
- identify some of the physiological changes that may affect the nutrition requirements of masters athletes
- identify general changes to the nutrition requirements with age
- describe how common nutrition-related chronic conditions may affect the nutrition requirements of masters athletes
- understand the role of supplements in the diet of the masters athlete.

THE CHANGING NUTRITION REQUIREMENTS OF THE MASTERS ATHLETE

The definition of masters athletes usually varies according to sport; competitions generally include those 35 years of age or older, but there are younger competitors in some sports (for example, gymnastics). The broad age range means that basic nutrition requirements can vary widely. There are no specific sports nutrition guidelines for masters athletes, so guidance may be based on sport-specific recommendations for younger athletes (Thomas et al. 2016), physiological changes associated with ageing (Reaburn et al. 2015) and general dietary guidelines for specific age groups (NHMRC 2013). This section provides a brief overview of the latter two.

The reduction in the metabolically active fat-free mass (FFM), including muscle tissue, that occurs with ageing, along with a potential reduction in activity or training, translates to a decrease in energy requirements for some masters athletes. However, the energy requirements for masters athletes will be higher than for their inactive peers due to their higher activity levels. If the amount of energy they consume is limited (for example, to achieve a particular physique), it may be more challenging to meet macronutrient requirements for activity, particularly for carbohydrate. For example, a 70 kilogram male endurance athlete exercising at moderate to high intensity would require 6–10 g/kg BM/day of carbohydrate (Thomas et al. 2016), equating to 6720–11,200 kJ/day. While carbohydrate uptake may not be affected by age (Elahi & Muller 2000), glycogen storage may be reduced, particularly in novice masters athletes (Meredith et al. 1989). This is a consideration for strategies, such as carbohydrate loading, often used to optimise performance in endurance events.

Similarly, digestion and absorption of protein does not appear to change significantly with age; however, protein requirements increase due to factors such as a decline in anabolic response to protein intake and disease processes (such as insulin resistance) (Bauer et al. 2013). Masters athletes may need ≥1.2 g/kg BM/day (Bauer et al. 2013) depending on their age, and 35–40 grams of leucine-rich protein following muscle-damaging exercise rather than the 20 grams usually recommended for younger athletes (Doering et al. 2016). However, protein intake does need to be lower for those with impaired kidney function (for example, as a result of diabetes). As with younger athletes, attention to timing of intake (in relation to resistance training and distribution of intake over the day), type (for example, leucine-containing, fast acting) and quality of protein are important considerations in nutrition advice to support exercise for masters athletes (see Chapters 3 and 5 and Bauer et al. 2013). Food sources of high biological-value protein, such as lean red meat, fish, poultry and dairy foods, are good protein choices for masters athletes.

Changes in gut function can affect the absorption and digestion of some micronutrients, increasing requirements for calcium, iron, zinc and B vitamins (Reaburn et al. 2015). However, iron requirements do reduce for women after menopause. Reduced skin capacity to synthesise vitamin D, reduced immune function, change in liver uptake of vitamin A and increased oxidative stress may increase the need for vitamins A, B6, C, D, E and zinc (Reaburn et al. 2015). Supplementation may occasionally be clinically indicated; however, increased needs can generally be met with a balanced diet, particularly with the increased food intake needed to meet the demands of sport.

Physiological changes which affect fluid needs should be considered in advice on hydration for the older athlete. Masters athletes may have a decreased thirst perception, reduced kidney function and altered thermoregulatory mechanisms (Reaburn et al. 2015; Soto-Quijano 2017). Reduced thirst perception may increase the risk of hypohydration via reduced fluid intake; however, slower water and sodium excretion may increase the risk of hyponatraemia and hypertension in some masters athletes (Soto-Quijano 2017). This latter risk is potentially greater for smaller and slower masters athletes exercising in cool conditions, since these factors lower fluid requirements. For masters athletes exercising for long durations and/or in the heat, commercial carbohydrate-electrolyte drinks (such as sports drinks) may be a useful fluid-replacement choice (Gifford et al. 2015). However, a fluid-replacement plan developed by an Accredited Sports Dietitian and tailored to the fluid and electrolyte losses of the athlete would be optimal for masters athletes given their potentially altered physiological and health status.

General guidelines across the food groups are the same for individuals across the 19–50 year age group, but there are small changes for both men and women from the age of 51 (NHMRC 2013) which should be taken into account in nutrition advice given to masters athletes. Specifically, in the grains group, recommended serves decrease from six to four (51–70 years), and then to three serves for women over 70 years old. Recommended serves for men decrease from 71 years and over (from six to 4.5 serves). Reduction in bone health frequently occurs with age, particularly for women; foods containing calcium are beneficial to bone health, and the recommended serves of dairy foods and alternatives therefore increase from 51 years (from 2.5 to four serves) for women and from 71 years for men (from 2.5 to 3.5 serves). There are minor changes in the lean meat and alternatives group (for women and men) and the vegetables group (for men only). Changes to the recommended servings of other food groups, including grains and dairy, and alternatives are important for masters athletes, since these foods are important sources of carbohydrate, protein and energy for physical activity and recovery, as well as micronutrients such as B vitamins. Balancing these foods within an energy budget (kJ/day) that may be lower due to the ageing process may seem challenging; however, a lower energy requirement and physiological changes for micronutrients has been taken into account in the development of general recommendations on food groups. When energy intake is more restricted, the quality of the diet is important so energy dense, nutrient-poor foods (such as cakes, takeaway foods and soft drinks) should be minimised.

CHRONIC HEALTH CONDITIONS IN OLDER ATHLETES

While the limited research that has been conducted on masters athletes suggests they may be healthier than their non-active counterparts, masters athletes may still need nutrition advice for conditions such as obesity, Type 2 diabetes, CVD and changes in musculoskeletal function that also aligns with performance goals.

The reduction in energy requirements with ageing can lead to weight gain in the form of fat mass (FM). There is no single dietary approach to guarantee weight reduction; however, an energy deficit created by reducing energy intake and/or increasing energy expenditure is necessary to affect a change in FM. Low glycaemic index, higher-fibre carbohydrates (such as wholegrains and fruits and vegetables) and protein foods (such as meat, dairy foods and nuts) increase the feeling of fullness and can be incorporated into weight management plans. For masters athletes, periodising energy requirements to support the needs of training and competition, and reducing energy intake on rest days or outside of competition, could accommodate both weight reduction and performance goals.

Increased overall and abdominal FM increases the risk of developing Type 2 diabetes and CVD. There is a further increased risk of CVD in people with Type 2 diabetes. Dietary management of Type 2 diabetes usually includes weight reduction, management of carbohydrate intake and strategies to reduce the risk of or manage concurrent CVD. For many masters athletes, carbohydrate is an important fuel source, particularly for moderate- to high-intensity training and events that last longer than 60–90 minutes (Thomas et al. 2016). Masters athletes with Type 2 diabetes are advised to consume good-quality (low glycaemic index, wholegrain, higher fibre and unrefined) sources of carbohydrates, such as dairy foods, wholegrains, fruit and low glycaemic index starchy vegetables (such as legumes) spread over the day and mapped around training and competition needs. In long training sessions or events, there may be a need for more refined carbohydrate sources such as sports (carbohydrate-electrolyte) drinks or gels to assist in the provision of sufficient glucose to maintain energy and blood glucose. Masters athletes who take glucose-lowering medications may need to adjust their dosage with the support of their physician or diabetes educator, as there is a higher risk of hypoglycaemia with exercise.

Reduction in weight, attention to quality of dietary fat and plant sterols, increase in soluble fibre and reduction in sodium are frequently used strategies to manage CVD for those with or without Type 2 diabetes. While fat is energy dense, inclusion of poly- and monounsaturated fats (PUFAs and MUFAs) and reduction of saturated fats (as in butter, palm oil and many processed foods) is important to manage blood fats and other CVD risk factors. Sources such as oily fish, nuts, margarines and most vegetable oils are good choices. Changes in endothelial function, including stiffening of artery walls with age, may contribute to hypertension; however, active individuals are more likely to have healthy arterial function. Diets that have plenty of vegetables (such as the Mediterranean or dietary approaches to stop hypertension (DASH) diets) may assist with lowering blood pressure due to their nitrate content, and nitrates may also enhance performance in some sports (Lidder & Webb 2013). Reduction in sodium intake to manage hypertension may conflict with sports nutrition advice to increase sodium intake for optimising fluid balance and should be managed by an Accredited Sports Dietitian.

Two common changes in musculoskeletal function with age are a decline in bone mineral density (BMD), leading to osteopenia or osteoporosis, and development of osteoarthritis (OA). Postmenopausal women may experience a deterioration in bone health leading to an increased fracture risk due to the decline in circulation of the protective hormone, oestrogen. History of amenorrhoea may also contribute to poor bone health in women; however, relative energy deficiency in sport or RED-S (which may cause amenorrhea) may also affect hormonal balance and bone health in men (Mountjoy et al. 2014). BMD increases with weight-bearing activity (walking, running, resistance training), so masters athletes with a history of participation in cycling and swimming may have lower BMD at certain sites (for example, the spine) than masters athletes with a history of sports such as running. Weight-bearing exercise and inclusion of calcium and vitamin D according to population recommendations are recommended for both female and male masters athletes for optimal bone health. With respect to OA, the principal nutrition strategy is weight reduction to reduce the load on affected weight-bearing joints. Supplement use is relatively common for the treatment of OA but is often ineffective.

Finally, medications taken to treat chronic disorders may impact physiological function, performance (Brun 2016) and nutrition advice. A fuller discussion of these, and nutrition to support masters athletes with chronic nutrition-related lifestyle conditions, can be found in previous reviews (Gifford et al. 2015; Brun 2016).

SUPPLEMENTS IN OLDER ATHLETES

Supplements can be categorised as medical supplements, specific performance supplements and sports foods such as sports drinks. Supplement use is common among athletes at all levels; however, type and reasons for use may be different for masters athletes versus their younger counterparts. This section focuses on medical and sports performance supplement use in masters athletes. Masters athletes commonly use supplements for injury or other health reasons, whereas younger athletes are more likely to use supplements for sports performance (Striegel et al. 2006). This pattern may partly reflect use of supplements in the general population. The last Australian Health Survey found that use of dietary supplements increased with age and was more common in females, that vitamin and mineral preparations were the most common dietary supplement, and that special dietary foods such as sport and protein beverages and powders were more commonly consumed by 19- to 30-year-old males (Australian Bureau of Statistics 2014).

Masters athletes may take medical supplements for a variety of health reasons, either self-prescribed or recommended by a health professional or others. Long-chain PUFAs such as omega-3 fatty acids (in fish oils) are known to have a positive effect on CVD risk factors; however, these may also be sourced from foods such as oily fish (as in the Mediterranean diet). Calcium and vitamin D supplementation may be taken, particularly by female masters athletes, to improve bone health; however, dietary sources of these nutrients are also available. Consuming good sources of calcium (dairy foods and calcium-fortified foods), with the dose divided over the day (more in the evening), will help to maximise absorption (Gifford et al. 2015). Vitamin D can be obtained from wild-caught oily fish, liver, eggs and fortified foods; however, prudent exposure to sunlight and/or medically supervised supplementation may be necessary to obtain adequate vitamin D (Gifford et al. 2015). Supplements for OA are some of the most investigated in older populations. Evidence for the use of substances with anti-oxidant activity (vitamins A, C and E, and selenium), fish oil supplements, glucosamine and chondroitin sulphate is not consistent or conclusive in relation to the management of OA (Gifford et al. 2015). Masters athletes may take vitamin and mineral supplements for the health benefits of some nutrients within a restricted energy budget; however, overconsumption of some nutrients could be harmful.

There are few studies specifically on the performance effects of supplements in masters athletes, so benefits for masters athletes are generally inferred from studies in younger athletes. However, physiological changes in nutrient absorption and metabolism in masters athletes may mean some supplements do not have the same effect as for younger athletes, and there is always the concern of harm to health or performance. For example, caffeine is known to enhance endurance performance in younger athletes but may acutely affect blood pressure, which could be problematic for masters athletes with hypertension. On the other hand, supplements such as creatine and whey protein may assist functionally in masters athletes, limiting muscle loss and promoting muscle gain in older individuals. Competing masters athletes should be cautious about taking any supplement, as some products may contain substances banned by the World Anti-Doping Agency (WADA) or may interact with medications. While checking the ingredients list of the product may seem a prudent safeguard, ingredients may be omitted from the list or the product may be inadvertently contaminated by substances during manufacture. Quality assurance programs are now available for testing products and some products will carry a logo as proof of testing (LGC Group 1999–2018).

SUMMARY AND KEY MESSAGES

Nutrition recommendations for the general population consider the physiological effects of ageing and should be used as a basic framework to map dietary plans of masters athletes. Guidance for specific sporting requirements can be taken from those of younger athletes, while considering the physiological changes that occur with age and any underlying chronic nutrition-related conditions.

Key messages
- The broad age range of masters athletes and differences in general health means that basic requirements can vary widely.
- There are no specific sports nutrition guidelines for masters athletes. Guidance may be inferred from general dietary guidelines for specific age groups, information on physiological changes with ageing and sport-specific recommendations for younger athletes.
- Potential changes in physiology and physiological function in the masters athlete include reduction in FFM, changes in glycogen storage capacity, reduction in absorption and digestion of some micronutrients, reduced immune function and increases in oxidative stress.
- General population guidelines consider physiological changes with ageing and can be used as a basic framework for the diet of masters athletes.

- Chronic nutrition-related lifestyle conditions may alter nutrition advice given to athletes; however, an Accredited Sports Dietitian can assist in tailoring advice for individual athletes around changes in energy, carbohydrate, protein and other nutrients to support health and performance.
- Masters athletes may take supplements for health conditions or to improve performance. Most of the information about performance supplements is inferred from studies in younger athletes. Professional guidance from an Accredited Sports Dietitian who understands individual clinical and sports performance needs would be beneficial to assist masters athletes in considering the use of dietary supplements.

REFERENCES

Australian Bureau of Statistics, 2014, *Australian Health Survey: Nutrition First Results—Foods and Nutrients, 2011–12* [Online], Australian Bureau of Statistics, <http://www.abs.gov.au/ausstats/abs@.nsf/Lookup/by%20Subject/4364.0.55.007~2011-12~Main%20Features~Key%20Findings~1>, accessed 29 January 2018.

Bauer, J., Biolo, G., Cederholm, T. et al., 2013, 'Evidence-based recommendations for optimal dietary protein intake in older people: A position paper from the PROT-AGE study group', *Journal of the American Medical Directors Association*, vol. 14, no. 8, pp. 542–59.

Brun, S., 2016, 'Clinical considerations for the ageing athlete', *Australian Family Physician*, vol. 45, no. 7, pp. 478–83.

Doering, T.M., Reaburn, P.R., Phillips, S.M. et al., 2016, 'Postexercise dietary protein strategies to maximize skeletal muscle repair and remodeling in masters endurance athletes: A review', *International Journal of Sport Nutrition & Exercise Metabolism*, vol. 26, no. 2, pp. 168–78.

Elahi, D. & Muller, D.C., 2000, 'Carbohydrate metabolism in the elderly', *European Journal of Clinical Nutrition*, vol. 54, suppl. 3, pp. S112–120.

Gifford, J., O'Connor, H., Honey, A. et al., 2015, 'Nutrients, health and chronic disease in masters athletes', in Reaburn, P. (ed.), *Nutrition and Performance in Masters Athletes*, Boca Raton, FL: CRC Press, pp. 213–41.

LGC Group, 1999–2018, *Informed-Sport.com* [Online], <www.informed-sport.com/>, accessed 11 February 2018.

Lidder, S. & Webb, A.J., 2013, 'Vascular effects of dietary nitrate (as found in green leafy vegetables and beetroot) via the nitrate-nitrite-nitric oxide pathway', *British Journal of Clinical Pharmacology*, vol. 75, no. 3, pp. 677–96.

Meredith, C.N., Frontera, W.R., Fisher, E.C. et al., 1989, 'Peripheral effects of endurance training in young and old subjects', *Journal of Applied Physiology*, vol. 66, no. 6, pp. 2844–9.

Mountjoy, M., Sundgot-Borgen, J., Burke, L. et al., 2014, 'The IOC consensus statement: Beyond the female athlete triad—Relative energy deficiency in sport (RED-S)', *British Journal of Sports Medicine*, vol. 48, no. 7, pp. 491–7.

National Health and Medical Research Council (NHMRC), 2013, *Australian Dietary Guidelines*, Canberra, ACT: Commonwealth of Australia.

Reaburn, P., Doering, T., & Borges, N., 2015, 'Nutrition issues for the masters athlete', in Burke, L. & Deakin, V. (eds.), *Clinical Sports Nutrition*, 5th edn, North Ryde, NSW: McGraw-Hill Education, pp. 619-646.

Soto-Quijano, D.A., 2017, 'The competitive senior athlete', *Physical Medicine and Rehabilitation Clinics of North America*, vol. 28, no. 4, pp. 767–76.

Striegel, H., Simon, P., Wurster, C. et al., 2006, 'The use of nutritional supplements among master athletes', *International Journal of Sports Medicine*, vol. 27, no. 3, pp. 236–41.

Thomas, D.T., Erdman, K.A. & Burke, L.M., 2016, 'American College of Sports Medicine Joint Position Statement. Nutrition and Athletic Performance', *Medicine & Science in Sports & Exercise*, vol. 48, no. 3, pp. 543–68.

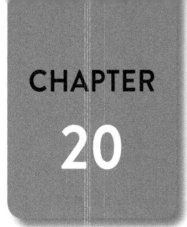

CHAPTER 20

Paralympic athletes

Michelle Minehan and Elizabeth Broad

Paralympic athletes compete with physical, visual or intellectual impairments. A classification system allows athletes with similar functional ability to compete against each other on an even playing field. Since the first Paralympic Games in Rome in 1960, the Paralympic movement has developed rapidly. Summer and Winter Paralympic Games now occur every four years and participation is consistently increasing. In 2016, 4333 athletes from 159 countries competed at the Rio Paralympic Games.

Working with Paralympic athletes can be challenging due to limited research and potentially complex interplay between athletes' clinical, life and sporting needs. Modern Paralympic athletes train and perform at an elite level with increasingly competitive standards, with some events won by fractions of a second or by a single point. In many cases, the nutritional needs of Paralympic athletes are very similar to able-bodied athletes. In other cases, nutrition recommendations need to be modified to suit individual circumstances.

LEARNING OUTCOMES

Upon completion of this chapter you will be able to:

- understand the range of physical, visual and intellectual impairments that may affect Paralympic athletes

- describe key factors driving the need for modification of nutrition recommendations for Paralympic athletes
- consider how sports nutrition recommendations might need to be modified for different types of Paralympic athletes.

CLASSES OF PARALYMPIC ATHLETES

To compete as a Paralympic athlete, at least one of the impairments in Table 20.1 must be present. Some sports cater for only one type of impairment, while others have classes for all impairments. For example, goalball is played exclusively by athletes who are visually impaired, whereas athletics offers a full spectrum of events. Within each sport, athletes are classified based on their level of impairment. For example, the T42 category in athletics is for track athletes with a 'lower limb affected by limb deficiency, leg length difference, impaired muscle power or impaired range of movement'. The goal of classification is to create an even playing field for competition. Discussion and recommendations in this chapter will focus on the needs of athletes with physical impairments.

Paralympic sports vary widely, from traditional events such as athletics to modified events such as boccia and goalball. Table 20.2 summarises the diverse mix of sports contested at summer and winter Paralympic games.

RESEARCH CHALLENGES

In 1993, the International Paralympic Committee (IPC) established a Sports Science Committee to advance knowledge of Paralympic sport across five central themes: (1) involving the academic world, (2) athlete health and safety, (3) classification, (4) socio-economic determinants of participation and success, and (5) Paralympic athlete, trainer and coach education. Research activity is increasing; to date, however, limited work has been done on nutritional issues for Paralympic athletes. Challenges to conducting research include:

- large variation in functional capacity of athletes
- athletes dispersed over large geographical distances
- medical contraindications to participation in experimental research (for example, use of particular medications)
- small athlete pool, which makes it difficult to set up designs with randomisation and control groups
- small number of scientists actively researching Paralympic athlete issues
- national focus, with many scientists working with Paralympic athletes having a mandate to help athletes from their own countries win medals, limiting opportunities for collaboration and sharing
- limited funding opportunities for sport-related research, especially Paralympic sport.

Table 20.1. Impairments in Paralympic sports

Impairment	Explanation
Impaired muscle power	Reduced force generated by muscles or muscle groups in one limb or the lower half of the body, e.g. spinal cord injury.
Impaired passive range of movement	Range of movement in one or more joints is reduced permanently. Joints that can move beyond the average range of motion, joint instability and acute conditions such as arthritis are not considered eligible impairments.
Limb deficiency	Total or partial absence of bones or joints, from birth or as a consequence of trauma or illness.
Leg length difference	Bone shortening in one leg from birth or trauma.
Short stature	Reduced standing height due to abnormal dimensions of bones of upper and lower limbs or trunk, e.g. achondroplasia.
Hypertonia	Abnormal increase in muscle tension and a reduced ability of a muscle to stretch, which can result from injury, illness or a health condition, e.g. cerebral palsy.
Ataxia	Lack of coordination of muscle movements due to a neurological condition, e.g. cerebral palsy.
Athetosis	Unbalanced, uncontrolled movements and a difficulty in maintaining a symmetrical posture, e.g. cerebral palsy.
Visual impairment	Vision impacted by a physical or neurological impairment.
Intellectual impairment	A limitation in intellectual functioning and adaptive behaviour as expressed in conceptual, social and practical adaptive skills, which originates before the age of 18.

Source: Adapted from www.paralympic.org/classification (accessed June 2017).

Table 20.2. Sports contested at Paralympic Games

Summer Paralympic Sports				Winter Paralympic Sports
Archery	Judo	Wheelchair basketball		Para alpine skiing
Para athletics	Para powerlifting	Wheelchair fencing		Para biathlon
Badminton	Rowing	Wheelchair rugby		Para cross-country skiing
Boccia	Shooting Para sport	Wheelchair tennis		Para ice hockey
Canoe	Sitting volleyball			Para snowboard
Cycling	Para swimming			Wheelchair curling
Equestrian	Table tennis			
Football 5-a-side	Taekwondo			
Goalball	Triathlon			

Source: Adapted from www.paralympic.org/sports (accessed August 2018).

In the absence of a large Paralympic specific research base, it is necessary to extrapolate knowledge gleaned from studies of able-bodied athletes. Budding researchers are encouraged to consider projects with Paralympic populations.

TRAINING AGE

Paralympic athletes compete across a wide age range. The youngest athlete at the Rio Paralympics in 2016 was 13 years old, while the oldest was 73. Many Paralympic athletes follow a traditional sports career path, playing a sport from a young age and gradually improving until they compete at an elite level. Others take up Paralympic sport later in life, after acquiring a disability due to traumatic injury or disease progression.

It is also relatively common for Paralympic athletes to cross-over between and within Paralympic sports. The events offered at major events such as world championships and major games can change to balance the total number of events and according to participation rates. This might require a 400-metre runner to switch to 1500 metres, or a javelin thrower to convert to shotput in order to gain a spot on a national team. As new competition opportunities arise, some athletes transfer to new sports. For example, Para-Triathlon was contested at the Paralympic Games for the first time in 2016, enticing athletes to swap from sports such as athletics, cycling and swimming. Australian athlete Dylan Alcott competed in both wheelchair basketball and wheelchair tennis at different Paralympic Games.

Consequently, athletes can compete at major events with relatively few years of sports specific training under their belt. It is important to consider the training 'age' of an athlete as well as their chronological age. Nutritional needs can be different for an athlete with a long training history compared to an athlete rapidly adapting to a training stimulus. Altering body composition might be a lower priority while an athlete focuses on building up sufficient strength and stamina to cope with training. It can be easy to assume that older athletes have acquired significant knowledge about how to manage their nutrition intake for their sport, but in reality they might be very new to the sport and on a rapid learning trajectory.

ENERGY NEEDS

Estimating energy expenditure is arguably the biggest challenge when working with Paralympic athletes. The physiological demands of most Paralympic sports are unmeasured and predictive equations have limited applicability to many Paralympic athletes. Direct measurement of resting metabolic rate (RMR) via indirect calorimetry is useful but not easily accessible for all athletes. In general, predictive equations based on muscle mass (for example, the Cunningham equation) are more useful than equations based solely on height and weight (such as the Harris-Benedict equation). A trial-and-error process based on estimated energy intake and weight changes may be needed to fully understand individual energy requirements.

Athletes with conditions such as spina bifida and cerebral palsy might have proportionally higher energy requirements due to inefficient ambulation and conditions such as athetosis (involuntary movements). Some individuals who walk with a prosthesis might have a higher energy expenditure due to inefficiency of movement caused by gait asymmetry. In most cases, this additional energy cost is small and possibly offset by factors such as reduced muscle and reduced daily activity.

Energy expenditure of individuals who use a wheelchair is typically reduced compared with able-bodied individuals. as daily movements use a smaller muscle mass. RMR is typically lower (up to 25 per cent) in athletes with spinal cord injuries (SCI) due to non-functioning muscle and subsequent muscle wasting. The impact is greater the higher the injury to the spinal cord but can vary according to how complete the injury to the spinal cord is and whether the individual experiences involuntary muscle spasms.

Like able-bodied athletes, many Paralympic athletes strive to keep their physique lean. A reduced RMR means they can have a limited kilojoule budget and have to prioritise nutrient density. It can be a fine balance between supporting performance goals while achieving a suitable physique.

ENERGY AVAILABILITY

Low energy availability has emerged as an important issue for athletes. Energy availability refers to the amount of energy available to support bodily functions once the cost of training has been met. If energy availability is low, metabolism can slow, leading to negative hormonal changes and reduced bone density (Blauwet et al. 2017). This can put athletes at risk of injury, illness and suboptimal body composition.

Currently, little is known about the prevalence of low energy availability in Paralympic athletes. While diagnostic criteria are available for able-bodied athletes (see Chapter 18), specific criteria for different types of Paralympic athletes are currently unavailable. However, there is reason to suspect that many Paralympic athletes could be affected, as low energy availability can arise from both intentional (restricting intake to maintain a lean physique) and unintentional (insufficient opportunity to eat all required food or lack of understanding of total energy requirements) under-eating.

Athletes who do not weight-bear typically have reduced bone density. The primary cause is reduced skeletal loading which may be related to their sport (for example, swimming, cycling) and/or their disability (for example, spinal cord injury, amputation). However, the influence of low energy availability should also be considered.

MACRONUTRIENT AND MICRONUTRIENT NEEDS

Carbohydrate requirements are primarily influenced by the type of training completed. As with able-bodied athletes, adequate carbohydrate availability is required for long (>90 mins) sessions or sessions where maximum work output is required (such as repeated sprints) (see Chapter 10). Rates of glucose utilisation in arm cycling and wheelchair events are largely unknown. However, the capacity to store glycogen in the arms is less than in the large muscles of the legs. Athletes competing in long duration arm cycling and wheelchair events might have a higher need for carbohydrate replacement during sessions to compensate for reduced storage capacity. This can prove challenging as athletes with SCI typically do not like to eat or drink while exercising.

The protein needs of Paralympic athletes have not been documented. However, it is widely accepted that able-bodied athletes have higher protein requirements than sedentary individuals, as additional protein is required for repair, recovery and muscle growth. In general, the same is expected for Paralympic athletes. However, it is expected that athletes with less functional muscle (SCI, amputees) require lower absolute amounts of protein than able-bodied athletes but likely the same intake relative to functional muscle mass. Some Paralympic athletes with SCI or congenital defects have altered kidney function, which may require modifications to protein recommendations. Timing and spread of high-quality protein is as important for Paralympic athletes as for other athletes and, as such, optimal intakes need to be tailored to each individual.

Requirements for micronutrients are generally expected to be similar for Paralympic athletes. Athletes with restricted intakes due to low energy budgets might have difficulty meeting needs from food alone. Athletes with SCI might be at increased risk of vitamin D insufficiency due to inadequate diet, anticonvulsant medication and reduced sunlight exposure. Supplementation might be warranted in some circumstances. In these instances, vitamin D levels should be monitored and supplementation discussed with a doctor or dietitian.

HYDRATION AND HEAT REGULATION

In general, Paralympic athletes are encouraged to start exercise sessions in a euhydrated state and to match fluid intake to sweat losses during exercise. Fluid balance monitoring (weighing before and after exercise) is useful to track fluid losses and plan for individualised fluid replacement (see Chapter 11).

Fluid requirements for athletes with SCI need additional consideration. The ability of the brain to control body temperature through dilation of blood vessels and increased sweating is altered in athletes with SCI if the injury is at or above the T8 vertebrae (top half of the spinal column). The extent of the impact depends on the severity and level of the damage to the spinal cord. The higher the lesion, the greater the impairment to thermoregulation. Furthermore, some medications (diuretics, thyroid medication, muscle relaxants) can hamper thermoregulation. Reduced sweating means fluid losses are often less for athletes with SCI but it also means that capacity to cool is impaired; hence, messages around hydrating effectively may need to be modified, with more focus on external cooling strategies.

Acclimatisation is important when athletes are competing in the heat (Price 2016). Generally, 7–14 days are required for adaptation to exercise in the heat. However, some Paralympic athletes with coexisting medical conditions might require longer. Paralympic athletes need to schedule travel to allow sufficient time for acclimatisation before competing, or to implement acclimatisation strategies such as use of heat chambers before departure. The potential for acclimatisation in athletes with high-level SCI is undocumented. These athletes might consider limiting their exposure to hot environments prior to competition.

Various cooling strategies, such as water immersion, cooling jackets, ice slushies and water sprays, have been tested in athlete populations. Current evidence is mixed as to the effectiveness of these strategies in Paralympic athletes. Athletes with SCI can also have impaired shivering mechanisms and hence have difficulty warming the body when required. A balance needs to be found to deliver the optimal level of cooling.

Many athletes with SCI have disrupted signals from the brain to the bladder and require catheterisation to manage bladder function. It is common for athletes to time fluid intake carefully around competition and travel to manage catheterisation around events. Some athletes may limit fluid intake to avoid having to empty catheter bags or devices. Catheterisation practices need to be considered when planning fluid intake strategies and conducting hydration assessment. Measures such as morning urine specific gravity (USG) and fluid balance might require modification in some circumstances. It may be important to discuss and trial new strategies, including the use of electrolytes, with athletes to find the optimal balance between appropriate hydration (especially for travel) to minimise risk of developing a urinary tract infection and better support training and recovery.

INJURY AND ILLNESS

Athletes perform best when they consistently complete all scheduled training sessions. Hence, a goal is to minimise loss of training due to injury or illness. Some evidence suggests injury rates are higher in Paralympic sports. This may be due to Paralympic athletes being more likely to have coexisting medical conditions, to biomechanical inefficiencies that increase susceptibility to injury, or to exposure to high training loads before they are physically ready. Poor nutrition and low energy availability may also increase susceptibility to injuries and illness.

Athletes who use catheterisation to manage bladder function are more susceptible to urinary tract infections (UTI). Recurrent UTI can result in significant loss of training days over a season. A variety of catheterisation systems are available but all have the potential to expose the bladder to bacteria, leading to UTI (Compton et al. 2015). Key measures to prevent UTI include maintenance of good hygiene when using catheters, frequent emptying of catheters (every 3–4 hours) and sufficient fluid intake. Cranberry juice is a popular preventative measure for UTIs, although evidence for efficacy is inconsistent.

BODY COMPOSITION ASSESSMENT

Many athletes find it useful to monitor body composition over time as it provides useful feedback on the effectiveness of training and nutritional regimes. Surface anthropometry (skinfolds) and dual energy X-ray absorptiometry (DXA) are the most common methods for assessing body composition in athletes. However, other methods are also available and it is important to understand the assumptions and limitations that influence their validity. It is often necessary to modify techniques for Paralympic athletes. For example, according to the International Society for Advancement of Kinanthropometry (ISAK), skinfolds are routinely taken on the right side of the body. However, it is more relevant to measure the left side if an athlete has hemiplegia (weakness) or is missing a limb on the right side. The standard ISAK skinfold protocol involves measures at seven or eight body sites. However, for athletes with SCI, measures are often limited to the biceps, triceps, subscapular and abdominal sites.

DXA is useful for measuring body fat and lean tissue changes over time in athletes with a variety of physical impairments. There is little value in comparing data to normative data derived from able-bodied reference groups; rather, the data obtained can be useful for monitoring changes within the Paralympic athlete over time. It is often necessary to adjust standard positioning to obtain the most useful information for Paralympic athletes. For example, in standard DXA protocols athletes lie on their back in standard anatomical position with legs straight and arms alongside the body. Some Paralympic athletes cannot lie in standard position within the scanning area. While it is possible to customise positioning and analysis of DXA scans, these adjustments are yet to be validated.

GASTROINTESTINAL ISSUES

Athletes with SCI, congenital abnormalities of the gastrointestinal tract, a history of gastrointestinal injury or medication use are more likely to experience gastrointestinal issues than other Paralympic athletes. Some athletes have altered transit time (for example, SCI) while others have various food intolerances or food aversions. Many athletes who compete in wheelchairs avoid eating before training or competing as the bent position in the chair is uncomfortable when the stomach is full.

As such, it is important to work with Paralympic athletes to gain a full understanding of gastrointestinal issues when providing dietary advice. The timing of food and fluid intake around sessions typically needs to be adjusted according to individual tolerance. Some athletes need to focus on eating more in the later part of the day to compensate for restricted intake in the earlier part of the day; this is contradictory to most nutrition guidelines. Experimentation with quickly absorbed forms of carbohydrate such as gels and confectionery is often needed. This can be challenging when energy budget is limited.

MEDICAL ISSUES AND MEDICATION

Many Paralympic athletes have coexisting medical conditions such as epilepsy, high blood pressure, kidney impairment, osteoporosis, reflux, diabetes and heart conditions (Johnson et al. 2014). Some athletes require multiple medications. The impact of medical conditions and medications needs to be considered when providing nutrition advice. Some Paralympic athletes have a very poor understanding of their medical conditions, so it is useful to work closely with other support staff specifically trained in managing these clinical conditions—doctors, dietitians, physiologists and physiotherapists—to gain an accurate understanding.

SUPPLEMENTS

A recent report utilising data from 399 athletes from 21 different nationalities and 28 different sports indicated that the frequency of supplement use is similar in Paralympic and able-bodied athlete populations (Graham et al. 2014). Paralympic athletes in this survey identified using a range of products, including nutritional supplements (vitamins, minerals) sports foods (gels, protein powders, sports drinks) and ergogenic aids (such as caffeine and bicarbonate).

All athletes, including Paralympic athletes, are encouraged to meet their nutrient requirements from food. However, there might be circumstances in which nutritional supplementation is warranted. For example, some athletes might need to supplement key micronutrients if their energy budget does not allow for all nutrients to be consumed from food choices.

Minimal research has been conducted on the effect of ergogenic aids on Paralympic athletes. However, it is reasonable to assume that, in the absence of contradictory medical conditions or functionality, similar ergogenic effects are likely. When advising on use of supplements, potential interaction with any medication and health conditions needs to be considered. Timing and doses might need to be adjusted if gastrointestinal function is altered or muscle mass is significantly lower than in able-bodied athletes. It is wise to test individual tolerance and response during training sessions before use in competition.

TRAVEL

Travel is an inevitable and uncomfortable experience for all athletes (see Chapter 21). However, some Paralympic athletes face additional challenges. Airlines typically ask people with impaired mobility to board planes first and exit planes last. This can substantially increase time spent sitting on the plane. Additionally, some athletes choose to limit fluid intake to avoid having to use the toilet or empty a catheter during a flight. It is useful to prepare a fluid intake plan for flights to minimise dehydration.

Large events such as Paralympic Games and world championships typically cater well for athletes with myriad disabilities. However, modification might be needed when eating at venues unfamiliar with Paralympic athletes. Trays are useful for athletes in wheelchairs when eating buffet-style, although they are not always available. Food serveries are typically at an inconvenient height for people in wheelchairs; this might cause some athletes to avoid dishes towards the back of the servery, as they are difficult to access. Support staff need to look out for challenges and request modifications if required (for example, a temporary servery set up on a lower table, or pre-plated meals). As some Paralympic athletes need to modify eating times according to their gastrointestinal tolerance, provision of takeaway containers is useful to allow flexibility for when meals are consumed.

SUMMARY AND KEY MESSAGES

After reading this chapter, you should have an awareness of the athlete diversity in Paralympic sports. Paralympic athletes compete in a wide range of events and with wide-ranging functionality. Some Paralympic athletes have very similar needs to athletes competing in corresponding able-bodied events. Others require bespoke modifications to suit their individual characteristics. As research regarding the nutritional requirements of Paralympic athletes is limited, an individual approach to nutrition planning should be used along with a trial and modification process to determine optimal nutrition support.

Key messages
- Paralympic athletes compete in a diverse mix of sports and have diverse physiological requirements—there are no generic nutrition recommendations for Paralympic athletes.
- Limited research is available regarding nutritional requirements for Paralympic athletes.

- Athletes with SCI are more likely to have altered heat regulation, gastrointestinal tolerance and increased illness risk compared to other Paralympic athletes.
- Theoretically, ergogenic aids should have similar effects in Paralympic athletes; however, individual testing and adjustment is needed.
- Sports dietitians working with Paralympic athletes need to work closely with other support staff (medicine, physiotherapy, physiology) to fully understand the requirements of each individual.

REFERENCES

Blauwet, C.A., Brook, E.M., Tenforde, A.S. et al., 2017, 'Low energy availability, menstrual dysfunction, and low bone mineral density in individuals with a disability: implications for the para athlete population', *Sports Medicine*, vol. 47, no. 9, pp. 1697–708.

Compton, S., Trease, L., Cunningham, C. et al., 2015, 'Australian Institute of Sport and the Australian Paralympic Committee position statement: Urinary tract infection in spinal cord injured athletes', *British Journal of Sports Medicine*, vol. 49, no. 19, pp. 1236–40.

Graham, T., Perret, C., Crosland, J. et al., 2014, *Nutritional Supplement Habits and Perceptions of Disabled Athletes*, World Anti-Doping Agency, <www.wada-ama.org/sites/default/files/resources/.../tolfrey-final-2012-en_0.pdf>, accessed 28 June 2017.

Johnson, B.F., Mushett, C.A., Richter, D.O. et al., 2014, *Sport for Athletes with Physical Disabilities: Injuries and Medical Issues*, USA: BlazeSports America, <www.blazesports.org/wp-content/.../BSA-Injuries-and-Medical-Issues-Manual.pdf>, accessed 28 June 2017.

Price, M.J., 2016, 'Preparation of Paralympic athletes: Environmental concerns and heat acclimation', *Frontiers in Physiology*, vol. 6, p. 415.

CHAPTER 21

Travelling athletes

Shona L. Halson, Georgia Romyn and Michelle Cort

Most athletes are required to undertake significant travel for competition. This can have consequences for both physiological and psychological status and has the potential to impair performance. Nutrition is one aspect of travel which requires careful planning to minimise the risk of illness and to ensure nutritional goals are met. Obtaining adequate sleep when travelling (especially if crossing multiple time zones) can also be problematic for many athletes, and there is emerging evidence that nutrition may influence sleep quality and quantity and, therefore, may be useful to the travelling athlete. The influence of carbohydrate, protein (tryptophan), alcohol and caffeine may be important to consider when managing travel and jet lag in athletes. This chapter will discuss the key nutrition-related considerations for travel, including jet lag, training and competition schedule, accommodation and meal arrangements, availability of food and drink at destination, hygiene issues, climate and venue facilities.

LEARNING OUTCOMES

Upon completion of this chapter you will be able to:
- understand the causes and consequences of jet lag
- identify strategies to minimise travel fatigue and jet lag
- plan, prepare and execute effective travel nutrition

- identify some of the nutritional issues athletes face when travelling
- understand why sleep is important to athletes
- identify strategies to enhance sleep
- understand how nutrition may influence sleep.

JET LAG AND THE IMPACT OF TRAVEL ON PERFORMANCE

The competition and training schedules of elite athletes often require them to undertake frequent long-haul air travel that negatively affects the **sleep–wake cycle**. Accordingly, air travel can interrupt training schedules and increase the physiological and perceptual loads of athletes prior to competition (Fowler et al. 2014). With performance often required within days of arrival in a new time zone, it is important to develop a plan to combat the detrimental effects of sleep disruption, **circadian process desynchronisation** and travel fatigue so athletes can return to optimal performance as soon as possible. This will reduce the days lost to training following travel and may help to optimise competition readiness and performance.

Sleep–wake cycle
Also known as circadian rhythm, a daily pattern that determines when it is time to sleep and when it is time to be awake.

Circadian process desynchronisation
Disruption of the sleep–wake cycle/circadian rhythm.

Jet lag is associated with rapid travel across time zones, such as flying east to west or west to east on an aeroplane (transmeridian travel). Circadian processes influence the physiological, mental and behavioural changes that occur daily on approximately 24-hour cycles. When circadian processes do not correspond with the external environment jet lag symptoms occur, and the severity of jet lag increases with the number of time zones crossed. The primary symptoms of jet lag are difficulty initiating and maintaining sleep at night, daytime sleepiness, impaired physical and mental performance, poor mood, appetite suppression and gastrointestinal complaints (Waterhouse et al. 2004).

Jet lag
A physiological condition experienced when circadian processes do not correspond with the new external environment.

Jet lag is not experienced with north-to-south or south-to-north long-haul travel as no time zones are crossed. However, this travel still involves exposure to mild **hypoxia**, cabin noise and cramped and uncomfortable conditions; some athletes may also experience anxiety (Youngstedt & O'Connor 1999). This leads to travel fatigue and sleep disruption, contributing to decreases in aerobic performance, reaction time, concentration, alertness, skill acquisition, mood, immune function, tissue regeneration and appetite regulation (Youngstedt & O'Connor 1999). A study of northbound long-haul travel on sleep quality and subjective jet lag in professional

Hypoxia
Deficiency in the amount of oxygen reaching the tissues.

soccer players found that sleep was disrupted due to flight and competition scheduling, causing travel fatigue (Fowler et al. 2015).

MINIMISING TRAVEL STRESS

Jet lag and travel fatigue are of concern to athletes as they can compromise physical and cognitive performance. Sleep hygiene recommendations before, during and after the flight may help alleviate the negative effects of travel on sleep. Under normal circumstances, internal circadian processes respond to external cues from the outside environment. These cues are called **zeitgebers** and the most influential is sunlight and the light–dark cycle. Food, exercise, sleep and pharmacological interventions that mimic hormones involved in circadian processes are also zeitgebers but are generally weaker than sunlight.

Zeitgebers
External or environmental cues which synchronises our biological rhythms to the Earth's 24-hour light–dark cycle.

One potential strategy to minimise jet lag is to use exposure to, and avoidance of, bright light. While natural sunlight has powerful phase-shifting properties, some laboratory-based research suggests that correct timing of artificial/indoor light exposure and avoidance can also be used to facilitate adaptation to a new time zone (Fowler et al. 2015). More research on the impact of scheduled artificial bright light exposure and avoidance on circadian process resynchronisation following long-haul aeroplane travel is required.

Melatonin is a hormone produced by the body at night, or under dark conditions, that signals night-time to the body. In normal circumstances, melatonin is secreted into the bloodstream between about 9 p.m. and 7 a.m. (Waterhouse et al. 2004), in line with the timing of the innate drive to sleep. Melatonin has several effects on the body, including dilation of blood vessels on the skin, which increases heat loss from the body, subsequently causing the drop in core body temperature required for sleep (Waterhouse et al. 2004). In the absence of melatonin, heat loss and the subsequent drop in core body temperature are affected and sleep onset and quality will be negatively impacted. Normally, melatonin is released in the body from approximately two hours before bedtime, provided there is limited light exposure at this time. When circadian processes are desynchronised with the external environment, melatonin secretion is incorrectly timed; this is one of the primary reasons for sleep disruption when jet-lagged. Therefore, melatonin may be used to treat jet lag, although the timing of ingestion is highly specific and individual. The dose of melatonin is also highly individual and, if the dose is too high, melatonin may remain in the bloodstream too long and act at the wrong time. Additionally, melatonin should be administered with caution in athletes as it is considered a medication, can only be prescribed by a doctor, is not readily available, and, in many cases, must be provided by a compound pharmacist.

It has been found that exercise lasting one to three hours can induce significant circadian phase shifts. Time of day at which exercise is completed, intensity of exercise, lighting conditions and age and gender of participants are complicating factors. Furthermore, most previous research in this area has been conducted on elderly patients, a population vastly different to elite athletes. However since athletes are highly likely to engage in training before and after travel, there is potential to schedule this training at the times most likely to correctly adjust circadian processes.

The strategies below may be used to minimise travel fatigue.

Box 21.1: Strategies to minimise travel fatigue

BEFORE TRAVEL

Sleep
- Sleep should be prioritised.
- Aim for at least eight hours of sleep per night in the two weeks leading up to travel.
- Bedtime and wake time should be kept consistent to give the best opportunity for good-quality sleep.
- Do not stay awake late at night before an early morning flight.

Planning
- Avoid intense training the day before and the day of travel to minimise muscle damage before flying.
- If possible, schedule long-haul flights to arrive at the destination late in the day so that the athlete does not need to stay awake all day before sleeping overnight.
- Book an aisle row or exit row to give more space and comfort, especially if the athlete is tall.
- Pack what is needed to be comfortable, such as a travel pillow, eye mask, earplugs, noise-cancelling headphones and blankets.
- Plan to bring entertainment.
- Pack as much as you can in advance and try not to leave this to the last minute.

Nutrition
- Fill your water bottle (after boarding) and drink enough water to stay hydrated.
- Does travel food meet your nutritional needs? Pack your own food for your flight and for the duration of your trip if required. Choose foods that fit with your nutrition plan for the current

phase of training and competition; be mindful of carbohydrate and protein foods to maintain requirements.

Compression
- Put medical-grade compression socks on before the flight and wear them during the flight and for as long as possible after the flight. Compression socks reduce swelling and promote blood flow, reducing the risk of developing deep-vein thrombosis (DVT) and helping you feel better on arrival.
- DO NOT wear compression tights or tops, as these will not stop swelling in the hands and feet.

DURING TRAVEL
Airport and flight
- Arrive with plenty of time to check in, get through security and board without rushing.
- At check-in, ask for the seat you want (aisle, window, exit row).
- Once on the plane, ask if there are any spare seats or rows you can move to to stretch out after take-off.
- Ask when meals will be served so you can plan when you will sleep.
- Adjust your watch to the destination time.

Sleep
- Sleep as much as possible. Spread out where possible and get comfortable. Use ear plugs, noise-cancelling headphones, eye shades and neck pillows to improve sleep and comfort during travel.
- ANY sleep/rest is beneficial! Take what you can get.

Aeroplane exercises
- Athletes may suffer from DVT due to injuries, bruises and damaged muscles.
- Complete stretching, self-massage and light exercises every 1–2 hours (when awake) to increase blood flow and promote relaxation.

Hydration and nutrition
- Drink enough fluid to stay hydrated. If possible, eat meals at the time you will at the destination. To help avoid disruption to sleep, avoid large amounts of caffeine (<1 cup of coffee per four hours) and stop drinking coffee, cola and other caffeinated beverages before 4 p.m.

AFTER TRAVEL

Compression
- Wear your compression socks for at least 1–2 hours (or as long as possible) after the flight. You may remove compression socks to do hydrotherapy or before sleeping at night.

Hydrotherapy
- If possible, use contrast showers (alternate between hot and cold water) or ideally a pool or beach hydrotherapy session on arrival to help reduce physiological stress.

Nutrition
- Avoid caffeine in the afternoon and evening.

The strategies listed below can be used to minimise jet lag.

Box 21.2: Strategies to minimise the effects of jet lag

SLEEP
- Prioritise sleep at night in the new time zone.
- Get to bed early and, if possible, sleep in the following morning.
- If you arrive early in the day, and feel you will not make it through the day without sleep, have a short (<90 minute) nap in the early afternoon.

LIGHT EXPOSURE
- Get outside and seek daylight in the new time zone. This can be coupled with some light exercise and stretching.

NUTRITION
- Eat meals at the usual time of day.

EXERCISE
- If possible, train at the time of day that you will be competing.

NUTRITION AND TRAVEL

Travel can heighten the risk of an athlete being unable to meet their nutrition goals or developing an illness. Unfortunately, this is often at a time when the outcomes

Table 21.1. An example of a travel nutrition risk management audit

Risk	Risk management strategy in place?	Further strategy development required?	Level of risk?	Level of risk with strategy in place?
Example: Unknown food supply on flight	Call airline and discuss food provided.	Plan to take own snacks on board if airline cannot provide special meal.	Moderate	Low

of training preparation and competition performance are of greatest importance. Athletes should seek personalised advice, as nutrition recommendations vary and will be specific to each destination and athlete.

Planning

Preparation prior to departure can mitigate many of these risks to performance and health. One strategy that is useful for athletes and support staff to undertake well in advance of departure is a travel nutrition 'risk management audit'.

Several questions must be answered within this audit, the first being, what are the risks to successful performance at the destination? Each 'risk' then needs to be further explored and a risk management strategy put in place. Table 21.1 shows an example of the audit process.

It is often useful to talk to other athletes, staff and coaches who have travelled to the destination previously. Their experiences can highlight issues that need to be considered during planning.

A timeline for strategy development and execution, along with allocation of roles and responsibilities, then needs to be developed.

Considerations that should be incorporated into the planning process include:
- itinerary
- training and competition schedule
- type of accommodation and meal arrangements
- familiarity with the destination—food and drink availability, hygiene issues, climate
- local dietary habits (for example, timing of meals)
- food and fluids provided by competition management/organisers
- distance between accommodation and training/competition venue(s)
- venue facilities (safe water supply, refrigerators, etc.).

An athlete's specific nutrition goals need to be central to all planning. While some adaptability will be needed, a nutrition action plan for training and competition days should be made before departure so that major issues are avoided.

Common travel nutrition issues

Many of the common nutrition-related issues experienced by athletes who travel are presented in the following section, along with suggestions for how these issues could be mitigated.

Flights

A number of stresses can take place in transit that are independent of the time zones crossed.

Dry, pressurised air in the cabin of an airplane results in a need for increased fluid intake during flight. This is especially the case for long-haul flights, where significant dehydration could occur.

- Carry an empty water bottle and use the onboard taps (located near the flight attendant stations) to refill.
- Request additional fluids beyond those provided at meal services (these are invariably very small containers).
- Alcohol can contribute to dehydration and avoidance should be considered.
- Caffeine-containing fluids are a suitable choice to add to fluid balance if they are a regular part of an athlete's diet.

Food supplied by airlines does not always meet the nutrition requirements of an athlete.

- Airlines tend to provide a limited range of foods. Special requests can be made, but airlines may not be able to meet an athlete's requirements.
- Special meal requests to airlines should be made well in advance of flights.
- Athletes should take their own snacks on board. These are useful if the food provided does not meet requirements, or if unexpected delays occur.
- If an athlete's energy requirements are high, they should take high-kilojoule snacks onboard to snack on, such as trail mix, muesli or energy bars.
- Alternatively, if the athlete has low energy needs they will need to be wary of snacking due to boredom. Taking some sugar-free chewing gum and drinking low-energy (kJ) fluids, such as water, can be a useful strategy to overcome this temptation.

Travel by road

If travelling via car or bus it is advisable to pack a small cooler or lunchbox with meals or snacks and fluids to ensure appropriate items are on hand. This will also be a more economical option than relying on over-priced service station items.

Illness

Gastrointestinal infections related to travelling are frequent among athletes and are often food- and fluid-borne.

- Education of athletes and support staff before travel is required.
- Many infections can be prevented by taking care with food and fluid choices, along with personal hygiene.
- Avoiding the local water supply in countries where potential pathogens could be consumed in this manner is essential. Care should be taken to avoid ice in drinks and to avoid brushing teeth with local water. Drinks should be consumed from sealed containers only.
- Beware that salads and peeled fruit may have been washed in local, contaminated water and are best avoided unless you are sure that they are safe.
- Unpasteurised dairy products should be avoided.
- Care should be taken to only eat meals that are either served very hot or cold.
- Using probiotics and prebiotics (see Chapter 23) both prior to departure and during the travel period can help minimise the risk of certain infections.

Additional food supplies

Packing a supply of food and sports foods from home will be useful if the food supply (type, quality, safety) is unknown, the athlete is a fussy eater, or if they rely on specific products around training sessions and competitions.

Always check ahead with customs/quarantine authorities to identify what foods are restricted.

Environment

An athlete's nutrition needs may be different at the destination due to the environment (for example, due to altitude or heat; see Chapter 22).

Develop a plan to counter any negative effects of these changes before leaving home.

Eating out

Eating out can be tricky in terms of meeting nutrition requirements.

- Try to check out menus online before selecting a restaurant.
- Special dietary needs should be organised ahead of time.
- If travelling with large groups of athletes, calling ahead and arranging for a certain number of specific meals to be ready to serve can help reduce wait times.

Buffets

Buffets offer a large variety of foods and it is easy to eat more than required in this setting.

- It is important that the athlete is familiar with their own nutrition goals.
- Athletes should be encouraged to do 'a lap' of the buffet or dining hall to gauge what is on the menu before plating their own meal.
- The athlete should be selective with their choices rather than taking some of everything on offer.
- Leaving the dining area as soon as the meal has been consumed helps to prevent the temptation to go back for more.

Self-catering

Staying in apartments that have cooking facilities allows for flexibility in meal times and food options.

- Using an online shopping service can be useful if ordering large quantities (for example, when cooking or ordering for a whole squad).
- Having 'go-to' recipes that require few ingredients and minimal cooking equipment (often sparse in rented accommodation) is suggested.

Hydration

Monitoring hydration using morning body weight or with urine specific gravity testing is advisable, especially after long-haul flights or in hot climates.

- In hot and humid countries and sporting venues, sweat rates can be significant.
- Regular body weights of individual athletes before and after exercise sessions are useful to determine hydration status.
- Drinking large volumes of water, especially during hard exercise, may lead to hyponatraemia. Use of a sports drink or electrolyte drink can help to address this problem.

Sleep

Sleep is increasingly recognised as one of the critical foundations of an athlete's training program. Sleep is considered the best recovery strategy available to athletes due to its physical and psychological restorative effects. Getting a good night's sleep can decrease injury risk, improve reaction time, coordination, concentration, memory, learning, motivation, mood and immunity and increase performance. Sleep also aids the repair and regeneration of muscles and tissues due to important hormonal release (growth hormone in particular) that occurs during sleep (Halson 2014).

Sleep studies with training athletes are an emerging area of research, and most studies have found that athletes have poorer-quality sleep and less time asleep than is recommended (Lastella et al. 2015; Leeder et al. 2012; Sargent et al. 2014). This effect is likely exacerbated by long-haul or frequent travel. Given the importance of sleep and the poor quality and amount of sleep experienced by many athletes, strategies to enhance sleep should be considered (see Box 21.3).

Box 21.3: Strategies for a good night's sleep

BEDROOM
- The bedroom should be cool (19–21°C is best), dark, quiet and comfortable.
- The bed and pillows used are important. They should be supportive and requirements will vary according to individual physical attributes.

ROUTINE
- Create a good sleep routine by going to bed at the same time and waking up at the same time every day (or as often as possible).
- A before-bed routine can help the body prepare for sleep. The routine should start about 30 minutes before bedtime and be consistent. This may include activities such as cleaning teeth and reading a book.

ELECTRONICS
- Avoid watching television or using smartphones/computers in bed. These can steal sleep time and form bad habits.

AVOID WATCHING THE CLOCK
- Many people who struggle with sleep tend to watch the clock too much.
- Frequently checking the clock during the night can wake you up (especially if you turn on the light to read the time) and may reinforce negative thoughts.

GET UP AND TRY AGAIN
- If you haven't been able to get to sleep after about 20 minutes, get up and do something calming or boring until you feel sleepy, then return to bed and try again.
- Sit quietly on the couch with the lights off (bright light will tell your brain that it is time to wake up).

FOOD AND FLUID
- Avoid the use of caffeinated food and fluids later in the day.
- Do not go to bed after consuming too much fluid; this may result in waking up to use the bathroom.

BE ORGANISED
- Utilise a 'to-do' list or diary to ensure organisation and prevent unnecessary over-thinking while trying to sleep.

RELAX
- Investigate relaxation or breathing techniques.

NUTRITION AND SLEEP

Although our knowledge of how nutrition impacts sleep is still somewhat sparse, it is an area of growing interest to researchers and athletes alike. Some nutrition strategies are known to impact both sleep onset and quality, and can be manipulated by athletes to achieve improved sleep outcomes.

Several brain neurotransmitters are associated with the sleep–wake cycle. Specific nutrition interventions can act on these neurotransmitters to influence sleep (Halson 2014). The rate of synthesis and function of the neurotransmitter 5-HT (which in turn stimulates the production of melatonin), is influenced by the availability of its precursor tryptophan (Grimmett & Sillence 2005). Tryptophan is an amino acid found in foods such as eggs, meat, poultry and dairy products.

Tryptophan must be transported across the blood–brain barrier for it to have its sleep-inducing impact, and carbohydrate is needed to support this process. Therefore, a drink, snack or meal that contains both tryptophan and carbohydrate could help induce sleep. Popular sleep-inducing snack options include a milk drink, yoghurt or tuna and crackers.

Alcohol may also help a person feel sleepy and fall asleep more quickly. However, once alcohol levels in the blood fall, sleep is disrupted and the amount of quality sleep is reduced (Ebrahim et al. 2013). Athletes should be made aware of this so that an informed choice around alcohol consumption can be made.

Caffeine has a role in the performance plan of many athletes, as well as being a regular feature in many athletes' habitual eating plans. Given caffeine can delay an athlete's natural signals to go to sleep, its use as an ergogenic aid in sport needs to be carefully planned. The athlete should identify the dose and timing of caffeine required to maximise performance and minimise sleep disturbances by trialling caffeine intake strategies in training (see Chapter 12).

SUMMARY AND KEY MESSAGES

Effective planning and preparation for travel in elite athletes is essential to optimise performance and reduce the risk of illness. Reducing the symptoms of jet lag can aid in reducing training days lost due to travel. Through careful planning and execution of travel, nutrition and sleep strategies, it is possible to minimise some of the negative influences of travel in athletes. This may have a positive influence on health, wellbeing, mood and, importantly, performance.

Key messages

- Jet lag can result in physiological and psychological symptoms that may impair performance.
- Light, exercise, caffeine and melatonin may be used to manage jet lag, although these need to be used with caution.
- Strategies such as sleep, planning, nutrition, exercise and compression garments can be used before and during travel to manage travel fatigue and jet lag.
- Nutritional considerations such as nutrition provisions in transit, food and fluid safety (hygiene), meal availability at the destination and food and fluid provided by the training or competition venue are important.
- Destination eating options (eating out, buffets and self-catering) have issues that need to be planned for prior to travel.
- Monitoring hydration after travel is recommended.
- Optimal sleep is important for athletes' performance as well as managing jet lag.
- The role of nutrition in enhancing sleep is likely to become an important area of future focus.

REFERENCES

Ebrahim, I.O., Shapiro, C.M., Williams, A.J. et al., 2013, 'Alcohol and sleep I: Effects on normal sleep', *Alcoholism: Clinical and Experimental Research*, vol. 37, no. 4, pp. 539–49.

Fowler, P., Duffield, R., Howle K. et al., 2014, 'Effects of northbound long-haul international air travel on sleep quality and subjective jet lag and wellness in professional Australian soccer players', *International Journal of Sports Physiology and Performance*, vol. 10, no. 2, pp. 648–54.

Fowler, P., Duffield, R., Morrow, I. et al., 2015, 'Effects of sleep hygiene and artificial bright light interventions on recovery from simulated international air travel', *European Journal of Applied Physiology*, vol. 115, no. 3, pp. 541–53.

Grimmett, A. & Sillence, M.N., 2005, 'Calmatives for the excitable horse: A review of L-tryptophan', *The Veterinary Journal*, vol. 170, no. 1, pp. 24–32.

Halson, S.L., 2014, 'Sleep in elite athletes and nutritional interventions to enhance sleep', *Sports Medicine*, vol. 44, suppl. 1, pp. S13–23.

Lastella, M., Roach, G.D., Halson, S.L. et al., 2015, 'Sleep/wake behaviours of elite athletes from individual and team sports', *European Journal of Sport Science*, vol. 15, no. 2, pp. 94–100.

Leeder, J., Glaister, M., Pizzoferro, K. et al., 2012, 'Sleep duration and quality in elite athletes measured using wristwatch actigraphy', *Journal of Sports Sciences*, vol. 30, no. 6, pp. 541–5.

Sargent, C., Lastella, M., Halson, S.L. et al., 2014, 'The impact of training schedules on the sleep and fatigue of elite athletes', *Chronobiology International*, vol. 31, no. 10, pp. 1160–68.

Waterhouse, A.J., Reilly, T. & Edwards, B., 2004, 'The stress of travel', *Journal of Sport Sciences*, vol. 22, no. 10, pp. 946–66.

Youngstedt, S.D. & O'Connor, P.J., 1999, 'The influence of air travel on athletic performance', *Sports Medicine*, vol. 28, no. 3, pp. 197–207.

CHAPTER 22

Environmental and climate considerations for athletes

Alan McCubbin

With the increasing connectedness of our planet, humans have found themselves testing their physical limits in almost every corner of the globe. A soccer player can find themselves in the searing heat of the Australian summer, or walking out into a snow-covered stadium in Europe. A triathlete can train all winter in the southern hemisphere, then fly halfway around the world to compete in the heat and humidity of Hawaii. There are also people exercising in environments where oxygen is in limited supply—explorers trekking to the peaks of the highest mountains, and those deliberately training at actual or simulated altitude.

Understanding the impact of environment on exercise physiology and nutrition requirements is crucial in helping athletes stay healthy and perform at their best. This chapter will explore the effects of heat and humidity, cold, altitude and hypoxia on the body during exercise, and nutritional strategies used to optimise performance in these environments.

LEARNING OUTCOMES

Upon completion of this chapter you will be able to:

- understand the impact of heat, cold, altitude and hypoxia on the body during exercise
- describe the effect of environmental extremes on nutritional requirements
- identify the challenges of maintaining optimal nutritional intake in extreme environments
- develop practical nutrition strategies to optimise athletic performance in different environmental conditions.

HEAT, HUMIDITY AND EXERCISE

Conduction
The transfer of heat from one object to another through contact. Heat is transferred from the warmer to the cooler object.

Convection
The transfer of heat through the movement of warmer liquids or gases towards areas that are cooler, usually due to air or water flow over the skin. The greater the flow of air or water, the greater the heat transfer.

Radiation
The transfer of heat through any medium, without contact, using thermal or infrared radiation.

Evaporation
Sweat from the surface of the skin accounts for the majority of heat transfer during exercise. The rate of sweating can increase significantly during exercise to increase the amount of evaporation and, therefore, the amount of heat transferred from the body.

During exercise, the production of energy for muscle contraction also produces heat as a by-product. This heat accumulates and causes a rise in core body temperature. Human body temperature is regulated within a narrow range; lower than 35°C or higher than 40°C places an individual at risk of serious health complications. Therefore, the heat produced during exercise must be dissipated into the environment to prevent core body temperature rising to dangerous levels. Initially, heat produced by the working muscles is transferred to the blood. The blood is preferentially circulated to the skin, so heat can exchange with the surrounding environment. Heat exchange occurs via several processes, including **conduction**, **convection** and **radiation** from the skin, and **evaporation** of fluid in the lungs and of sweat on the skin surface.

It is not surprising that heat exchange is less effective in hot and humid environments, resulting in higher core body temperatures for the same exercise bout. For example, when two hours of moderate intensity (60 per cent VO_{2max}) treadmill running was performed in 35°C, rectal temperature rose 2.4°C from the start to finish of the exercise bout. The same exercise performed in 22°C caused a rise of only 1.4°C (Snipe et al. 2018).

Exercise performance in hot and humid environments

Exercise performance in one-off sprint events is usually improved in hot weather, whereas performance in prolonged efforts or repeated sprint efforts (such as in team sports) is reduced (see Figure 22.1) (Guy et al. 2015). The exact mechanisms by which

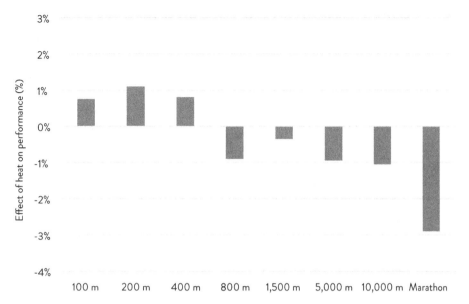

Figure 22.1. Effect of heat (<25°C compared to >25°C) for running events in IAAF World Championship events held between 1999 and 2011

Source: Data from Guy et al. 2015 (Note: average of male and female data; positive effects indicate faster finish time; negative effects indicate slower finish times).

heat affects prolonged exercise performance are not well understood, but it is known that increased core temperature limits performance and increases the body's perceived level of effort at any given exercise intensity. Exercising in the heat reduces activity of working muscles, resulting in less power generated, even before core temperature begins to rise (Tucker et al. 2004). When core body temperature does rise, sweat glands also become increasingly active, increasing the rate of sweating. This results in greater losses of fluid and electrolytes, particularly sodium and chloride. While electrolyte losses are not believed to negatively impact on performance, dehydration from the loss of fluid is well established as a performance-limiting factor. For more information on hydration and performance, refer to Chapter 11.

Athletes in sports where significant metabolic heat is generated usually produce better performances in cooler and less humid conditions. For example, an increase from 23°C to 32°C reduced power output by 6.5 per cent in elite road cyclists (Tatterson 2000). The optimal temperature chosen by scientists supporting the Nike Breaking 2 project (an attempt to break the two-hour barrier for the marathon) was 7–12°C, in order to maximise heat exchange. An increase in relative humidity from 24 per cent to 80 per cent reduced the time cyclists could ride to exhaustion at 70 per cent VO_{2max} by 22 minutes, even when the temperature remained constant (Maughan et al. 2012).

Health consequences of exercising in hot and humid environments

More concerning is the potential health consequences of exercise in hot and humid environments. Heat exhaustion occurs when significant dehydration has caused a reduction in circulating blood volume and blood pressure. Symptoms including nausea and vomiting, rapid heart rate, significant fatigue, dizziness or fainting are associated with core body temperatures lower than 40°C. If core body temperature exceeds 40°C, **exertional heat stroke** is more likely. This is a potentially life-threatening condition in which the central nervous system, major organ systems and skeletal muscles can be affected. Rapid cooling and urgent medical attention are required in this scenario.

Because the rise in core body temperature causes a significant shift of blood flow to the skin, there is a proportional reduction in blood flow to other organs, including the gastrointestinal tract. In addition, exercise in the heat increases the body's **sympathetic nervous system** activity. Because of both these factors, exercising in the heat has been shown to significantly increase the risk of both gastrointestinal symptoms and intestinal damage, known as **exercise-induced gastrointestinal syndrome** (Snipe et al. 2018). In some cases, it is believed that intestinal damage and the resulting immune system response is a major contributor to exertional heat stroke. For more information on exercise-induced gastrointestinal syndrome, refer to Chapter 23.

Although dehydration is an obvious potential consequence of exercise in the heat, what is less intuitive is an increased risk of **exercise-associated hyponatraemia** (EAH), which is typically caused by fluid overload and dilution of blood sodium concentration. This may be due partially to fluid retention, because the blood plasma volume expands during exercise in the heat. But EAH has also been shown to occur in situations where an individual deliberately consumes large amounts of fluid during exercise for fear of dehydration, often above thirst and at a rate equal to or greater than sweat losses. It is also believed that, while less common, there are cases of hyponatraemia that have developed from large, unreplaced sweat sodium losses, without over-hydration (Hew-Butler et al. 2015). Regardless of the cause, the consequences of EAH are severe. Fluid can accumulate around the

Exertional heat stroke
An elevated core temperature associated with signs of organ system failure due to overheating.

Sympathetic nervous system
Often termed the fight or flight response. It accelerates heart rate, dilates bronchial passages, decreases motility of the digestive tract, constricts blood vessels, increases sweating.

Exercise-induced gastrointestinal syndrome
A term used to describe disruption to the structure and function of the gastrointestinal tract during exercise. This can result in gastrointestinal symptoms during exercise. Physical damage can also occur to the gut lining, allowing movement of bacteria and their by-products from the gut into the bloodstream. This causes a significant response from the immune system, which can further raise core body temperature, increasing the risk of exertional heat stroke (Costa et al. 2017).

Exercise-associated hyponatraemia
Also called low blood sodium, and defined as 'hyponatraemia occurring during or up to 24 h after physical activity. It is defined by a serum, plasma or blood sodium concentration ([Na+]) below the normal reference range of the laboratory performing the test. For most laboratories, this is a [Na+] less than 135 mmol/L' (Hew-Butler et al. 2015).

lungs and brain, causing shortness of breath and altered conscious state. To date, at least ten people have died as a result of hyponatraemia, including some exercising in hot environments.

During exercise in hot conditions, electrolyte—particularly sodium—losses are significantly increased compared to cooler conditions. The rate of sweat production increases in the heat, and the sweat sodium concentration itself increases with increasing sweat rate. This occurs because sweat flows faster through the sweat duct to the skin surface, reducing the ability of the duct to reabsorb sodium and chloride and prevent it leaving the body. The total amount of sodium that can be lost during exercise is probably not significant for shorter exercise bouts, even in the heat. A very high rate of sodium loss of 1000 milligrams per hour, for two hours, represents a change in sodium stores of less than three per cent. This is less than the typical sodium losses in a day from urine, and in this case the kidneys simply respond by reducing urinary sodium excretion to compensate. However, in ultra-endurance sports participants can be exercising continuously for ten hours or more. In this case, the total theoretical sodium loss could accumulate to more than 20 per cent of the body's total sodium if not replaced. There is currently no research to show whether sweat glands act to conserve sodium when such a large deficit occurs, but specifically replacing sodium would seem prudent in this scenario. The exact health consequences of large sodium deficits during exercise have not been well studied, but the potential complications include whole-body muscle cramping, exercise-associated hyponatraemia and a loss of bone minerals (Eichner 2008; Hew-Butler et al. 2013; Hew-Butler et al. 2015).

Because of the potentially significant health consequences of exercising in hot environments, many sports have adopted policies to shorten, postpone or cancel events in the event of extreme heat. The Australian Open tennis tournament has an extreme heat policy to move matches indoors and close the stadium roof where possible, at the discretion of match referees. The Cycling Australia Road National Championships in 2018 were shortened, and the mass participation support event cancelled due to temperatures forecast to exceed 40°C. And soccer matches in the A-League and W-League, played during the Australian summer, have been postponed from daytime to evening to reduce the impact of extreme heat, in response to several players vomiting at half-time during matches played in 38°C.

Effect of heat and humidity on nutrient metabolism and nutritional requirements during exercise

The use of carbohydrate for fuel is increased, and fat reduced, during exercise in the heat. In particular, muscle glycogen appears to be the source of increased carbohydrate use, with the use of blood glucose as a fuel not altered by heat exposure. Two potential reasons have been proposed to explain this. Firstly, increased blood flow to the skin and reduced blood flow to muscles results in less oxygen, fatty acids and glucose being delivered, and this may favour the use of fuels already stored in the muscle—particularly carbohydrate, which needs less oxygen for the same ATP output. Secondly, there is often an increase in the hormone epinephrine during exercise in the heat, which has been shown to increase muscle glycogen use as a fuel source. Total oxidation of carbohydrate during exercise is at least 15 per cent greater in the heat than in cooler conditions, with some studies finding greater differences (Hargreaves et al. 1996; Fink et al. 1975).

Heat acclimatisation and acclimation

Heat acclimatisation
The process of adaptation by living and training in a naturally hot environment.

Heat acclimation
The process of adaptation from completing specific training sessions in artificially induced heat, such as a climate chamber or heated room.

The responses already mentioned assume that the person exercising in the heat is not already adapted to hot environments. However, if an athlete undergoes heat **acclimatisation** or **acclimation**, several processes occur that improve the body's ability to transfer heat. These reduce the detrimental effects of heat on performance and health to some extent. Among the range of adaptations that occur over a one- to two-week period of exercising in the heat:

- blood volume expands, increasing stroke volume and reducing heart rate
- skin blood flow increases, improving the ability for heat exchange
- sweating begins at a lower core body temperature, and sweat rate is significantly higher
- sodium and chloride concentrations become significantly lower
- total carbohydrate oxidation is reduced and fat oxidation increased at the same exercise intensity.

Overall, these adaptations result in increased fluid needs but decreased carbohydrate needs compared to someone exercising with no previous heat exposure. Sodium needs are about the same; while the sodium concentration decreases with acclimation, the total volume of sweat produced increases.

Nutritional interventions in the heat

In addition to increased requirements for carbohydrate, fluid and sodium, for which strategies to optimise intake are covered in previous chapters, sports nutrition practitioners have sought to reduce the effect of heat on core body temperature to improve health and performance in the heat. One common method is the use of ice slushies in the 30 minutes before exercise as a pre-cooling strategy. This approach was used by the Australian Institute of Sport in preparation for hot temperatures expected at the 2008 Beijing Olympic Games. Pilot testing showed a reduction of 0.25°C in rectal temperature after consuming 500 grams of an ice slushie made from sports drink, with a 0.6°C reduction after consuming 1000 grams of ice slushy (Ross et al. 2011). This reduction remained constant after warm-up for a simulated cycling time-trial, so that the athlete began exercise at a lower core body temperature. The final strategy used at the Beijing Olympics combined the consumption of an ice slushie and covering the legs in towels that had been soaked in ice-cold water. This reduced core body temperature by 0.72°C, and improved performance in a simulation of the Olympic time-trial by 66 seconds, or 1.3 per cent, compared to drinking 4°C water and not using iced towels (Ross et al. 2011).

Other researchers and practitioners have attempted to use ice slushies or cold water as a cooling strategy during exercise, with some success. Slushies can be given during half-time in some team sports, for example; however, in many sports this is not affordable or practical. Icy-poles can also be used, but the total fluid quantity is usually smaller. As shown in Figure 22.2, large fluid volumes are an important factor in precooling, outweighing the effectiveness of a food that is slightly colder but contains less total fluid.

The effect of cold water has also been investigated as a strategy to reduce the effects of exercise-induced gastrointestinal syndrome. Participants ran at 60 per cent VO_{2max} on a treadmill for two hours in 35°C heat, drinking water at 0.4°C, 7.3°C or 22.1°C. The cold water was successful in reducing rectal temperature but had minimal impact on gastrointestinal symptoms or damage (Snipe & Costa 2018).

Practical issues affecting nutrition in hot and humid environments

Keeping food and fluids cool can be a potential challenge depending on the environment in which exercise is taking place. It is easy to have an ice chest or tub of ice for storing drinks, or electric refrigeration, by the side of a team sport field or racquet sport court. But for longer training sessions, or competitions where the exercise takes place far from a single base of support, keeping food and fluids cool becomes more challenging. In multistage ultramarathons in desert environments, for example, the heating of sports drinks and gels in the sun can make them so unpalatable that athletes no longer consume them (McCubbin et al. 2016). Where practical, partially or completely freezing fluids prior to prolonged exercise can be useful, with fluid being consumed cold as it thaws. Ensuring foods and fluids are shaded from the sun where possible and avoiding direct contact with the body will also prevent heat exchange that warms the food product. Care should also be taken regarding food safety for non-packaged foods consumed during exercise. For example, rice cakes—a mixture of

(a)

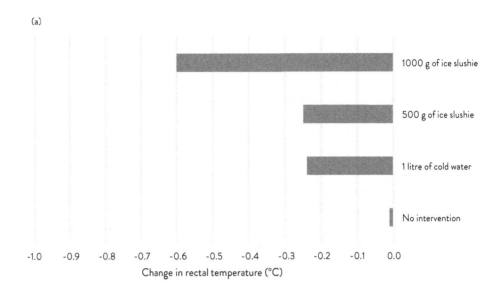

(b)

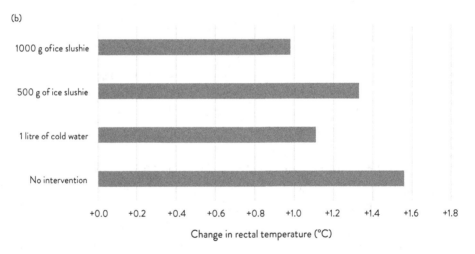

Figure 22.2. Effect of cold water and ice slushie ingestion on rectal temperature: (a) 30 minutes after commencing consumption; (b) following a 30-minute warm-up in preparation for competition

Source: Data from Ross et al. 2011.

cooked and cooled sushi rice combined with other ingredients—is a popular staple among road cyclists but is a high-risk food for contamination, especially on a hot day. Storing them refrigerated as long as possible and consuming early during exercise will minimise the risk of food poisoning.

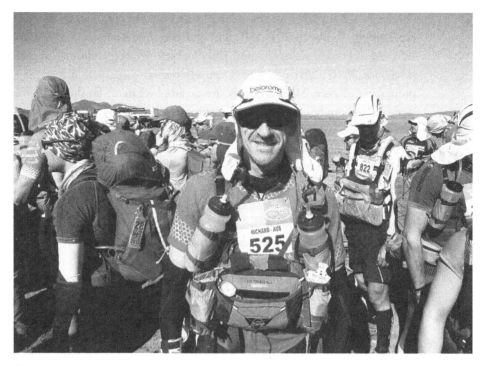

Figure 22.3. Athletes with extra fluid storage at the Marathon des Sables, Morocco

Source: Richard Bettles (used with permission).

As well as food temperature, increased fluid requirements can create a challenge in ensuring adequate fluid is available to athletes. The requirement to carry all food and fluids in desert ultramarathons like Marathon des Sables in Morocco can make it difficult to keep items cool and out of the sun. In addition, the amount of protective clothing (including gaiters around the ankles to prevent sand entering a runner's shoes) reduces the ability to transfer heat away from the body. With an understanding of an athlete's expected fluid losses, enough fluid can be organised to meet their expected needs.

COLD ENVIRONMENTS AND NUTRITION REQUIREMENTS DURING EXERCISE

Exercise in environments near or below freezing temperatures presents another challenge for athletes, whether specifically participating in snow sports or not. Energy requirements can increase in very cold weather, particularly if skin and core body temperature cannot be maintained either through protective clothing or heat production from exercise

(Meyer et al. 2011). The weight of additional protective clothing can also increase energy expenditure (Ocobock 2016). If skin and core body temperature is allowed to fall, shivering can occur, which can more than double energy expenditure compared to resting (Ocobock 2016), although this is unlikely during participation in most sports. The proportion of energy that is derived from carbohydrate or fat during exercise does not change significantly in colder weather, provided the exercise is undertaken at sea level. However, many sports undertaken in extreme cold do so at altitude, and this will influence fuel use independent of temperature, as described later in this chapter.

Although sweat rates are often assumed to be lower in cold environments, this may not always be the case. Excessive protective clothing will maintain skin and core body temperature while reducing heat transfer from the skin (O'Brien et al. 1998). Therefore, a lower sweat rate should not be assumed. In addition, increased fluid losses can occur from the lungs in cold weather, due to less moisture being present in the air (O'Brien et al. 1998), and the sensation of thirst can be impaired, reducing the motivation to drink (Meyer et al. 2011). Fluid balance assessment and the calculation of fluid needs should still be undertaken in cold environments, as in any other climatic condition.

As cold environments are usually associated with winter, it is common for athletes in winter sports to be exposed to less sunlight, and have lower vitamin D status, than athletes who train and compete outdoors in the summer months. This is especially true of athletes who travel between northern and southern hemispheres to continue training and competing year-round. For more information on vitamin D status, needs and supplementation, refer to Chapters 5 and 12.

Practical issues affecting nutrition in cold environments

Many of the impacts of cold environments on nutrition strategies are practical issues. Athletes in cold environments can be reluctant to drink due to the limited availability of toilets and the time and inconvenience of removing several layers of clothing. If thick gloves are worn, dexterity is often reduced, making opening food packaging or using drink bottles more difficult. Wrapping food in aluminium foil that can easily be torn open, and using drink bottles that can be opened with the teeth, can avoid these issues. Some sports foods and fluids also become too hard to chew, and may freeze in cold environments. Storing these close to the body can help keep them warm, and the use of disposable heat packs can prevent food and fluids stored in containers from freezing. Alternative foods that provide carbohydrate, fluid and sodium—such as dried fruit, hot soup, and tea or hot cocoa with added sugar or maltodextrin—can be used, particularly in the immediate pre- and post-exercise period. Hot foods are particularly useful if athletes are required to wait around in the snow with minimal protective clothing, risking hypothermia.

Altitude and hypoxia

Altitude exposure is generally considered to occur at 2000 metres or more above sea level (Thomas et al. 2016). Athletes often exercise at altitude, either as a deliberate training strategy before competing at sea level, or because competition occurs there (as with most snow sports). At altitude, although the percentage of oxygen in the air is the same as at sea level, air is less dense, meaning there are fewer oxygen molecules available. This reduces the amount of oxygen brought into the lungs with each breath. Commercial altitude tents or chambers attempt to simulate altitude while the athlete is at sea level. Although these devices lower the availability of oxygen (as occurs at altitude), they achieve it by filling the space with air that has a lower oxygen percentage, without changing air density.

There are several unique features of exercise at altitude that impact on nutrition. Firstly, fluid losses are greater at altitude, due to both lower humidity and the increased breathing required to deliver the same amount of oxygen to the blood (Thomas et al. 2016). Secondly, because carbohydrate produces energy with less oxygen, there is a shift to more carbohydrate and less fat use for the same exercise bout (Koehle 2014).

Perhaps most importantly, there is an increase in red blood cells as an adaptation to altitude, which is why endurance athletes often use altitude training to improve performance at sea level. This effect, however, draws considerably on iron stores in order to produce haemoglobin for the new blood cells; iron levels will usually fall after two weeks at altitude. It is recommended that athletes travelling to altitude have their iron status checked beforehand, and supplementation provided as required, before the altitude exposure.

SUMMARY AND KEY MESSAGES

After reading this chapter, you should be able to describe the key challenges that athletes face, from both a physiological and practical perspective, in achieving optimal nutritional intake when exercising in environments of extreme heat, cold and altitude.

Key messages

- Exercise in the heat results in a greater increase in core body temperature compared to exercise in cooler conditions.
- Exercise performance in sprint events is often improved or unaffected by heat; however, performance is reduced in more prolonged exercise.
- Elevated core body temperature can lead to heat-related illnesses and increase the risk of exercise-associated hyponatraemia and exercise-induced gastrointestinal syndrome.
- Exercise in the heat increases fluid and sodium losses from sweating and increases the use of muscle glycogen as an energy source.

- Nutrition strategies to improve performance in the heat include pre-cooling with ice slushies or very cold water, ensuring that drinks to be consumed during exercise are kept as cold as possible, and ensuring adequate fluid to meet the athlete's needs.
- Exercise in the cold can increase energy and fluid requirements, and can make the consumption of food and fluids more practically difficult.
- Athletes training and competing in winter year-round are at increased risk of vitamin D deficiency and should be monitored and supplemented as required.
- Altitude exposure increases carbohydrate and fluid requirements, and can draw significantly on iron stores.
- Assessing the iron status of athletes prior to prolonged altitude exposure is important to ensure deficiency does not develop, preventing the beneficial adaptations to training at altitude.

REFERENCES

Costa, R.J.S., Snipe, R.M.J., Kitic, C.M. et al., 2017, 'Systematic review: Exercise-induced gastrointestinal syndrome-implications for health and intestinal disease', *Alimentary Pharmacology & Therapeutics*, vol. 46, no. 3, pp. 246–65.

Eichner, E.R., 2008, 'Genetic and other determinants of sweat sodium', *Current Sports Medicine Reports*, vol. 7, no. 4, pp. S36–40.

Fink, W.J., Costil, D.L. & Van Handel, P.J., 1975, 'Leg muscle metabolism during exercise in the heat and cold', *European Journal of Applied Physiology*, vol. 34, no. 3, pp. 183–90.

Guy, J.H., Deakin, G.B., Edwards, A.M. et al., 2015, 'Adaptation to hot environmental conditions: An exploration of the performance basis, procedures and future directions to optimise opportunities for elite athletes', *Sports Medicine*, vol. 45, no. 3, pp. 303–11.

Hargreaves, M., Angus, D., Howlett, K. et al., 1996, 'Effect of heat stress on glucose kinetics during exercise', *Journal of Applied Physiology*, vol. 81, no. 4, pp. 1594–7.

Hew-Butler, T., Rosner, M.H., Fowkes-Godek, S. et al., 2015, 'Statement of the 3rd International Exercise-Associated Hyponatremia Consensus Development Conference, Carlsbad, California, 2015', *British Journal of Sports Medicine*, vol. 49, no. 22, pp. 1432–46.

Hew-Butler, T., Stuempfle, K.J. & Hoffman, M.D., 2013, 'Bone: An acute buffer of plasma sodium during exhaustive exercise?', *Hormone and Metabolic Research*, vol. 45, no. 10, pp. 697–700.

Koehle, M.S., Cheng, I. & Sporer, B., 2014, 'Canadian Academy of Sport and Exercise Medicine Position Statement: Athletes at high altitude', *Clinical Journal of Sports Medicine*, vol. 24, no. 2, pp. 120–7.

Maughan, R.J., Otani, H. & Watson, P., 2012, 'Influence of relative humidity on prolonged exercise capacity in a warm environment', *European Journal of Applied Physiology*, vol. 112, no. 6, pp. 2313–21.

McCubbin, A.J., Cox, G.R. & Broad, E.M., 2016, 'Case Study: Nutrition planning and intake for Marathon des Sables—A series of five runners', *International Journal of Sport Nutrition & Exercise Metabolism*, vol. 26, no. 6, pp. 581–87.

Meyer, N.L., Manore, M.M. & Helle, C., 2011, 'Nutrition for winter sports', *Journal of Sports Science*, vol. 29, suppl. 1, pp. S127–36.

O'Brien, C.Y., Young, A.J. & Sawka, M.N., 1998, 'Hypohydration and thermoregulation in cold air', *Journal of Applied Physiology*, vol. 84, no. 1, pp. 185–9.

Ocobock, C., 2016, 'Human energy expenditure, allocation, and interactions in natural temperate, hot, and cold environments', *American Journal of Physical Anthropology*, vol. 161, no. 4, pp. 667–75.

Ross, M.L., Garvican, L.A., Jeacocke, N.A. et al., 2011, 'Novel precooling strategy enhances time trial cycling in the heat', *Medicine & Science in Sports & Exercise*, vol. 43, no. 1, pp. 123–33.

Snipe, R.M.J. & Costa, R.J.S., 2018, 'Does the temperature of water ingested during exertional-heat stress influence gastrointestinal injury, symptoms, and systemic inflammatory profile?', *Journal of Science and Medicine in Sport*, vol. 21, no. 8, pp. 771–6.

Snipe, R.M.J., Khoo, A., Kitic, C.M. et al., 2018, 'The impact of exertional-heat stress on gastrointestinal integrity, gastrointestinal symptoms, systemic endotoxin and cytokine profile', *European Journal of Applied Physiology*, vol. 118, no. 2, pp. 389–400.

Tatterson, A.J.H., Hahn, A.G., Martin, D.T. et al., 2000, 'Effects of heat stress on physiological responses and exercise performance in elite cyclists', *Journal of Science and Medicine in Sport*, vol. 3, no. 2, pp. 186–93.

Thomas, D.T., Erdman, K.A. & Burke, L.M., 2016, 'American College of Sports Medicine Joint Position Statement. Nutrition and Athletic Performance', *Medicine & Science in Sports & Exercise*, vol. 48, no. 3, pp. 543–68.

Tucker, R., Rauch, L., Harley, Y.X. et al., 2004, 'Impaired exercise performance in the heat is associated with an anticipatory reduction in skeletal muscle recruitment' *Pflügers Archiv: European Journal of Physiology*, vol. 448, no. 4, pp. 422–30.

CHAPTER 23

Gastrointestinal disturbances in athletes

Dana M. Lis and Stephanie K. Gaskell

We have now established the importance of good nutrition for health and performance. However, for some people gastrointestinal disturbances can impact on their ability to consume a healthy diet and can also have a substantial impact on their exercise performance. This chapter will highlight the prevalence of gastrointestinal disturbances such as bloating, pain and diarrhoea in athletes. The primary causes, modulating factors and common symptoms involved in exercise-associated gastrointestinal disturbances will be discussed alongside nutrition strategies to help manage symptoms.

LEARNING OUTCOMES

Upon completion of this chapter you will be able to:
- appreciate the prevalence rates of gastrointestinal disturbances in athlete populations
- recognise the common symptoms of gastrointestinal disturbances
- understand the primary causes and modulating factors of exercise-associated gastrointestinal disturbances
- identify nutritional strategies to help manage exercise-associated gastrointestinal disturbances.

PREVALENCE OF GASTROINTESTINAL SYMPTOMS

Gastrointestinal symptoms are common, estimated to occur in approximately 30–70 per cent of athletes (Costa et al. 2017), particularly endurance athletes. In events such as ultramarathon running events (>42 kilometres) up to 85 per cent of athletes have reported gastrointestinal symptoms (Costa et al. 2016). In shorter events, serious gastrointestinal symptoms are reported by ~31 per cent of ironman competitors and to a lesser extent in marathon and road cycling races (Pfeiffer et al. 2012). The severity of gastrointestinal symptoms varies and is usually associated with three main triggers: physiological, mechanical and nutritional. Athletes may also be genetically predisposed to experience gastrointestinal symptoms. There are several training and nutrition strategies that can be implemented to reduce the potentially detrimental impact of moderate and more severe gastrointestinal symptoms on training capacity, nutritional intake and performance.

COMMON GASTROINTESTINAL SYMPTOMS

When examining the effects of exercise on organs and system function, the gastrointestinal system is commonly divided into two sections. The upper gastrointestinal section comprises the buccal cavity (mouth), pharynx, oesophagus, stomach and duodenum (beginning of small intestine). The lower gastrointestinal section includes the small intestine (duodenum, jejunum, ileum), where the majority of digestion occurs, and the colon (for more information on the anatomy and physiology of the digestive system, see Chapter 3). In both the upper and lower gastrointestinal areas mechanical forces, altered gastrointestinal blood flow, nutritional intake and **neuroendocrine** changes associated with strenuous endurance exercise can trigger or augment gastrointestinal symptoms.

Neuroendocrine
Relating to interactions between the neural and endocrine system, particularly relating to hormones.

Exercise-associated gastrointestinal symptoms may be experienced during exercise or the few hours afterwards, with the cause not being entirely understood. Symptoms range in severity, type and duration. Preventing and managing symptoms is challenging because episodes of distress are short-lived and difficult to replicate. Most symptom occurrences are reported as mild to moderate in severity with a likely negligible impact on training capacity or performance. Symptoms of greater severity, such as diarrhoea or debilitating cramps during a race, are more likely to have a detrimental effect on athletic performance than is minor bloating. The most commonly monitored and reported symptoms include:

Upper gastrointestinal:
- belching
- bloating

- gastroesophageal reflux disorder (GORD)
- nausea
- vomiting.

Lower gastrointestinal:
- abdominal cramps
- side ache
- flatulence
- urge to defecate
- diarrhoea (runner's trots)
- intestinal bleeding (indicated by blood in the stool).

FUNCTIONAL GASTROINTESTINAL DISORDERS

Several exercise-associated gastrointestinal symptoms are similar to symptoms experienced in functional gastrointestinal disorders (FGIDs). Although FGIDs are primarily managed by clinical dietitians and other relevant medical professionals, a basic understanding of these conditions is important as some athletes may have these conditions, diagnosed or undiagnosed. It is also possible that repeated and persistent stress placed on the gut during strenuous exercise may compromise normal gastrointestinal system functioning resulting in abnormalities similar to FGID.

FGIDs are considered disorders of gut–brain interaction and are classified by a range of recurrent or persistent gastrointestinal symptoms. Diagnosis is made by identification of structural and physiological abnormalities, often presenting in a combination of abnormal intestinal contractions, **visceral hypersensitivity** and alterations in the gut lining, **gut microbiota**, immune function and central nervous system functioning. In clinical settings, psychological therapy such as cognitive behavioural therapy may be a component of the overall FGID treatment plan.

Visceral hypersensitivity
Heightened sensation of pain in the internal organs.

Gut microbiota
Microbe population living in the large intestine.

Irritable bowel syndrome (IBS) is one of the most common FGIDs and is estimated to affect 15 per cent of the Western population. More common in females, IBS is a chronic condition that can occur at any age, with episodes that vary in frequency and severity. Symptoms of IBS may include abdominal pain, bloating, abnormal/delayed bowel movements, constipation or diarrhoea, with no obvious structural or physiological abnormalities in the gut. Several IBS symptoms are very similar to exercise-associated gastrointestinal symptoms such as bloating, cramping and diarrhoea.

PATHOLOGY OF GASTROINTESTINAL SYMPTOMS

Exercise-associated gastrointestinal symptoms are primarily related to physiological, mechanical and nutritional triggers. **Exercise-associated gastrointestinal syndrome** describes the physiological responses and symptoms that occur due to exercise and may subsequently impair gastrointestinal system function. There are two main pathways thought to be involved in this syndrome: **splanchnic hypoperfusion** and neuroendocrine-gastrointestinal changes.

Physiological

Exercise intensity, duration and load

Several physiological changes that occur in the gastrointestinal system during exercise are dependent on exercise intensity. More strenuous and longer-duration exercise generally results in greater alterations in gastrointestinal function and subsequent symptoms. At exercise intensities ranging from 70–80 per cent of maximal intensity or higher, physiological changes such as reduced splanchnic blood flow, impaired nutrient absorption and delayed gastric emptying occur. Damage to the **epithelial barrier** increases permeability, allowing bacterial endotoxins to enter the gut (Dokladny et al. 2016). Gastrointestinal injury can further compromise nutrient absorption, which has been shown in athletes running for one hour at 70 per cent VO_{2max} (Lang et al. 2006). In addition, delayed gastric emptying may reduce intestinal fluid absorption and absorption of nutrients.

Longer endurance events are associated with a higher incidence and severity of gastrointestinal disturbances. Athletes competing in ultra-endurance events, compared with relatively shorter events such as the marathon, report greater rates of gastrointestinal symptoms. For example, in a 24-hour continuous ultramarathon race 85 per cent of participants reported gastrointestinal complaints (Costa et al. 2017). Although methodological differences in studies make it difficult to quantify and compare rates of gastrointestinal symptoms, symptom rates and severity seem to be lower in shorter events. It is important to understand that most symptoms experienced by athletes are minor or moderate and, although uncomfortable, do not have detrimental implications for performance. Severe symptoms may have a more substantial impact on performance.

Gastrointestinal disturbances occur not only in competition but also in training for many athletes, and can compromise their training capacity. Strategies for reducing the

Exercise-associated gastrointestinal syndrome
Describes the physiological responses that occur due to exercise, which may compromise gastrointestinal system function and gastrointestinal barrier integrity and trigger adverse symptoms.

Splanchnic hypoperfusion
Splanchnic circulation refers to blood flow through the stomach, small intestine, colon, pancreas, liver and spleen. Hypoperfusion refers to *low* or *decreased* flow of fluid through the circulatory system. During exercise, blood flow to the splanchnic area (gastrointestinal organs) is decreased and instead shunted to working muscles.

Epithelial barrier
Surface cells lining the gastrointestinal tract.

impact of this are outlined below. However, it is important to consider that athletes with a high training load and multiple training sessions each day may experience recurrent gastrointestinal disturbances. The reason for this may be that the time between strenuous training bouts is less than the 4–5 days required for intestinal epithelial repair. More research is needed to identify whether repeated exercise stress impairs gastrointestinal function in a prolonged manner, or increases susceptibility to dietary triggers.

Splanchnic hypoperfusion

During exercise, particularly endurance-type exercise at higher intensity, blood flow is redistributed to the working muscles and away from the gastrointestinal organs. Blood flow to the gut can be reduced by up to 80 per cent during strenuous exercise (Rehrer et al. 2001), which causes epithelial barrier injury and increased permeability. Further, alterations in the movement of endotoxins across the epithelial barrier can initiate an inflammatory response.

Factors that contribute to splanchnic hypoperfusion include:

- exercise intensity
- duration of exercise
- dehydration during exercise
- heat stress.

Neuroendocrine

Exercise stress activates the sympathetic nervous system—this is the part of the nervous system that initiates the fight-or-flight response, in which blood flow is shunted from the gastrointestinal tract to working muscles. This then activates the neuroendocrine-gastrointestinal pathway, where hormones are secreted that impact on gut function. There is an increase in stress hormone secretion, which may alter gut motility and function. An important interplay between exercise-associated stress response and gut microbiota is increasingly recognised as a contributing factor in exercise-associated gastrointestinal disturbances and overall gastrointestinal health.

Environment

The risk of intestinal injury and increased permeability is greater in hot climatic conditions (>37°C). Exercising in the heat increases total body water loss (see Chapter 22), leading to a decrease in plasma volume and a further reduction of blood flow to the gut. Heat stress and dehydration may exacerbate intestinal injury, increasing the risk of gastrointestinal symptoms. In one study, the incidence of gastrointestinal symptoms increased when runners lost 3.5–4 per cent of body weight (Rehrer et al. 1990). While exercise in the heat and accompanying dehydration may worsen gastrointestinal injury and permeability, it is not known whether this is a direct cause of gastrointestinal symptoms.

To minimise the impact of heat on gastrointestinal stress during exercise, a carefully planned hydration regime should be implemented based on measured sweat rates and calculated fluid requirements. It is also important to note that hyperhydration, or over-hydrating, may cause an uncomfortable 'sloshing' sensation in the stomach. For this reason, too much fluid consumption is also ill-advised. Exercise-associated hyponatraemia—where too much water is ingested and blood sodium concentrations become abnormally low—has been linked to gastrointestinal symptoms, particularly nausea and vomiting. Beginning exercise in a euhydrated state and aiming to maintain a fluid loss of less than two per cent of body weight is ideal.

Mechanical

Gastrointestinal disturbances, particularly lower gastrointestinal symptoms, are more common in exercise that has a greater mechanical impact, such as running or triathlon (Pfeiffer et al. 2012). The mechanical jarring (up-and-down motion) of running is a possible trigger for gastrointestinal symptoms. Upper gastrointestinal symptoms seem to be more common in cycling due to the bent-over body position, which places pressure on the abdominal area. Technique-related breathing in swimming may result in swallowing air. It is normal to swallow small amounts of air; however, in swimming, air may be gulped and, combined with a horizontal body position, can be difficult to expel, causing certain upper gastrointestinal symptoms (bloating, burping, stomach pain).

Nutrition

Athletes trial various nutrition strategies around training and competition with the aim of individualising and optimising fuelling as well as to reduce the risk of gastrointestinal disturbance. Common pre-emptive nutrition strategies to prevent or minimise gastrointestinal symptoms include reduced dietary fibre intake, decreased fat and protein intake, adjusting food timing and training the gut to tolerate greater carbohydrate and fluid loads.

Athletes are advised to 'train race-day nutrition'. Ideally, competition nutrition strategies should be similar to those used in specific training sessions. Competition-specific strategies aimed at reducing race-day gastrointestinal disturbances may include a short-term **low-residue diet**, avoiding lactose the day before a competition, or modifying carbohydrates by increasing or reducing intake or changing the carbohydrate type. For example, athletes may avoid fructose or choose formulated sports nutrition products with multitransporter carbohydrates (maltodextrin, glucose, fructose blends). It is important to consider that, in some events, feed stations may offer a variety of foods

Low-residue diet
Diet limiting higher-fibre foods.

and fluids an athlete may not be familiar with. A less-experienced athlete may consume fuel options that they have not tried before or may overfuel due to inexperience or a fear of 'bonking'. Competition nutrition plans should be tested in training sessions of similar intensity and in similar climatic conditions. Logistical challenges and the additional stress of race situations may alter even the best-laid nutrition plans. The following sections elaborate on nutrition strategies for exercise to reduce the risk of gastrointestinal symptoms around and during training and competition.

Bonking
An athletic term describing a sudden and overwhelming feeling of running out of energy—often also termed 'hitting the wall'—during endurance events.

Fibre, fat and protein

Conclusive links between gastrointestinal symptoms and intakes of dietary fat, protein and fibre have not been drawn, even though several studies have attempted to connect exercise-associated gastrointestinal symptoms with certain macronutrients, quantities and timing. One of the first studies investigating dietary habits and the prevalence of gastrointestinal symptoms during endurance competition found that athletes who consumed foods high in dietary fibre, fat or protein before competition reported a higher prevalence of gastrointestinal symptoms, notably vomiting and reflux (Rehrer et al. 1992). However, this data was collected retrospectively so there is potential error associated with athletes' recall (refer to Chapter 7 for more information about dietary assessment). More recently, protein hydrolysate intake before and during exercise has been shown to be poorly tolerated and associated with higher rates of gastrointestinal disturbance (Snipe et al. 2018). Conversely, a prospective study in triathletes found no association of fibre, fat or protein intake with gastrointestinal symptoms during the cycle and run leg of a 70.3 triathlon (Rehrer et al. 1992). Due to the transient nature of gastrointestinal symptoms, and large individual variation in dietary intakes, it is difficult to draw firm conclusions about the effects of fibre, protein and fat on exercise-associated gastrointestinal symptoms. However, in the field practitioners will generally advise low fibre, low fat and moderate protein intakes around competition. Tailored, individualised nutrition is likely the key to successful macronutrient choices before, during and after exercise when aiming to moderate gastrointestinal disturbances.

Meal timing

Limited information exists linking meal timing with gastrointestinal symptoms. Several studies have attempted to explore how meal timing influences gastrointestinal symptoms and, based on these, it is suggested that solid food consumed close to the start of endurance exercise may increase upper gastrointestinal symptoms. Based on limited research and anecdotal evidence it can be suggested that athletes aiming to reduce gastrointestinal disturbance may have better success with easier-to-digest liquid fuelling options ingested closer to the start of exercise, rather than solids. However, ideal meal timing generally requires testing and individualisation.

Gluten-free diet

In recent years gluten-free diets (GFDs) have become popular among athletes, with a prevalent belief that this diet reduces gastrointestinal symptoms, improves overall health and even offers an ergogenic benefit, although supportive evidence is lacking. Briefly, a GFD restricts a family of gluten-related proteins found mainly in food or constituents derived from wheat, rye and barley. While it is interesting to consider that perhaps endurance athletes training and competing frequently at high intensities may develop an increased susceptibility to dietary triggers, such as gluten, this has not been shown in research. A greater awareness and improved diagnostics for clinical gluten-related conditions (**coeliac disease, non-coeliac gluten/wheat sensitivity**) may also influence the increasing number of athletes going gluten-free. Self-prescription of a GFD is common—partly due to the lack of a definitive biomarker for non-coeliac gluten/wheat sensitivity—and is also a contributing factor to the increased uptake of this diet in healthy athletic populations. It is imperative to consider any clinical necessity for a GFD, but it is also important to be aware of other dietary changes that can happen alongside a GFD as well as the belief effect, which may influence gastrointestinal symptom perceptions. While a strict GFD may provide less fibre and fewer micronutrients, Lis et al. (2015) found that after switching to a GFD subjects exhibited increased consumption of fruit, vegetables and gluten-free wholegrains, and an overall greater awareness and implementation of a healthy eating pattern. One distinct dietary change that may naturally take place alongside the adoption of a GFD is a subsequent reduction in short-chain rapidly fermentable carbohydrates (fermentable oligosaccharides, disaccharides, monosaccharides and polyols, or FODMAPs), specifically fructans and galactooligosaccharides.

Coeliac disease
Autoimmune disease in which the immune system reacts abnormally to gluten, causing damage to the small intestine.

Non-coeliac gluten/wheat sensitivity
A condition characterised by adverse gastrointestinal and/or extra-intestinal symptoms associated with the ingestion of gluten- or wheat-containing foods, in the absence of coeliac disease or wheat allergy.

FODMAPs

In athletes reporting symptomatic improvement after implementing a GFD, it may be the subsequent reduction in some FODMAPs (rather than in gluten) that is actually alleviating symptoms. FODMAPs are a family of short-chain fermentable carbohydrates that are slowly or poorly absorbed in the upper intestinal tract and rapidly fermented by colonic bacteria. In the upper intestine in particular, unabsorbed

FODMAPs may exert an **osmotic effect**, which means more fluid is drawn into the bowel. Combined with rapid fermentation of FODMAPs by gas-producing colonic bacteria, fluid and gas distend the bowel. As a result, bloating, abdominal pain, flatulence and alterations in bowel movement occur. A low-FODMAP diet, developed by researchers at Monash University (Melbourne, Australia), has shown promising results for the effectiveness of FODMAP restriction and reintroduction in clinical patients, such as those with IBS.

Many athletes avoid foods high in FODMAPs (Lis et al. 2015), such as milk or legumes, with the aim of reducing gastrointestinal symptoms, and there is a high rate of perceived symptom improvement. Repeated exercise stress placed on the gut, combined with high carbohydrate intakes and high FODMAP loads present in many sports foods, may create the perfect storm for FODMAPs to exacerbate exercise-associated gastrointestinal symptoms. Healthy endurance athletes with exercise-associated gastrointestinal symptoms do not intrinsically require a low-FODMAP diet, but it may be a tool that can be used to reduce symptoms in susceptible individuals.

Osmotic effect
The movement of water molecules from a higher water potential to a more negative water potential.

Fructose

Athletes, particularly endurance athletes, may have higher than average dietary intakes of fructose. Elevated energy requirements may be partially met through increased consumption of fruit, juice, honey and sports foods (gels, beverages), all of which are high in fructose. Fructose is normally absorbed in the small intestine by intestinal transporters, low-capacity facilitated diffusion GLUT 5 and a glucose-activated more rapid diffusion, GLUT 2. Malabsorption of fructose can occur when the activity of one of these transporters, GLUT 5, becomes saturated. Some individuals have a condition known as fructose malabsorption, in which fructose is not fully absorbed, exerting an osmotic effect and then being fermented by colonic bacteria and influencing gastrointestinal symptoms. It is possible that athletes ingesting large amounts of high-fructose foods may experience some fructose malabsorption, resulting in gastrointestinal symptoms. Fructose absorption can be improved by ingesting less of this monosaccharide, and also by consuming it as a component of foods or meals containing other nutrients.

Osmolality, carbohydrate intake and type

Ingestion of carbohydrate solutions with a high osmolality (that is, having a high concentration of molecules in a solution, also known as hyperosmolar) has been associated with gastrointestinal symptoms during exercise. Gastric emptying and intestinal fluid absorption are reduced when carbohydrate concentration in solution is greater than six per cent.

The ingestion of multiple carbohydrate types increases the oxidation of ingested carbohydrate, improving fuel availability and also possibly decreasing gastrointestinal symptoms. Large amounts of carbohydrate consumed during exercise may be incompletely absorbed, particularly if the carbohydrate load is only from one carbohydrate type (such as glucose). Leftover carbohydrate remaining in the intestine can exacerbate gastrointestinal symptoms through osmotic actions. Some examples of multiple transportable carbohydrates include a blend of glucose:fructose at a 2:1 ratio, maltodextrin and fructose, or glucose, sucrose and fructose. A series of studies have shown that—provided there are multiple carbohydrate types ingested, such as glucose and fructose—high rates of carbohydrate (90 g·h^{-1}) can be fairly well tolerated. Although a higher reported incidence of nausea occurred when the athletes ingested 90 g·h^{-1} compared to 60 g·h^{-1}, the exercise was relatively short in duration (running for 70 minutes) and conducted in mild environmental conditions (Pfeiffer et al. 2009). The amount and type of carbohydrate consumed by an athlete needs to be individually

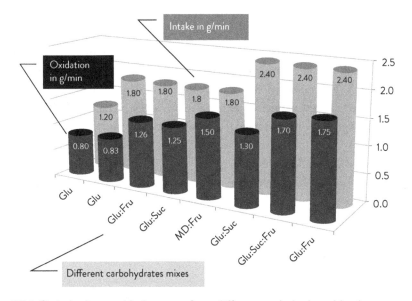

Figure 23.1. Carbohydrate oxidation rates from different carbohydrate blends

Note: Data are extrapolated from a number of studies. Increasing the intake of one carbohydrate type will plateau oxidation at approximately 1 g/min and increasing the intake of multiple transportable carbohydrate types increases oxidation up to 1.75 g/min.

Source: Asker Jeukendrup, SSE#108 Multiple Transportable Carbohydrates and Their Benefits (www.gssiweb.org/en-ca/Article/sse-108-multiple-transportable-carbohydrates-and-their-benefits).

assessed, although, importantly, tolerance to carbohydrate can be trained, as the gut is somewhat adaptable.

Figure 23.1 shows the peak carbohydrate oxidation that can be achieved proportional to the ingested amount. Practically, athletes can mix and match carbohydrate sources from drinks, gels, bars and jelly lollies based on preferences and fuelling logistics. For solid foods consumed during exercise, low-fat, fibre and protein content is important so that these macronutrients do not slow the delivery of carbohydrate and fluids.

Eating during exercise

Nutrient intake during exercise with impaired gastrointestinal function may increase the risk of adverse symptoms. However, frequent and consistent carbohydrate intake during exercise may also be a protective strategy for epithelial injury (Costa et al. 2017).

Trainability of the gut

Gastrointestinal symptoms are more frequent in novice athletes with less training. Training lessens the reduction of splanchnic blood flow, improving gut barrier function and likely reducing the risk of symptoms. This was recently demonstrated in a study where two weeks of a repetitive gut challenge involving the ingestion of high intakes of carbohydrate during running (ten days of ingesting 90 $g{\cdot}h^{-1}$ for one hour of 60 per cent VO_{2max} running) reduced the incidence of gastrointestinal symptoms experienced by recreational runners compared to a placebo (Miall et al. 2017). This point further highlights the importance of 'training race-day nutrition'.

Belief (placebo) effect

The belief/placebo effect is where the belief in a positive effect of an intervention improves a range of outcomes, such as perceived gastrointestinal symptoms. Several studies have shown that the placebo effect decreased symptoms in patients with IBS. Similarly, studies on athletes have shown the placebo effect (the belief that an intervention will improve performance) to have beneficial outcomes.

History of gastrointestinal symptoms and genetic predisposition

There appears to be a genetic predisposition to gastrointestinal symptoms, and those with a history of gastrointestinal symptoms are more susceptible to recurrent gastrointestinal disturbance.

Chronic low energy availability

Clinical and anecdotal data suggest that athletes experiencing chronic low energy availability report a high incidence of gastrointestinal disturbances. This area has not been well studied but, theoretically, limited nutrient intake may compromise the ability to absorb or tolerate nutrients and increase susceptibly to adverse symptoms.

Medications and supplements

Particular medications and supplements can interfere with the gastrointestinal system and influence symptoms. Non-steroidal anti-inflammatory drugs (NSAIDs) are commonly used by athletes to manage pain and swelling and reduce the impact of injury on performance. There is an associated three- to fivefold increased risk of upper gastrointestinal disturbances such as GORD and gastritis, mucosal bleeding or perforation when using anti-inflammatory drugs compared to no medication (Van Wijck et al. 2012). It is recommended that prolonged use of NSAIDs and use prior to exercise be avoided.

Nerve and muscle activity of the large intestine can be affected by supplements such as high-dose iron, leading to constipation. Antibiotics and high doses of magnesium can cause diarrhoea and high doses of vitamin C can cause digestive symptoms, including abdominal cramps, pain and diarrhoea.

Psychological stress

Stress, fatigue and mood disturbances commonly occur alongside gastrointestinal disturbances in athletes. Often, athletes experience gastrointestinal disturbances only around race situations, where stress and anxiety levels are higher compared to training. The psychological demands of intense exercise can initiate a stress response, resulting in stress and the release of hormones initiating a fight-or-flight response. Additionally, a complex interplay between these biochemical changes and gastrointestinal microbiotia is thought to reciprocally influence gastrointestinal symptoms. In some cases, mental training to address stress and coping mechanisms may be part of an athlete's toolbox to treat gastrointestinal disturbances.

NUTRITION ADVICE FOR ATHLETES WITH GASTROINTESTINAL DISTURBANCES

Gastrointestinal disturbances in athletes is multifactorial in nature and its dietary management requires individualisation. The following table outlines several dietary strategies to treat gastrointestinal disturbances in athletes. These tools may be helpful; however, the advice of an Accredited Sports Dietitian with specialised training in gastrointestinal nutrition is recommended. Furthermore, in cases of persistent gastrointestinal symptoms, both at rest and during exercise, the advice of a medical professional should be sought to determine possible underlying clinical conditions.

Table 23.1. Dietary management tools to prevent gastrointestinal symptoms*

Dietary and/or other management recommendations	Gastrointestinal symptoms that may be avoided
Avoid gulping fluids during training or competition. Use breathing techniques that avoid swallowing air. Avoid carbonated beverages.	Belching
Avoid agents that relax the lower oesophageal sphincter, such as caffeine, mint, chocolate and alcohol.	Belching GORD
Aim to eat ~2–4 hours prior to training or competition. Shorter times between eating and exercise start may increase risk of adverse gastrointestinal effects. As a general rule, the closer nutrition is taken to the start time the smaller the amount of food or fluid that should be ingested. Liquid nutrition options, such as meal supplements, may be better tolerated than solids.	GORD Vomiting Bloating Side ache / cramp Urge to defecate Diarrhoea, runner's trots
Consume easy-to-digest, low-fibre, low-fat and low- to moderate-protein meals/snacks prior to exercise and as much as 24 hours leading up to competition.	GORD Vomiting Bloating Side ache / cramp Urge to defecate Diarrhoea, runner's trots Flatulence
Choose carbohydrate solutions with a lower concentration or osmolality along with ingesting sufficient water.	GORD Vomiting Bloating Flatulence Nausea
Start exercise euhydrated and aim to minimise body weight loss (to within <2% body weight). Avoid over-hydrating.	Vomiting Bloating Nausea
Avoid over-nutrition prior to and during exercise by having an individualised and tested nutrition plan based on energy and nutrient demands.	Vomiting Bloating Nausea Flatulence
Gut training: The gastrointestinal system is adaptable and its capacity to uptake fluid and nutrients can be increased with training. Train with carbohydrate and fluid during exercise to improve absorption and identify individual tolerances. A focused carbohydrate challenge protocol, with increasing amounts, may improve gastrointestinal tolerance and reduce related symptoms. It is best to seek advice on such a protocol from a qualified sports nutrition practitioner.	Vomiting Bloating Nausea Flatulence Belching Side ache / cramp Diarrhoea, runner's trots

Dietary and/or other management recommendations	Gastrointestinal symptoms that may be avoided
Consume low-fibre or low-residue foods for 1–2 days leading up to the event.	Bloating Flatulence Side ache / cramp Urge to defecate Diarrhoea, runner's trots
Allow time for toilet stops before competition or training.	Urge to defecate
Consume a low-FODMAP diet for at least 24 hours before strenuous training or competition. High-FODMAP foods eaten before or during exercise may have a detrimental additive effect on gastrointestinal symptoms.	Osmotic diarrhoea Bloating Flatulence
Some may benefit from cognitive behavioural therapy; see an allied health professional trained in this technique.	Diarrhoea, runner's trots
Special situations	
Heat	Heat stress is known to increase gastrointestinal injury, splanchnic hypoperfusion and hypoxia, which may worsen symptoms. Heat acclimation, external and internal pre-exercise/during-exercise cooling may also improve gut health, although to date research is limited and conflicting.
Limited fluid access during exercise	Recent research suggests that some adaptation may occur to training dehydrated.
Caffeine	Caffeine can increase colon motility (movement of food), which could be additive to the mechanical impact of running leading to diarrhoea.
Nitrate	May improve splanchnic perfusion.
Other recommendations: Ingesting sufficient water and nutrients during prolonged exercise can help maintain splanchnic blood flow and reduce the risk of gut symptoms. Consumption of solutions with multiple carbohydrate types (glucose, maltodextrin, fructose) may reduce the risk of gastrointestinal symptoms.	

*Recommendations are based on limited research and may or may not be dietary triggers for individuals.

SUMMARY AND KEY MESSAGES

After reading this chapter you should understand that gastrointestinal symptoms are common among athletes and that although most are minor or mild in severity, some can be severe and impact negatively on exercise performance. Exercise-associated gastrointestinal symptoms can occur during or after exercise and although the cause is not entirely understood symptoms are primarily related to physiological, mechanical and nutritional factors. Nutrition can play a key role in reducing the risk of common gastrointestinal symptoms.

Key messages

- Gastrointestinal disturbances are a common occurrence among athletes and severe symptoms are likely to compromise training capacity and performance.
- The main triggers of gastrointestinal disturbances in athletes are physiological, mechanical and nutritional.
- Strenuous exercise, particularly endurance-based exercise, stresses the gastrointestinal system, causing reduced blood flow which initiates alterations in gut integrity. Impaired gastrointestinal function is a result of increased permeability, motility changes, alterations in endotoxin movement and subsequent systemic inflammatory response, triggering gastrointestinal symptoms.
- An important interplay between the gut–brain axis influences gastrointestinal symptoms and, in some athletes, may be the reason symptoms are hard to replicate and only occur in race situations or may be influenced by psychological stress.
- Exercise-associated gastrointestinal disturbance is multifactorial, requiring an individualised and multidisciplinary approach for successful treatment.
- Based on current knowledge, the key nutrition strategies that may reduce the risk of gastrointestinal disturbances include:
  - Eating a low-fibre or low-residue diet in the 1–2 days leading up to the event.
  - Pre-fuelling strategies such as eating the pre-event meal ~2–4 hours prior to exercise. It should be easy to digest, low fibre, low fat and low to moderate in protein.
  - Starting exercise euhydrated, aiming to minimise body weight loss during exercise and avoiding over-hydrating.
  - Avoiding over-nutrition (eating or drinking too much) prior to and during exercise by implementing an individualised and tested nutrition plan based on energy and nutrient demands.
  - Undertaking gut training to adapt the gut and its capacity to uptake fluid and nutrients.
  - Consuming solutions with multiple carbohydrate types, such as glucose, maltodextrin and fructose.

REFERENCES

Costa, R.J.S., Snipe, R., Camões-Costa, V. et al., 2016, 'The impact of gastrointestinal symptoms and dermatological injuries on nutritional intake and hydration status during ultramarathon events', *Sports Medicine Open*, vol. 2, no. 1, p. 16, doi:10.1186/s40798-015-0041-9.

Costa, R.J.S., Snipe, R.M.J, Kitic, C.M. et al., 2017, 'Systematic review: Exercise-induced gastrointestinal syndrome—implications for health and intestinal disease', *Alimentary Therapeutics & Pharmacology*, vol. 46, no. 3, pp. 246–65.

Dokladny, K., Zuhl, M.N. & Moseley, P.L., 2016, 'Intestinal epithelial barrier function and tight junction proteins with heat and exercise', *Journal of Applied Physiology*, vol. 120, no. 6, pp. 692–701.

Lang, J.A., Gisolfi, C.V. & Lambert, G.P., 2006, 'Effect of exercise intensity on active and passive glucose absorption', *International Journal of Sport Nutrition & Exercise Metabolism*, vol. 16, no. 5, pp. 485–93.

Lis, D., Stellingwerff, T., Shing, C.M. et al., 2015, 'Exploring the popularity, experiences, and beliefs surrounding gluten-free diets in noncoeliac athletes', *International Journal of Sport Nutrition & Exercise Metabolism*, vol. 25, no. 1, pp. 37–45.

Miall, A., Khoo, A., Rauch, C. et al., 2017, 'Two weeks of repetitive gut-challenge reduce exercise-associated gastrointestinal symptoms and malabsorption', *Scandinavian Journal of Medicine & Science in Sports*, vol. 20, no. 2, pp. 630–40.

Pfeiffer, B., Cotterill, A., Grathwohl, D. et al., 2009, 'The effect of carbohydrate gels on gastrointestinal tolerance during a 16km run', *International Journal of Sport Nutrition & Exercise Metabolism*, vol. 19, no. 5, pp. 485–503.

Pfeiffer, B., Stellingwerff, T., Hodgson, A.B. et al., 2012, 'Nutritional intake and gastrointestinal problems during competitive endurance events', *Medicine & Science in Sports & Exercise*, vol. 44, no. 2, pp. 344–51.

Rehrer, N.J., Beckers, E.J., Brouns, F. et al., 1990, 'Effects of dehydration on gastric emptying and gastrointestinal distress while running', *Medicine & Science in Sports & Exercise*, vol. 22, no. 6, pp. 790–95.

Rehrer, N.J., van Kemenade, M., Meester, W. et al., 1992, 'Gastrointestinal complaints in relation to dietary intake in triathletes', *International Journal of Sports Nutrition*, vol. 2, no. 1, pp. 48–59.

Rehrer, N.J., Smets, A., Reynaert, H. et al., 2001, 'Effect of exercise on portal vein blood flow in man', *Medicine & Science in Sports & Exercise*, vol. 33, no. 9, pp. 1533–37.

Snipe, R.M.J., Khoo, A., Kitic, C.M. et al., 2018, 'The impact of exertional-heat stress on gastrointestinal integrity, gastrointestinal symptoms, systemic endotoxin and cytokine profile', *European Journal of Applied Physiology*, vol. 118, no. 2, pp. 389–400.

van Wijck, K., Lenaerts, K., Van Bijnen, A.A. et al., 2012, 'Aggravation of exercise-induced intestinal injury by Ibuprofen in athletes', *Medicine & Science in Sports & Exercise*, vol. 44, no. 12, pp. 2257–62.

CHAPTER 24

Nutrition support for injury management and rehabilitation

Rebekah Alcock and Greg Shaw

Injuries are an unfortunate reality of both recreational and professional sports. In 2011–12, the Australian Institute of Health and Welfare (AIHW) reported that 36,000 people aged over 15 years were hospitalised as a result of a sporting injury (AIHW 2014), with the annual cost of sporting injuries in Australia estimated to be over \$1.5 billion (Medibank 2003). At an elite level, the impact of sporting injuries can be significant, often having various physical, psychological, professional and economic consequences for both the athlete and the organisation that contracts them. Injuries range from minor (cuts and abrasions), through moderate to severe (such as musculoskeletal and connective tissue injuries), including the small number that have life-long implications (for example, concussion). Depending on the type and severity of injury, the consequences may range from immediate but short-term cessation of sport to weeks, months or even years away from training and competition.

While rehabilitation strategies have been developed in physical therapy, medicine and psychology, nutrition interventions are often focused predominantly on controlling body composition. However, nutrition interventions outside of body composition management can play an important role during the rehabilitation phase for an injured athlete, and can influence their ability to return to training and competition. Nutrition strategies for injury rehabilitation should focus on supporting tissue regeneration, attenuating the effects of immobilisation on the musculoskeletal system and minimising unnecessary body composition changes associated with reduced training loads. Finally, and most importantly, any rehabilitation program should ensure the athlete is returned to competitive sport in a state that is similar to or better than pre-injury functioning where possible. The following chapter will give an overview of nutrition considerations in the management of injuries.

LEARNING OUTCOMES

Upon completion of this chapter you should be able to:
- understand the influence adequate nutrition has in preventing load-related injuries
- understand the timeline of injury rehabilitation and the nutrition considerations at each time point of the rehabilitation timeline
- understand nutrition support for assisting the athlete in 'return to train and then play'
- have an awareness of emerging nutrition interventions related to injury prevention and rehabilitation.

TYPES OF INJURIES

The types of injuries that occur within a sport are generally related to the characteristics of that particular sport. For example, contact sports, including rugby union, rugby league and Australian football, commonly result in injuries as a result of body contact and/or sudden directional changes, often involving musculoskeletal and/or connective tissues. Sports such as boxing commonly result in injuries as a result of a direct 'hit' or 'blow' to the body and may result in skin lacerations, fractures, dislocations or concussions. Athletes participating in endurance sports, such as long-distance running and triathlon, are often faced with injuries such as **tendinopathies**, which may be attributable to poor load management and over-use of a specific tissue. We will focus here on the most common injuries occurring in sport. These include injuries to the bone (fractures), soft tissues (including cartilage, ligaments, tendons and muscle) and 'other' injuries (including injuries to the head and skin). It should be noted that injuries rarely occur in isolation and often involve multiple components of the body.

Tendinopathies
Diseases of the tendons, which may arise from a range of internal and external factors.

Bone injuries

The term 'fracture' encompasses any injury in which a bone becomes cracked or broken, and fractures are the most common type of sports injury requiring hospitalisation, accounting for almost 50 per cent of injuries within Australia (AIHW 2012). Fractures can occur as an acute injury—due to a sudden impact such as contact with another person, obstacle or a fall—or as a result of repeated stress to the bone, as is the case for stress fractures. Acute fractures can occur in almost any sport where there is some form of direct contact with another person or object, or if there is a risk of a fall, such as in football, cycling, running, combat sports, snow and water sports, equestrian activities and motor sports. While stress fractures tend to occur over time, they are common in sports where loading can change quickly, such as watercraft sports (rowing, kayaking), running, gymnastics, ballet, basketball and volleyball. While it is important to focus on the adequacy of key nutrients (such as calcium and vitamin D) that may assist with bone healing, preventing nutrient deficiencies and ensuring adequate energy intake (see section on RED-S and energy availability below) is an important consideration for the prevention of bone injuries.

Soft-tissue injuries

Soft-tissue injuries refer to injuries to the musculoskeletal and connective tissues, whether acutely, such as a sprain/ strain or tear, or chronically, as in the case of tendinopathies. Soft-tissue injuries were the second most common type of injury requiring hospitalisation, according to the AIHW 2011–12 report. Sports characterised by high-speed movements and change of direction have a high incidence of soft-tissue injuries resulting from tears, ruptures and strains. These types of injuries are typically sustained while undertaking high-speed running—with or without a quick change of direction—which places significant strain on tissues incapable of handling the load. The duration of recovery can range from days to a year, depending on the severity of the injury. However, in sports where athletes increase load rapidly over days or weeks, more chronic conditions like tendinopathies develop. Specifically, the pain and dysfunction resulting from a tendinopathy can significantly interfere with the capacity to train and compete. Tendinopathies are complicated and do not have a common **pathology**, so the treatment of tendinopathies will often be specific to the tendon and the athlete's injury history. Consequences of soft-tissue injuries can range from reduced load for a period of a few days to inability to complete certain types of exercise for the rest of an athlete's life.

Pathology
A field in medicine which studies the causes of diseases.

Other injuries

Head injuries are frequently reported in contact sports. Symptoms can be as minor as short periods (minutes) of memory loss to long-term impairment in brain function.

Recently, this long-term impairment in brain function has been linked to multiple acute head injuries and **subconcussive** impacts. Researchers are investigating numerous interventions, including the influence specific nutrients (important for brain function) can have on helping the brain regenerate or cope with these types of injuries. Other injuries, such as skin lacerations (deep cuts) are also common in sport and present significant concern in sports where dietary adequacy may influence wound healing or in events where treatment options may be limited, such as multi-day ultra-endurance running events.

Subconcussive
A hit to the head that does not meet the clinical criteria for concussion, but is hypothesised to have long-term adverse effects.

Special interest area: Concussion

Concussion is a type of traumatic brain injury (TBI) generally caused by a violent blow to the head and resulting in temporary impairment of cognitive function, including loss of consciousness, vision, memory and equilibrium (balance). Short-term symptoms include diminished reaction times, headache, irritability and sleep disturbances. Repeated concussive injuries have been linked to chronic traumatic encephalopathy (CTE), a progressive degenerative disease of the brain. Often referred to as 'punch drunk syndrome' in retired boxers, it can eventually result in dementia. Under normal conditions, the human brain accounts for around 20 per cent of the oxygen and 25 per cent of the glucose utilised by the body (Belanger et al. 2011). However, after a concussion there is a cascade of functional disturbances within the brain, including alterations in energy, glucose and lactate metabolism, increased oxidative stress and inflammation, which may make the brain more susceptible to secondary injury and/or lead to future complications (Giza & Hovda 2014). Presently, the only treatment for concussion is physical and cognitive rest until acute symptoms are resolved.

Although nutrition interventions for TBI are still being explored, research to date suggests that antioxidants and anti-inflammatory agents may be of benefit. Emerging evidence suggests that omega-3 fatty acids (n-3 FA), particularly **docosahexaenoic acid** (DHA) (see Chapter 4) may play a role in both prevention and treatment of TBI. In animal models, depletion of DHA within the brain impairs recovery from TBI. Additionally, supplementing with n-3 FA prior to sustaining a concussion has been shown to protect against impact sustained from a concussion. Athletes at risk of frequent head collisions should regularly include cold-water fatty fish in their diets at least three times per week. Other nutrients that may play a role in the treatment of TBI include vitamins C, D and E, through the reduction of oxidative damage, and creatine, whose levels decrease within the brain after concussion.

Docosahexaenoic acid
A long-chain n-3 fatty acid with 22—carbons and six double bonds, found in fatty fish and breast milk.

Although further research is needed in athletic populations, the nutrients suggested as beneficial are easily obtained from dietary sources. Therefore, athletes competing in contact sports should be encouraged to consume foods high in the above nutrients as part of their well-planned sports-specific intake (Ashbaugh & McGrew 2016).

PHASES OF NUTRITION INTERVENTIONS FOR INJURIES

Typically, acute injury begins with the process of acute inflammation, followed by a potential period of immobilisation and a varying period of rehabilitation before returning to training and subsequently competition. Nutrition plays a critical role in each phase of this injury rehabilitation process, as outlined below. Although it is tempting to suggest nutrition will have a large impact on injury rehabilitation, its key role is in supporting the rehabilitation program designed by a physician, physical therapist or rehabilitation specialist. Nutrition will boost the repair process but the interventions will only be as successful as the program they are designed to support; thus, a multidisciplinary approach to support rehabilitation of the injured athlete is essential.

Injury prevention

While nutrition support plays an important role in injury rehabilitation, it is also important to consider that adequate nutrition plays a critical role in the prevention of injuries. It has long been known that significant acute changes in training load can lead to a range of injuries. It is not known whether the primary issue is the increase in load or the inability of athletes to change their dietary intake to meet the requirements of the increased load. An International Olympic Committee (IOC) working group has suggested that the inability to match energy intake to account for variations in the energy cost of exercise contributes to injury risk (Mountjoy et al. 2014). It is therefore essential that energy intake rises and falls in tight response to training load. Additionally, special focus should be given to ensure adequate nutrient availability necessary for the significant increase in remodelling that is associated with increased training load. Adequate intake of protein, carbohydrate, and calcium, timed closely to heavy training, has been shown to positively influence the remodelling process, reducing the breakdown of tissues such as bone that occurs after heavy training sessions. Nutrition recommendations for athletes undertaking increased load should focus on adequate energy availability combined with purposeful nutrient availability, to aid in the prevention of load-related injuries.

Special interest area: RED-S and energy availability
As previously discussed in Chapter 18, appropriate energy availability (EA) is particularly important for athletes. Reports suggest a healthy adult has a typical EA of

188 kJ/kg of fat-free mass (FFM). However, when EA drops below a threshold of 125 kJ/kg FFM (low energy availability), insufficient energy is available after exercise is accounted for to maintain key functions such as the immune system, bone remodelling, protein synthesis and hormonal functioning.

Relative energy deficiency in sport (RED-S), as a consequence of long-term low energy availability (LEA), has a range of implications for athlete health and a particularly large effect on bone remodelling, mostly due to the influence LEA has on oestrogen and its flow-on effect of reducing IGF–I (Mountjoy et al. 2014). IGF–I is a hormone that is essential for stimulating remodelling cells in the muscle, bone and connective tissue. It has also been shown that muscle protein synthesis is reduced during periods of LEA, but increasing the amount of protein consumed around exercise minimises those reductions (Areta et al. 2014). This highlights that LEA influences the remodelling of proteins in both bone and muscle tissues, potentially increasing the risk of injuries in these tissues. More work is needed to understand whether improving nutrient availability around exercise while in a state of LEA can potentially reduce the negative impact of LEA on bone, muscle and connective tissue synthetic processes. This complex and wide-reaching area of nutrition should be closely monitored and not discounted in the prevention of injuries. The primary focus of nutrition interventions as training loads increase should be ensuring that adequate EA is maintained to reduce the risk of injury.

The initial phase of injury (immobilisation)

After any injury the body's natural response is to increase inflammation (swelling), signalling the requirement for repair and remodelling. The management of chronic low-grade inflammation has been a major focus of lifestyle disease prevention in recent times; however, acute inflammation associated with injury is an important process that helps signal and stimulate remodelling. Evidence to support the use of anti-inflammatory nutrients to suppress inflammation, and hence improve injury rehabilitation, is lacking (Tipton 2015). In fact, in the short term (the period of the first few hours to days of an injury) it may be detrimental to reduce a response that is necessary for the healing and repair of damaged tissue.

Most injuries require some form of disuse, or even immobilisation, with acute tears and ruptures often requiring immobilisation for days to weeks. This immobilisation leads to significant reductions in energy expenditure. Often the first instinct of athletes is to reduce energy intake proportionally. However, during the initial phases of any injury, energy requirements may actually be increased due to energy demands for the proliferation and remodelling of injured tissue (Tipton 2015). This could be combined with the increased energy cost of abnormal movement patterns, especially with lower leg injuries. Therefore, severe energy restrictions leading to poor nutrient availability (especially protein) should be avoided, particularly in the first five days following injury and immobilisation. During this phase of injury, athletes are recommended to not actively restrict dietary intake, maintaining energy intake between 146 and 188 kJ/kg/FFM. They should focus on reducing carbohydrate intakes to the lower end of the guidelines (~3 g/kg BM/day) and maintain protein intake at 2–2.5 g/kg BM per day, spread evenly over all meals and snacks.

If immobilisation is expected for extended periods (>5 days) athletes are advised to implement nutrition strategies that help offset muscle wasting associated with disuse. Recent studies in this area have found that it is necessary to maintain an exercise stimulus when providing additional nutrition support to minimise muscle wasting associated with disuse or immobilisation. Recommendations should be to include high-**leucine** (~3 grams) protein sources (>16 grams of essential amino acids) at all meals and snacks over the day. This is especially important with exercise regimes capable of maintaining a stimulatory effect (such as electrical muscle stimulation) and can be effective at reducing muscle wasting (Dirks et al. 2017). Although traditionally the focus has been on minimising loss of muscle mass and function, connective tissue volume and function has also been shown to deteriorate rapidly when immobilised. Recently, novel nutrition interventions, such as gelatin, have been suggested to help support these tissues during immobilisation; however, more research is needed before definitive interventions can be recommended (Baar 2017).

Leucine
An essential amino acid, which is required for muscle protein synthesis.

Other nutritional interventions targeted at overcoming the anabolic resistance that occurs with disuse—such as omega-3 fish oils, creatine, b-Hydroxy-b-methylbutyrate (HMB, an active metabolite of the branch chain amino acid leucine), and other chemicals that play a key role in the muscle protein synthetic pathway (such as phosphatidic acid)—may be useful; however, the evidence for their use requires more investigation (Wall et al. 2015). Nutrition recommendations for injuries that require periods of immobilisation should be focused on ensuring adequate energy availability in combination with optimal total protein intake (>2 g/kg BM). High-leucine protein sources should be consumed every 2–3 hours throughout the day to maximally support optimal protein synthesis, especially in the early stages of injury. These interventions will be most effective when combined with sufficient exercise of the injured tissue to maintain at least a modest amount of protein synthesis.

Special interest area: Nutrition for chronic inflammation
While acute inflammation is a necessary and natural process of the body's immune system in response to initial tissue injury, chronic inflammation can lead to persistent

pain and has the potential to contribute to long-term damage within the tissue. Dietary sources of anti-inflammatory nutrients are highly effective at maintaining inflammatory processes within manageable ranges. It has been suggested that a low ratio of omega-3 (n-3) fatty acids (found predominantly in marine sources) to omega-6 (n-6) fatty acids (found in processed foods and some seeds, nuts and oils) leads to an imbalance in the control of inflammation within the body. Recommendations to manage this imbalance are to limit processed foods and seeds/nuts/oils high in n-6 while increasing intakes of dietary sources of n-3, such as oily fish (Simopoulos 2002). There is also an increasing focus on the bioactive components of plant-based foods that may assist in reducing inflammation, such as **polyphenols**. Polyphenols of interest include epigallocatechin (EGCG) (found in green tea), curcumin (found in turmeric) and rutin (found in a wide variety of plants, including apples and citrus fruits). While research is continuing to develop and evolve around the bioactive components of food, athletes may be able to help manage unwanted inflammation by ensuring that they consume a diet rich in plant-based foods.

Polyphenols

A group of over 500 compounds that are found in plants. They are important as they provide protection against disease.

The second phase of injury (return to train)

After the initial phase of disuse is completed and athletes are able to use and train the injured muscles or limb, nutrition focus should shift. Nutrition in this phase of injury rehabilitation will focus on maximally supporting the training stimulus to rebuild muscle and connective tissue to pre-injury levels. If nutrition and training strategies have been strategically implemented, muscle wasting as a result of disuse should have been minimised to no more than a few hundred grams. As per traditional training nutrition strategies, nutrition should firstly be targeted at meeting energy availability. During the initial weeks of this phase of rehabilitation, energy intake will still be lower than normal as total training load is still low. However, depending on the injury, this phase of rehabilitation may still include full-load resistance training of uninjured tissue and aerobic training using uninjured muscles and limbs (bike for upper body injury, grinder or similar for low body injuries). Therefore, careful thought should be given to energy intake as over- or underestimating energy expenditure during this period of rehabilitation can lead to suboptimal changes in body composition (fat mass increase, lean mass loss).

Rehabilitation periods are often utilised as opportunities to address physique insufficiencies. Although it may seem intuitive to manipulate body composition during extended rehabilitation periods, athletes and practitioners should ensure any gains in lean mass are achieved concurrently with appropriate increases in training loads.

Macronutrient goals should be re-aligned with typical training recommendations, with protein intakes between 1.4 and 2 g/kg BM per day; carbohydrate intakes matched to the training undertaken on a day-to-day basis; and fat intake from quality sources focused on meeting energy requirements. Dietary supplements such as creatine, caffeine, beta-alanine and sports foods, if used, should be focused on supporting training capacity and enabling athletes to improve training performance, hence retraining injured muscles quickly back to pre-injury strength and metabolic capacity.

The third phase of injury (train to play)

Once an injured muscle, joint or limb has returned to pre-injury function and size, the nutrition focus should shift from synthesis and regeneration to amplifying the adaptive signal of exercise. Over the last ten years, significant research has demonstrated that the provision or restriction of specific nutrients can help amplify the biochemical signalling of exercise. For those athletes looking to fast-track aerobic adaptations, manipulating carbohydrate availability around training has been shown to be a potent stimulator of aerobic adaptation. Strength, power and team sport athletes may benefit from dietary interventions focused on enhancing high-intensity training volumes. Small, purposeful carbohydrate intakes prior to exercise, combined with supplements that enhance training capacity (such as creatine, beta-alanine, nitrates and caffeine) can enhance work completed during training if used strategically, hence fast-tracking the physiological adaptations achieved from training (see Chapters 12 and 15).

The fourth phase of injury (return to competition)

Athletes who have completed a rehabilitation program through the above stages and are deemed ready to compete should no longer require additional or specific nutrition requirements. Nutrition recommendations should follow those of healthy non-injured athletes. Injured limbs or muscles should be returned to similar, if not enhanced, muscle size and function prior to return to competition and should not require ongoing nutritional support.

However, injuries, especially to joints, can often place significant strain on both the injured and other non-injured joints, leading to degenerative conditions such as **osteoarthritis**. Although numerous nutrition interventions have been suggested to either treat or alleviate the symptoms of these conditions (glucosamine, fish oils, curcumin, hydrolysed collagen) the evidence for their use is still equivocal and requires more research. Athletes should maintain an appropriate body weight throughout the rest of their career and then throughout their adult life, to avoid placing unnecessary load on the injured joint and increasing the risk of developing a degenerative joint condition.

Osteoarthritis
A degenerative condition of the joints that occurs when the cartilage in the joint degenerates, which leads to loss of function.

Table 24.1. Overview of rehabilitation and nutrition planning for the injured athlete

	Time (week)			
Stage/aims	Disuse 1 day to 12 weeks	Return to train 3 days to 10 weeks	Train to compete 2 to 10 weeks	Competition
Physical	Minimise muscle atrophy	Retrain muscle Optimise physique	Enhance adaptation to training	Train for competition intensity
Fitness	Minimise loss of aerobic fitness	Re-develop aerobic fitness	Retrain aerobic/anaerobic capacity	
Nutrition	Energy availability: 146–188 kJ/kg FFM Protein: >2 g/kg BM/day HBV protein sources high in leucine (>3 g) (every 2–3 hrs) Supplements: Fish oils: 4 g/day, HMB: 3 g/day.	Energy availability: 188 kJ/kg FFM Protein: 1.4–2 g/kg BM/day HBV protein sources high in leucine (>3 g) (every 2–3 hrs) CHO: to meet training requirement 3–8 g/kg BM Supplements: creatine (load 20 g/day x 5 days then 5 g/day for return to train)	Energy availability: 146–188 kJ/kg FFM Protein: 1.8–2.4 g/kg BM/day CHO: vary CHO availability Supplements: to increase work completed/physiological adaptation	As per traditional sports nutrition guidelines

Notes: FFM: fat-free mass, BM: body mass, HBV: high biological value, HMB: b-Hydroxy-b-methylbutyrate, CHO: carbohydrate.

THE ROLE OF SUPPLEMENTATION IN REHABILITATION

While whole foods provide an opportunity for the athlete to meet multiple goals at once and should always be the first choice, supplements may further assist by filling in any gaps within the diet and/or providing concentrated or convenient sources of specific nutrients that may be of benefit. A supplement such as **whey protein isolate** (WPI) may provide a convenient low-energy (kJ) source of protein during a low-energy requirement period like disuse. Alternatively, other supplements, such as high-strength fish oils, may provide a convenient, and relatively low-cost, option to obtain the large amounts of omega-3 fatty acids needed to attenuate anabolic resistance or inflammation. Finally, conditionally essential amino acids such as **arginine** have been shown to

Whey protein isolate
A by-product of cheese production, which contains a high percentage of pure protein and is virtually lactose-free, carbohydrate-free, fat-free and cholesterol-free.

Arginine
A conditionally essential amino acid that has been shown to have benefits in wound healing.

aid in wound healing (Stechmiller et al. 2005) while more recently there is promising evidence that amino acids abundant in collagen-containing tissues (including bone, tendons and ligaments) may play a role in the regeneration and repair of these tissues (Baar 2017). However, the source and quality of any supplement should be carefully considered with athletes; a recent study in New Zealand found 69 per cent of 32 omega-3 fish oils tested contained less than two-thirds of the amount of omega-3 stated on the label (Albert et al. 2015). Additionally, the risk of contamination with the use of supplements should always be considered by athletes governed by the WADA code (refer to Chapter 12). Therefore, supplementation should be only used as a supportive dietary option and, in most instances, the purposeful use of whole foods and fluids can meet the nutrition requirements of injury rehabilitation.

SUMMARY AND KEY MESSAGES

After reading this chapter, you should understand that strategic and targeted nutrition has the potential to support the rehabilitation process of the injured athlete. This occurs mainly by minimising wasting of essential tissue during disuse and fast-tracking the retraining of injured tissue back to pre-injury levels.

Key messages

- Injuries range from moderate to severe and are related to the characteristics of the sport, with both immediate and potentially long-term consequences for athletes.
- It is important to consider the different phases of the injury/rehabilitation process, from prevention through to 'return to play', when considering nutrition interventions.
- It is important to achieve a balance between consuming a sufficient amount of energy to support the body in the healing and regeneration process, and preventing unwanted increases in fat mass.
- The purposeful timing of macro- and micronutrients can significantly influence the adaptations achieved during the rehabilitation process.
- Supplements may be warranted in some circumstances; however, meeting nutrient goals should be achieved through the intake of whole foods where possible.

REFERENCES

Albert, B.B., Derraik, J.G., Cameron-Smith, D. et al., 2015, 'Fish oil supplements in New Zealand are highly oxidised and do not meet label content of n-3 PUFA', *Scientific Reports*, vol. 5, pp. 7928.

Areta, J.L., Burke, L.M., Camera, D.M. et al., 2014, 'Reduced resting skeletal muscle protein synthesis is rescued by resistance exercise and protein ingestion following short-term energy deficit', *American Journal of Physiology, Endocrinology & Metabolism*, vol. 306, no. 8, pp. E989–97.

Ashbaugh, A. & McGrew, C., 2016, 'The role of nutritional supplements in sports concussion treatment', *Current Sports Medicine Reports*, vol. 15, no. 1, pp. 16–9.

Australian Institute of Health and Welfare (AIHW), 2012, *Australian Sports Injury Hospitalisations*, AIHW, <www.aihw.gov.au/reports/australias-health/australias-health-2012/contents/table-of-contents>.

—— 2014, *Australian Sports Injury Hospitalisations*, AIHW, <www.aihw.gov.au/reports/australias-health/australias-health-2014/contents/table-of-contents>.

Baar, K., 2017, 'Minimizing injury and maximizing return to play: Lessons from engineered ligaments', *Sports Medicine*, vol. 47, suppl. 1, pp. 5–11.

Belanger, M., Allaman, I. & Magistretti, P.J., 2011, 'Brain energy metabolism: Focus on astrocyte-neuron metabolic cooperation', *Cell Metabolism*, vol. 14, no. 6, pp. 724–38.

Dirks, M.L., Wall, B.T. & Van Loon, L.J.C., 2018, 'Interventional strategies to combat muscle disuse atrophy in humans: Focus on neuromuscular electrical stimulation and dietary protein', *Journal of Applied Physiology*, vol. 125, no. 3, pp. 850–61.

Giza, C.C. & Hovda, D.A., 2014, 'The new neurometabolic cascade of concussion', *Neurosurgery*, vol. 75, suppl. 4, pp. S24–33.

Medibank, 2003, *Sports injuries in Australia now costing $1.5 billion a year in new report finding* [Online], <www.medibank.com.au>, accessed 9 August 2018.

Mountjoy, M., Sundgot-Borgen, J., Burke, L. et al., 2014, 'The IOC consensus statement: Beyond the female athlete triad—Relative energy deficiency in sport (RED-S)', *British Journal of Sports Medicine*, vol. 48, no. 7, pp. 491–7.

Simopoulos, A.P., 2002, 'The importance of the ratio of omega-6/omega-3 essential fatty acids', *Biomedicine & Pharmacotherapy*, vol. 56, no. 8, pp. 365–79.

Stechmiller, J.K., Childress, B. & Cowan, L., 2005, 'Arginine supplementation and wound healing', *Nutrition in Clinical Practice*, vol. 20, no. 1, pp. 52–61.

Tipton, K.D., 2015, 'Nutritional support for exercise-induced injuries', *Sports Medicine*, vol. 45, suppl. 1, pp. S93–104.

Wall, B., Morton, J.P. & Van Loon, L.J., 2015, 'Strategies to maintain skeletal muscle mass in the injured athlete: Nutritional considerations and exercise mimetics', *European Journal of Sport Science*, vol. 15, no. 1, pp. 53–62.

CHAPTER

25

Cultural perspectives

Frankie Pui Lam Siu and Evangeline Mantzioris

Athletes often travel abroad for training and competition. Their usual dietary habits and eating plans may be affected when they face new environments with different cultures. Additionally, with globalisation and the ease of international travel, many countries now have teams that are composed of athletes with different ethnic, cultural and religious backgrounds, as well as different philosophical approaches to choosing food. Although the principles of healthy dietary intake and the nutrition goals of sports performance are similar across different cultures, there is an infinite variety of food combinations that athletes may choose to meet their nutritional goals. An understanding of different cultural perspectives is important for athletes and the sports nutrition professionals who work with them to appreciate how foods from different countries of the world may contribute to their dietary plan for exercise and performance.

In this chapter, you will be presented with an overview of the dietary customs of different ethnic, cultural and religious groups, as well as the typical eating patterns and food availability in different countries across Asia, the Middle East, Australia and New Zealand.

LEARNING OUTCOMES

Upon completion of this chapter you will be able to:
- describe the different religious and philosophical approaches to food selection
- understand the different food cultures and customs in different countries
- identify foods available to support sports performance in different countries.

RELIGIOUS, CULTURAL AND PHILOSOPHICAL DETERMINANTS OF EATING

Many religions prescribe a set of guidelines for eating; for some religions they are prescriptive, while for others they are recommendations. Just how closely individuals choose to adhere to the guidelines will be determined by their devotion to their religion, as well as cultural and family influences. As culture strongly influences the foods we consume, it is important to be aware of an athlete's cultural background and personal philosophy before translating sport-specific nutritional guidelines into food-based dietary advice for exercise performance. Here, we look in more detail at the dietary practices of religions with prescribed or recommended dietary restrictions or fasting.

Vegetarianism features in a number of religions, and it is important to understand that there are a number of types of vegetarianism, and that athletes may choose a vegetarian diet based on any number of religious or philosophical beliefs.
- Vegans avoid the consumption of any food that is derived from animals, including dairy, eggs and animal fats that may be used in the food industry.
- Lacto-ovo vegetarians avoid the consumption of any foods that are derived from the flesh of the animal that requires the animal to be slaughtered. They will consume eggs and dairy products. A lacto-vegetarian will consume dairy products but avoid meat and eggs. An ovo-vegetarian will consume eggs but avoid dairy and meat.
- Pescetarians incorporate fish into a vegetarian diet.
- Flexitarians will usually consume eggs and dairy products, and sometimes fish, but will tend to consume meat less than once per week.

Hinduism

Diet in Hinduism varies with its diverse traditions. Hinduism does not explicitly prohibit the consumption of meat; rather, it strongly advocates *ahimsa*—non-violence against all life forms, including animals. As such, many Hindus prefer a vegetarian or lacto-vegetarian diet which incorporates food production that is aligned with a respectful consideration of nature that is compassionate and respectful of all life forms. Although the majority of Hindus are vegetarian, a significant number still consume meat. However, given the respect for the cow as part of the Hindu belief system, they do not consume beef. Among meat-eating Hindus the preference is to consume chicken, fish, lamb and goat. There may also be periods of the year in which Hindus may fast, such as the Festival of Navratri, when the devout may abstain from many types of food and only eat one meal per day.

Islam

Islamic dietary law is in the interest of health and cleanliness as well as in obedience to God. It distinguishes between food that is good (halal) and those foods that are prohibited by God (haram). The dietary law allows prohibited foods to be consumed under the 'law of necessity' under certain circumstances, such as if no viable alternative exists. With this in mind the following foods are haram.

- 'Dead' meat (the carcass of an already-dead animal that was not slaughtered by appropriate means).
- The meat of an animal that has been sacrificed to idols.
- The meat of an animal that died from electrocution, strangulation or blunt force.
- Meat from which wild animals have already eaten.
- Blood.
- The flesh of swine (pork, bacon and ham).
- Intoxicating drinks. For devout Muslims, this even includes sauces or food-preparation liquids that might include alcohol, such as soy sauce.

There are also fasting periods within the Islamic calendar. Ramadan, the ninth month in the Islamic calendar, which varies from year to year, is considered the most sacred month. Under Islamic law, followers do not eat or drink (and in some cases will not swallow their own saliva) from dawn to dusk. All adult Muslims are required to fast except for pregnant, lactating and menstruating women, women who have given birth in the last 40 days, people with short-term illnesses, those who are seriously ill and travellers. However, it is expected that they will fast to make up the days they have lost before the next Ramadan period.

Buddhism

The Buddhist laws concerning diet are based, like those of Hinduism, on *ahimsa*—avoidance of harm to any living thing—and many Buddhists are vegetarians. Dietary laws apply more strictly to Buddhist monks and nuns and even those who live in monasteries will adapt their diet based on food availability and their personal need. Additionally, East Asian Buddhist cuisine differs from vegetarianism in its avoidance of killing plant life. Therefore root vegetables (potato, carrots, onion and garlic), which require the plant to be pulled up, are forbidden. The ultimate goal of Buddhist practice is to eliminate suffering by limiting attachment to worldly goods, which leads to the cuisine becoming quite simple in taste as well. Meals are relatively simple and are based on ingredients such as tofu, legumes, rice and vegetables (excluding root vegetables). Buddha bowls are becoming increasingly popular, containing grains, greens, other vegetables, legumes and topped with nuts and seeds and a dressing.

Judaism

Kashrut is the body of Jewish law that considers the foods that can and cannot be eaten. Foods that meet the standards set in the kashrut and may be eaten are referred to as kosher. Briefly the general rules of kashrut are as follows.

- Certain animals (hare, hyrax, camel, pig and shellfish) may not be eaten at all—this includes the flesh (meat), organs, eggs and milk of these forbidden animals.
- Of the animals that may be eaten, the birds and mammals must be killed in accordance with Jewish law. There are strict guidelines on the way the animal should be killed and it must be performed by a pious (devoutly religious) Jew.
- All blood must be drained from meat and poultry or broiled out of it before it is eaten.
- Certain parts even of permitted animals may not be eaten (sciatic nerves and surrounding vessels; chelev (suet), which is the fat surrounding vital organs and liver).
- Fruits and vegetables are permitted but must be inspected for insects (which cannot be eaten).
- Meat (the flesh of birds and mammals) must not be eaten with dairy. Eggs, fruits, vegetables and grains can be eaten with either meat or dairy. According to some views, fish may not be eaten with meat.
- Utensils, pots and pans and other cooking surfaces that have come into contact with meat may not be used with dairy, and vice versa. Utensils that have come into contact with non-kosher food may not be used with kosher food. This applies only where the contact occurred while the food was hot.
- Grape products, including wine, made by non-Jews may not be consumed.

Mormonism

The dietary restrictions in Mormonism are based on the belief that people should care for their bodies. The Mormon Church prescribes exercise, sleep, cleanliness and dental hygiene as well as dietary restrictions. The dietary restrictions include abstinence from coffee, tea, hot drinks, energy and carbonated drinks that contain caffeine, alcohol and tobacco. Mormons are allowed to eat animal products, but they are advised to choose them in smaller quantities. Fasting is expected for one day per month and the money that would have been spent on food is donated to the poor.

Seventh Day Adventism

The dietary guidelines prescribed for Seventh Day Adventists are based on the belief that God calls them to respect and care for their bodies. A vegetarian diet is promoted along with exercise and avoidance of harmful substances such as tobacco and alcohol. No meat or fish is allowed; however, eggs and dairy in moderation are acceptable.

Rastafarianism (or Rastafari)

Rastafarianism, developed in Jamaica in the 1930s, advocates eating food that is natural. Often this relates to food being produced organically and locally. Based on Judaism, they avoid eating pork or crustaceans, while many Rastas remain vegetarian and avoid the addition of additives, sugar and salt to their food. They also avoid alcohol. Rastas typically avoid eating food which has been produced by non-Rastas or other unknown sources.

Christian—Catholic, Eastern Orthodox

There are many different Christian denominations, but only two have dietary guidelines and fasting restrictions; these are the Eastern Orthodox Church and the Roman Catholic Church.

Eastern Orthodox Church

While commonly referred to as Greek Orthodox (due to the use of the Greek language in all of its theological writings and its heritage with the Byzantine Empire), Eastern Orthodox Christians are also of Russian, Eastern European, Caucasus, African and Middle Eastern background.

The set fasting periods in the Eastern Orthodox Church are Lent (eight weeks before Easter), Dormition (1–15 August), Apostles (varying number of days before 29 July) and Nativity Fast (six weeks before the Feast of the Nativity), the Eve of Theophany, the Beheading of St John the Baptist and the Elevation of the Holy Cross. Eastern Orthodox Christians also fast every Wednesday and Friday, except for the week after Easter Sunday and between Christmas and the Eve of Theophany. As a result, devout observers can be fasting for up to 180 days per year. The guidelines state that during fasting no alcohol, olive oil, animal products (including eggs and dairy products) or fish with backbones can be consumed, although shellfish and fish roe are permitted. Children, pregnant and lactating women, the elderly and those that are sick (physically or mentally) are not expected to fast.

Roman Catholic Church

The Roman Catholic Church did have a dietary restriction which prohibited the consumption of meat on Fridays, but this was abolished in 1966 in the Apostolic

Constitution of Pope Paul VI. Due to its relative recency, some devout Roman Catholics will still not eat meat on Fridays and the meat is replaced with fish—hence the 'Friday Fish Fry'. That is why in some catering facilities (hospitals, boarding schools and pubs) in Western countries fish is routinely available on the menu on Fridays. However, Roman Catholics are still required to abstain from meat (except fish) on Ash Wednesday and Good Friday.

Religion and ethical belief systems can play a large role in the type of foods that athletes will eat. However, perhaps a bigger influence is a person's cultural identity as identified by their country of birth, or that of their parents or grandparents. The next section provides an overview of foods consumed by cultures in different geographic locations around the world. It is important to remember that within these regions, there may be a number of different religious and cultural influences.

THE DIETARY CULTURE IN DIFFERENT PARTS OF THE WORLD

Asia

Asia is the largest and most populous continent in the world. Asian cuisines vary greatly, from the delicacies of Japan to the strong flavours of Vietnam and Thailand and the hot and spicy flavours of India. Rice and noodles are staple foods consumed in almost every meal and feature heavily in all Asian cuisine. Portion sizes are relatively small compared with portion sizes in Western countries.

Eastern Asian Cuisine

East Asian cuisine includes Chinese, Japanese, Korean, Taiwanese and Mongolian food.

China

China is the world's most populous country and the world's second largest by land area, with different climates, ethnicities and religions. As a result there are many distinctive styles of cuisine which form an important part of Chinese culture.

In the northern part of China (Beijing, Hebei), wheat is the staple crop and people eat noodles, dumplings, wheat buns and pancakes. Due to the large proportion of Muslims in the northwest of China, mutton is popular. Garlic, scallions, leeks and chillies are also used heavily in seasoning meals. With cold weather in the north, fresh vegetables are less available so preserving vegetables is common.

In the eastern part of China (Shanghai, Jiangsu), the cuisine is often lighter, mellower and slightly sweet in taste compared to other cuisines. This is attributed to the use of sugar, wines, vinegars and soy sauces while retaining the original flavours of the raw ingredients.

In southern China (Guangzhou (Canton) and Hong Kong), much of the region is subtropical and is green year-round, allowing year-long production of foods such as rice, fruits and vegetables. Reflecting the great variety in produce grown in this subtropical region, any one dish in Cantonese cuisine will contain many fresh ingredients, usually cooked by either steaming, broiling or stir-frying.

From western China (Sichuan, Yunnan), we have one of the most popular cuisines, Sichuan (Szechuan) style. The typical Sichuan dishes are spicy, hot and oily. Sichuan peppercorn, the most common ingredient in Sichuan cuisine, has a very strong numbing effect on the mouth and face when eaten. Mushroom, bamboo shoots and rice are also prominent ingredients in dishes, and goat's milk, lamb and mutton are staple foods in this area.

Chinese people usually like to eat their meals together and share their dishes whether eating in restaurants or at home. Food is always cooked in bite-size pieces, facilitating easy serving with chopsticks.

Dessert is not a common feature in Chinese dining, although westernisation of these countries has led to increased availability of sweets in the country.

Japan

Japanese cuisine is based on the staple foods: rice, miso soup and seasonal produce, with rice being consumed 2–3 times a day. The common phrase *ichijū-sansai*, which means 'one soup, three dishes (one main dish and two side dishes)' refers to the make-up of a typical meal. This is based on rice with miso soup and one main dish, such as fish, meat, poultry or egg, which is mainly a source of protein. The two side dishes are vegetables, either fresh or pickled, and commonly include seaweed and mushroom. In general, Japanese cuisine is light, less spicy and healthy. The exception to this is tempura and other deep-fried foods.

Before Japanese people start to eat, they say *Itadakimasu* which literally means 'I humbly receive', reflecting Japan's Buddhist origins of thanking the plants and animals that have been sacrificed, as well as those involved along the steps required to produce the meal. Traditionally this can be witnessed as people (either alone or as a group) put their palms together and slightly bow in front of their meal. At the end of a meal they say *Gochisosama deshita* with a bow again, which means 'Thank you for the food'.

Japanese people use chopsticks for eating. They use soy sauce sparingly, particularly with sushi.

Korea

Korean cuisine is quite similar to Chinese and Japanese cuisines. With Korea's extensive coastal and mountainous regions, there is a wide variety of foods consumed in the diet.

The most characteristic flavour of Korean food is spiciness; strong flavour is imparted with seasonings including red pepper, green onion, bean paste and garlic.

A traditional Korean meal consists of a bowl of rice, meat and a number of side dishes. Side dishes include spicy fermented cabbage (kimchi), seasoned soybean sprouts (kongnamul muchim), seasoned spinach (sigeumchi namul), steamed eggplant (gaji namul), and braised tofu (dooboo jorim). When having Korean style barbeque or hot pot, athletes who need to limit energy intake should limit the common fatty meats (pork belly, spare ribs) and sauces that contain fat in them. Heated stone rice (dolsot) is a popular and healthy dish because it contains rice with meat and vegetables.

Before eating, Korean people usually say to the cook, serving staff or food *Jal mukgesseubnida*, which literally means 'I will eat well' or 'I will enjoy this meal'; after eating, they say *Jal muhguhsseubnida*, which means 'I ate well'. Unlike other Asian countries, Korean chopsticks and other dining utensils are made from stainless steel. While Chinese and Japanese people use chopsticks to eat rice, Koreans normally consume rice with a spoon instead of chopsticks (as eating rice with chopsticks is considered rude). It is also not usual to lift a rice or soup bowl while eating.

Southeast Asia

Southeast Asian cuisine includes the foods of Thailand, Vietnam, Indonesia, Malaysia and Singapore. The traditional Southeast Asian cuisines have a strong aromatic component using different spices and herbs, such as mint, coriander, basil and lemon grass. Many Southeast Asian cuisines use fish sauce as a substitute for soy sauce. Commonly used cooking methods are stir-frying, steaming and boiling.

Vietnam

The ideal Vietnamese cuisine has a balance of the five taste elements—spicy, sour, bitter, salt and sweet—which provides distinctive flavour by using herbs (lemongrass, mint and basil) and sauces (fish sauce and shrimp paste), as well as fresh seasonal ingredients, minimal oil and a variety of textures.

There are some regional variations in Vietnamese cuisine. In northern Vietnam, the cuisine is influenced more by neighbouring China and the colder climate which limits the production and availability of spices, contributing to the light taste of Vietnamese cuisine. Black pepper is used in place of chilli to produce spicy flavours. The use of meat, pork, beef and chicken was relatively limited in the past, but is now increasingly commonplace in northern Vietnamese cuisine. Seafood is widely used in the northern area. In the central area there is an abundance of spices produced by the mountainous terrain, and this is reflected in the local cuisine, which has hot and spicy flavours. Chillies, black peppers and shrimp sauces are among the widely used ingredients. The dishes in this area are served in small portions, making them ideal for shared meals. The warm weather and fertile soil of southern Vietnam create ideal conditions for growing a wide variety of fruits, vegetables and livestock. As a result, foods in southern Vietnam are often vibrant and flavourful, with liberal uses of garlic, shallots, and fresh herbs. Rice is a staple food in Vietnamese cuisine and appears at breakfast, lunch, dinner and dessert. People eat rice or 'made-from-rice' dishes such as rice porridge, rice noodle (Pho), and square rice cake (Banh chung) in every meal.

Thailand

Although Thai food has a reputation for being spicy, traditional Thai cuisine, like Vietnamese cuisine, is based on the balance of five different flavours—spicy, sour, sweet, salty and bitter. Each Thai dish includes at least three or four different tastes by using herbs or seasoning such as lemongrass, basil, coriander and kaffir lime leaves.

Thai cuisine can be described based on four different regional cuisines. Not surprisingly, the variations tend to reflect the local geography and climate as well as the influence of neighbouring countries. In the northern area, the taste is generally milder than other areas. Due to the influence of neighbouring Myanmar and Laos, people prefer glutinous rice (sticky rice); it is rolled into a ball, and dipped into dishes and sauces. Noodle-based dishes are popular in northern Thailand. One such regional dish which is popular in Chiang Mai is Khao soi, a coconut milk-based curry seasoned with curry powder and served with egg noodles. The food in the northeast of Thailand is influenced by Laos; the food is highly spiced, and sticky glutinous rice is the preferred staple for northeastern dishes. Food in the southern area of Thailand is renowned for being strong in taste—very hot, salty and sour, with coconut milk used in many dishes. Because the south has a huge coastline, fish and seafood are a major part of the everyday diet and are often grilled, flavoured with chillies and lime, roasted in a pot filled with salt, boiled in curries, stirred into salads or simply deep-fried. The central region offers a melting pot of tastes from the north and south. Jasmine rice (non-sticky rice) is a staple food. Tom yam kung (hot and sour soup) and Tom kha kai (chicken soup in coconut milk) originate from the central region. However, due to strong Chinese influence in the central region, plain soups that usually include tofu, ground pork and green squash are also common. Curries are also popular in Thailand and there are four main types of curries (based on colour); the hottest is green curry followed by red, yellow and orange curry, the mildest.

Street food in Asia

Street food is very popular and tempting in most Asian countries. However, caution must be exercised as there is a possible risk of food poisoning. When athletes want to

> ## Box 25.1: How do Thai curries differ from other Asian curries?
>
> Generally, Thai curries use a lot of coconut milk and more liquid than Indian curries. Thai curries use a lot of vegetables and even meat and seafood and contain local ingredients such as chilli peppers, lime leaves, lemon grass and coconut which makes them more aromatic than Indian curries. Japanese curry is usually thicker, sweeter (apple, carrots and potatoes are common ingredients in Japanese curries) and not as hot as Thai and Indian curries. In India, curries commonly use lentils as their featured ingredients.

have street food, they should purchase it from reliable street vendors. Reliable street vendors can be identified by having the food stored below 4°C and raw food separated from cooked food and protected by containers. Athletes should also be wary of high-risk foods such as undercooked or raw meats and seafood.

Middle East

The countries of the Middle East include Afghanistan, Iran, Iraq, Israel, Kuwait, Syria and the United Arab Emirates. In general, Middle Eastern cuisine includes an extensive range of spices such as cumin, cinnamon and cloves. Rice and wheat products—such as bread, flat breads (naan, pita bread, matzo), burghul, whole wheat and couscous—are staple foods and served with most dishes. Most countries in the Middle East are primarily Islamic; certain dietary rules are observed, as described earlier in this chapter. Alcohol is prohibited in many countries, as are pork products. Chicken, beef and lamb are popular protein choices and often served as kebabs, where chunks of meat are cooked skewered with vegetables. Soups and side dishes include lentils, beans, capsicum, eggplant and other vegetables. Yoghurt and olive oil are common accompaniments with meals as well as being used in the cooking. Butter or oil is heavily used when cooking many Middle Eastern dishes. Ensure you discuss with athletes suggestions for healthier options, such as olive oil, canola oil, avocado oil, etc., and discuss cooking methods that use less oil if there is concern over their kilojoule intake. In the Middle East, people consider eating an important socialising event and they put a lot of food on the table. Therefore, it is easy to go for second and third helpings. If athletes need to control body weight, you should encourage them to serve their dishes on smaller plates and to place leftovers in the fridge right away; also remind them that it takes 20–30 minutes for satiety to set in.

Iran

Iranian (also known as Persian) cuisine is gaining popularity in many countries. Rice and wheat products (whole wheat, burghul, couscous) are also staple foods in Iran. Although beef and poultry are consumed in Iran, sheep and goat are the preferred meat sources. For Iranians living near coastlines, fish is their main protein source. Other plant-based protein sources, such as beans, chickpeas and lentils, are consumed on a daily basis as an addition to stews, or mixed with rice and bread. Because Iran is a Muslim country, pork and some seafood such as shellfish, molluscs and lobster are considered unclean. Saffron, dried lime, cinnamon and coriander are common ingredients in Iranian cuisine.

Israel

Israeli cuisine comprises local dishes of the native Israeli people as well as foods brought by immigrants to Israel. The Mediterranean diet also has an influence on Israeli cuisine, with olives, wheat, chickpeas, dairy products, fish and vegetables such as tomatoes, eggplants and zucchini featuring in Israeli cooking. Fresh fruits and vegetables are plentiful in Israel and are cooked and served in many dishes. As the majority of people in Israel are Jewish, they follow Jewish dietary law (Kashrut) regarding foods consumed, food preparation and cooking methods. In addition, Jewish festivals or special occasions influence the cuisine. For example, in Passover, unleavened bread (Matzah) and other unleavened foods are eaten. In Hanukkah (festival of light), fried food such as sufganiyah (jelly-filled doughnuts) and latkes (potato pancakes) are served. Eating dairy foods such as cheese, cheesecake and blintzes (cheese-filled crepes) is also popular and is a newer food tradition for Hanukkah.

Lebanon

Lebanese cuisine has evolved and been influenced through its long history of successive invasions by the Egyptians, Babylonians, Greeks, Turks and French. The Lebanese diet focuses on herbs, spices and fresh ingredients such as mint, parsley, garlic, allspice and cinnamon. Bread such as marqouq (mountain bread) or Syrian bread is a staple food in Lebanon and is served with almost every meal. Although meat is not a major ingredient in Lebanese cuisine, poultry and lamb make up the most popular Lebanese dishes. Mezzes, an array of small hot and cold dishes which are shared, is another popular part of Lebanese cuisine.

Turkey

While partly situated within Europe, Turkish dietary patterns have similar features to Middle Eastern cuisine. Turkish cuisine varies across the country and each region has its own food culture. In the central, eastern and southern parts of Turkey, oily, spicy meat dishes, kebabs and dishes made with grains and legumes are famous. The cuisine of the Black Sea region is composed predominantly of fish, particularly anchovies, and corn. In Marmara, the Aegean and Mediterranean regions are rich in vegetables, legumes, beans, fish, olive oil, lemon juice, yoghurt and feta cheese. Turkish people consume the highest amount of bread in the world. Rice, pilaf, couscous and börek (filo dough stuffed with vegetables or meat) are common meals. Mutton, lamb and beef are basic components of Turkish cuisine. Organ meats such as brain, liver and kidney are also popular. Kokoreç, a dish of Balkan origin made of skewered lamb intestines barbecued over slow heat, is sold in many places in Turkey.

Arabian Peninsula

The Arabian Peninsula includes Bahrain, Kuwait, Oman, Qatar, Saudi Arabia, the United Arab Emirates and Yemen. Arabic cuisine consists of lamb, mutton, chicken, beef, milk, dates, squash, radishes and okra. Common spices used in cooking include turmeric, garlic, cumin, coriander, fenugreek, black lemon and saffron. Rice is also a staple food in the Arabian Peninsula. In the coastal regions, fish and seafood are more heavily offered. Whole fried fish is preferred, served with spring onions. Arabians prefer fermented forms of dairy products.

Australia and New Zealand

The food and cuisine of Australia and New Zealand is wide and diverse, reflecting the many different cultures that now live in these countries. However, traditionally the food is based on the modest, often plain and hearty British (Anglo-Saxon) diet, which reflects the first line of migration into these countries. This cuisine is typified by the 'meat and three vegetables', representing the typical meal in Australian and New Zealand dining rooms up to the 1970s. However, the influence of Southern European migrants from Greece and Italy from the 1950s to the 1970s introduced a more diverse diet with the use of olives, olive oil and a greater variety of vegetables—often cooked in tomato-based sauces—pasta and rice dishes, as well as the use of cured and spicy meats. Italian cuisine still remains a popular meal choice and there are many Italian-style restaurants and cafes. Since the 1980s, it has been Asian immigration that has influenced cuisine, with the widespread appearance of stir-fries using fresh herbs and sauces with noodles or rice, while curries have continued to grow and feature in the cuisine of Australia and New Zealand.

While the influx of different migrant groups has contributed greatly to the cuisine, there has been increasing incorporation of Indigenous foods such as kangaroo, small marsupials, emu, crocodile, turtle and witchetty grubs along with native plants such as quandong, kutjera, muntries, riberry and finger lime in Australia. In New Zealand, the kumara (sweet potato) and taro are now staples of the diet.

In both Australia and New Zealand, fusion cuisine has become very popular. This involves the combination of elements from different culinary traditions, including fusion of traditional British cuisine and Asian influences, as well as fusion with Indigenous ingredients. The fusion of Mediterranean dishes with Asian and Middle Eastern influences has also become popular in the restaurant industry, as well as in home cooking. This has led to a diet and selection of foods that truly represent the multicultural nature of the Austral-Asian and Middle Eastern regions.

For the athlete travelling to Australia and New Zealand, it is highly likely they will find their favoured traditional cultural or religious cuisine in restaurants, cafes, fast-food and foods available for self-catering. Bakeries are another popular eating spot, providing a range of breads, rolls, wraps and baked pies and pasties (meat and vegetable fillings encased in pastry). Ensuring adequate intake of carbohydrates at each meal is not difficult as dishes can be ordered with bread and pizza, pasta, rice, noodles, couscous and starchy vegetables are all common components in meals from most restaurants and cafes. Eating at Italian, Asian and Middle Eastern style restaurants will ensure most meals on the menu contain carbohydrate (noodles, rice, pasta, couscous). Most of the meals listed in Tables 25.1 and 25.2 are also available in Australia and New Zealand.

SUMMARY AND KEY MESSAGES

Previous chapters have focused on the specific nutritional requirements to support the needs of performance and activity for athletes. An equally important aspect is the cultural, religious and philosophical food choices that affect an athlete's dietary intake. It is important to take this into consideration when assessing and making recommendations to athletes.

Key messages
* Athletes and teams come from a variety of dietary backgrounds which affect food choices.
* It is important to prepare athletes for the foods available in different countries so that they are able to meet their nutrient recommendations for sports performance.
* Athletes should also be warned about countries in which food hygiene needs to be considered to avoid gastrointestinal illness.
* Athletes should also be provided with education about suitable high-carbohydrate (and, where relevant, low-fat) food choices to meet their requirements in the countries they are visiting.
* Different religions set dietary laws that can affect the type of foods that are consumed, as well as the timing of food consumption.

Table 25.1. Summary of healthy food options in Asian countries

	China (including Hong Kong, Macau and Taiwan)	Japan	Korea	Vietnam	Thailand	Singapore, Malaysia
Main and entrée Carbohydrate source	• Steamed rice • Noodle in soup • Steamed plain bun • Congee/rice porridge	• Gohan (steamed rice) • Okyau (congee) • Soba (buckwheat noodle) or Udon in soup • Sushi (made with cooked ingredients only)	• Bap (steamed rice) • Juk (congee) • Bibimbap (mixed rice with vegetables and meat) • Dolsot (heated stone bowl rice) • Guksu jangguk (noodle in clear broth)	• Com (steamed rice) • Chao (congee) • Pho (rice noodle in soup) • Banh mi (Vietnamese baguette)	• Khao (steamed rice) • Jok (congee) • Khao tom (Thai-style rice soup)	• Nasi (steamed rice) • Bubur (congee) • Nasi lemak (rice cooked with coconut milk and pandan leaves) • Mee (noodles) • Lemang (glutinous rice, coconut milk and cooked in a hollowed bamboo stick) • Kaya toast • Nasi goreng • Hainanese chicken rice
Desserts Carbohydrate source	• Sweet soybean curd • Red/green bean sweet soup • Mixed beans sweet soup • Sweet potato soup	• Anmitsu (agar jelly with red bean paste and fresh fruit) • Mochi (Japanese rice cake) • Shiruko (red bean sweet soup)	• Tteok (rice cake) • Jeonggwa (boiling sliced fruits, roots or seeds in honey) • Patjuk (hot red bean porridge)	• Chè Trôi Nước (sweet glutinous rice dumplings) • Chè Sương Sa Hạt Lựu (rainbow dessert)	• Kanome maw gaeng (sweet potato pudding) • Coconut juice	• Thick Apam Balik (Malaysian peanut pancake turnover) • Kuih pisang (banana cake) • Penang cake

	China (including Hong Kong, Macau and Taiwan)	Japan	Korea	Vietnam	Thailand	Singapore, Malaysia
Main and entrée Protein source	• Steamed meat bun • Stir-fried/ steamed/boiled meat, fish and seafood • Steamed tofu and egg	• Teriyaki meat or vegetable • Shabu/Sukiyai (hot pot dish with meats) • Nikujaga (stewed meat and potato) • Nizakana (poached fish) • Steamed or cold tofu • Chawanmushi (steamed egg custard) • Oden (stewed fishcake, eggs, daikon) • Kushiyaki (skewered meat)	• Gimbap (Korean-style sushi) • Samgyetang (ginseng chicken soup) • Haemultang (seafood stew) • Oden (skewered fishcake)	• Goi cuon (steamed spring roll) • Gà nóng sả (roasted chicken with lemongrass) • Chả lụa (pork sausage) • Bò Lúc Lắc (sautéed diced beef) • Nem nguội (meatball)	• Tom Yam (hot and sour soup) • Pla pad priew wan (sweet and sour fish) • Som tum (Thai papaya salad)	• Ikan bakar (grilled fish) • Satay chicken, beef or pork • Sup Kambing/Spo Kambing (mutton soup) • Otak-otak (grilled fishcake)

Table 25.2. Summary of healthy food options in Middle East countries

	Iran	Israel	Lebanon	Turkey	Arabian Peninsula
Main and entrée Carbohydrate source	• Rice – Polo/Chelo (rice cooked in broth) – Kateh (sticky rice) – Doodi (smoked rice) • Zereshk polow (bareberry rice) • Naan bread • Lavash bread • Sangak bread • Qandi bread • Komaj	• Pita bread • Bagel • Challah • Sabich (pita bread served with eggplant, boiled eggs, Israeli salad, amba, parsley, tahini sauce and hummus) • Ptitim (Israeli couscous)	• Flat breads • Rice • Lahma bi Ajeen (Arab pizza) • Laban Immo (cooked yoghurt and lamb with rice) • Riz bil-Foul (rice and Fava beans) • Riz bi-Djaj (chicken with rice)	• Rice • Bazlama • Gözleme • Misur ekmeği (corn bread) • Yufka • Sade pilav (plain rice pilaf) • Pathicanli pilav (rice with eggplant)	• Aish (rice) • Bukhari rice • Khoubz bread • Maqluba (rice, eggplant and meat casserole) • Semolina • Murtabak (pan-fried bread or pancake stuffed with vegetables and minced meat)
Dessert Carbohydrate source	• Bastani Akbar Mashti (saffron ice cream) • Fereni (Persian rice pudding) • Sholezard (saffron rice-based dessert) • Halva Ardeh (semolina-based dessert)	• Fazuelos • Tahini cookie • Rugelach	• Baklava • Date pastry • Nammourah (Lebanese semolina cake)	• Baklava • Sütlaç (rice pudding) • Tavuk göğsü (gelatinous, milk pudding dessert) • Turkish delight	• Zardah (sweet rice pudding) • Mahalbiah (rice or starch-based milk pudding)

	Iran	Israel	Lebanon	Turkey	Arabian Peninsula

Main and entrée Protein source	• Kebab (lamb or beef)
	• Dolma (stuffed grapevine leaves)
	• Khoresh (stew dishes)
	  – Baghala ghatogh (stewed fava beans, dill and eggs)
	  – Dizi (mutton stew with chickpeas and potatoes)
	  – Khoresh e alu (stewed prunes and meat)
		• Kebab
		• Tilapia
		• Moussaka (oven-baked dish of ground meat with eggplant or potato and béchamel sauce)
			• Kebbe Lakteen (meatballs)
			• Shish Barak (dough balls stuffed with ground beef and cooked in yoghurt)
			• Deleh Mehshi (stuffed rib cage of lamb)
			• Kafta Bithine (spiced meat with sesame concentrate)
				• Kuzu güveç
				• Ankara tava (pilav with lamb)
				• Köfte (meatball)
				• İncik (lamb shank cooked in the oven)
				• Etli bamya (okra with meat)
					• Kubbah (wheat balls stuffed with mince wheat)
					• Falafel
					• Kababs (skewered minced meat)

FURTHER READING

Liu, J., 2011, *Introduction to Chinese Culture*, 1st edn, New York, NY: Cambridge University Press.

Edelstein, S., 2010, *Food, Cuisine, and Cultural Competency for Culinary, Hospitality, and Nutrition Professionals*, 1st edn, Sudbury, MA: Jones & Bartlett Learning.

CHAPTER 26

Working with athletes

Anthony Meade

The preceding chapters have provided us with an overview of the key concepts in sports nutrition. While there are common themes, concepts and athlete goals, there are also individual challenges in translating these concepts into meaningful, practical sports nutrition advice. In this chapter, we will explore how to turn theoretical sports nutrition information and food knowledge into practical, individualised sports nutrition advice in various settings. We will also look at the roles of sports dietitians as well as other sport and nutrition professionals in providing nutrition advice and support for athletes.

LEARNING OUTCOMES

Upon completion of this chapter you will be able to:
- understand the role of a sports dietitian within the team of support people for an athlete
- describe the skills needed to work as a sports dietitian with individual athletes
- describe the skills needed to work as a sports dietitian with team sport athletes and within a team sport environment
- recognise the various roles of support staff in the implementation of team sports nutrition practices.

THE ROLE OF A SPORTS DIETITIAN: MORE THAN JUST DIETARY ADVICE

Sports dietitians are highly trained and specialised nutrition professionals. In Australia, accreditation as a sports dietitian requires completion of at least a four-year university degree in dietetics, additional training in sports nutrition and several years of practical experience. The environments in which sports dietitians work are varied and include private clinics, sports institutes, sports teams, universities, research and industry. In this chapter, we will focus on the two most common environments: private clinical practice and team sports.

There are many challenges to working as a sports dietitian, but the need to work independently, often as a sole practitioner, is perhaps the most common.

Communication and organisational skills are as important as clinical knowledge and skills. High-level communication skills are critical for building rapport with the athlete, as well as for detailed nutrition assessment and implementation of plans, and, perhaps even more importantly, for involving other members of the athlete support team in these processes. While there are equipment and technologies that can enhance what a sports dietitian does, none can replace good communication skills.

The ability to manage time, prioritise workflows and adjust to unexpected situations are skills common to many professional people, but critical to success as a sports dietitian, as we will explore below.

NON-TEAM ENVIRONMENT

One of the biggest challenges working in the private clinical setting is being remote from the other members of the athlete support team.

There are advantages to working within a sports medicine clinic, where the other professionals in the clinic are also involved with the same or similar athletes or sporting teams. However, this is not always possible so a thorough training history, medical history, analysis of goals, objectives and timelines, and body composition assessment are as important as a diet history (see Chapters 7 and 8 for more detail about dietary assessment and dietary counselling).

Understanding the roles of the other clinicians and being able to ask questions about non-nutritional management is helpful when planning nutrition interventions. For example, liaising with the athlete's physiotherapist during injury rehabilitation can guide periodisation of energy and protein intakes during the different phases of the rehabilitation program. In addition, including other members of the multidisciplinary team in the nutritional planning conversation can increase the athlete's support and adherence, as well as being a valuable source of insight into the athlete's progress and challenges, particularly between consultations.

Importantly, the athletes who come to private clinical practice are often highly motivated, even if they do not compete at an elite level. In fact, some age group and recreational athletes may be more motivated to optimise their nutrition practice than elite or professional athletes, and may come with unique needs not seen in elite athletes.

Where possible, it is useful to encourage the athlete to come to their appointment prepared with training diaries or plans and even a multi-day food record. Unfortunately, in private clinical practice it is not always possible to know much about a client until they walk through the door; however, it pays to research the athlete's chosen sport/event in advance, if possible. If it is a sport with which you are unfamiliar, it is far better to recognise the limitations of your knowledge and invest time asking questions of the athlete (or spending time doing some research) than to pretend to know (and demonstrate your lack of knowledge) and lose the client.

Take time to understand what it is that the athlete wants from you. It may be a complete nutrition assessment and eating pattern overhaul; it may be some targeted questions or a competition or race-day plan; or it may be a new clinical issue (such as diagnosis of diabetes or other health concern) that requires reassessment of current training nutrition strategies.

When working in private practice, it is highly recommended to get involved with the local sports medicine community. Being visible within the sports medicine community has many advantages. Involvement in professional meetings, conferences and professional development sessions can raise your profile and lead to increased referrals and other opportunities with athletes, teams and organisations that other sports medicine professionals are involved with, as well as providing a better understanding of the roles of other members of the athlete support team. Having professional networks for support is critical to effective private practice so that you know who to call or email when you need support. Another benefit is gaining insights into training, medical and nutritional practices from other sports and other practitioners, which can often be applied or adapted to other athletes.

TEAM ENVIRONMENT

There are common elements to working in private clinical practice and working in sporting teams, institutes or sporting organisations, but there are also many additional considerations and roles when providing support to a team or squad. The individual client/athlete nutrition assessment and advice are essentially the same regardless of the setting; however, the structures in place in a team or organisation add both advantages and complexity to the implementation.

Access to other members of the athlete support team is likely to be easier, or at least more clear and consistent, in a team environment, but communication is essential for success. Within a sporting team environment, a sports dietitian would commonly interact with many other individuals including:

- players and athletes
- administrators and administrative staff
- sponsorship and marketing staff
- coaches
- physical performance staff/sports science staff
- support staff (team managers, trainers, volunteers)
- medical staff
- other allied health professionals (physiotherapy, psychology, massage)
- food service and catering suppliers, food companies
- supplement companies, representatives
- universities and academic researchers.

Starting in a new team environment can be daunting, particularly if there has been a lack of nutrition services provided previously. The team is likely to have expectations of the role, although these may not necessarily align with your own expectations, skills and abilities. In many situations, budget constraints may mean there is a specific focus area while other aspects of nutrition are considered less important or optional extras. When starting out, it is important to get a clear role description and familiarise yourself with governance structures, communication and reporting lines and the areas considered high priority. Then you need to identify who everyone is, what their roles are, where everything is and how everything is currently working. Oh, and as quick as you can please!

Box 26.1: Tips for sports dietitians starting out in a new team

- Make as many friends as you can by listening to all of the people involved and understanding the team dynamics.
- Make as many notes as you can and be prepared to report back.
- Pick off low-hanging fruit as far as problems go—look for easy fixes and efficiencies that can quickly build your credibility.
- Be prepared to be flexible and deal with issues at short notice. It is not uncommon to be asked to change a plan after a team loss or a coaching observation, even though it may not always appear rational or a high priority.

Unless you're starting out with a newly created club, there are likely to be established systems and structures that have developed over many years. Some of these may have evolved over time, others remain unchanged because no one remembers why things are done a certain way, and others are compromised due to limited resources, personnel, skills or time. Be prepared to invest time in observation, thinking about how you see an ideal set up and assessing what is and what is not working. Talk to as many of the support staff as you can to gather information about how well they think systems work, and be prepared to explore the history of how the team/club/organisation has evolved to better understand how things work.

WORKING WITH PLAYERS AND ATHLETES

Invest time learning who the players are, their experience levels, those perceived to be good at what they do and those who need work. With this knowledge in mind, remain objective and be prepared to assess.

In any team there will be leaders and influencers who other athletes will look to, observe or aspire to be. Invest time figuring out who the 'influencers' and 'early-adopters' are and get to know what they do that can be used to guide other players/athletes. If you are trying to implement a new strategy or change an existing practice, you can make good use of the 'early-adopters' to help sell what you are trying to do. The dietitian's role is often linked with weight reduction or the need to reduce skin-folds, and in some teams it is seen as a negative or 'being in trouble' to get a dietitian's input. Being seen to work with the 'good' athletes who others consider not to need your input is a valuable way to build credibility and reduce anxiety of 'having to see the dietitian'!

Ultimately, the sports dietitian's goal is to create an environment in which athletes feel comfortable asking for nutritional advice to improve their performance.

It is important to learn the player schedules to find times to fit in appointments. These may be small windows of opportunity, sometimes just to complete an assessment before a training session with a plan to follow up after the training session. These conversations may be in an office or quiet room, changerooms, corridors, warm-up areas, the gym, the race, recovery stations, over lunch or with a coffee or on the training ground. Some players may be quite comfortable having a discussion in front of teammates, others may only be comfortable in a quiet room away from prying eyes. It is always a good idea to offer a quiet space and ask what the player would prefer. There are many factors that may affect a player's ability on a daily basis to keep an appointment time, so be flexible, reschedule as needed, remind (and remind again), be in a place the players can easily find you and let other staff know you have an appointment so they can also remind the player.

Importantly, when setting up appointments, ask or learn how the players prefer to be contacted or notified, as this is likely to vary. Phone calls, text messaging and social media applications may be more effective than emails. Appointment times on a prominent noticeboard can be helpful if the players know to look there, but useless if not. It is prudent not to assume a player will remember their appointment.

Not every conversation is formal or takes place in a consultation room. While appointments generally make life easier to perform more detailed assessments and provide education, it is equally important to be visible and to 'float' around so as to be available to ask questions. Being at training, or key positions such as recovery stations, often leads to conversations that develop rapport and allow you to demonstrate what you do in a more 'public' space. Sometimes overhearing player conversations (or players overhearing your conversations) encourages other individual or group discussions, initiated by the players or the dietitian.

Obviously, individual nutrition assessment and education are a major part of a sports dietitian's responsibilities, but there are many other aspects to the role that may take up as much or more time.

The amount of time dealing directly with administrators and administrative staff will vary from role to role and the size of the club/team/organisation. There are likely to be meetings and committees set up to deal with budgets and expenditure, policy and procedural issues, and often integrity issues, which are now commonplace in major sporting competitions. You may be asked to complete accreditation procedures before being employed or to work in specific competitions. Where teams travel for competition, a good working relationship with the person organising the travel is essential to ensure that arrangements for meals are consistent with the principles you are applying in individual consultations, and that individual needs (intolerances, beliefs, goals) and team philosophies are appropriately catered for.

WORKING WITH ADMINISTRATIVE AND COACHING STAFF

Sponsorship and marketing is a key role in any major sporting organisation. There are times when sponsorship opportunities arise that may be beneficial to the nutrition program and the club, but there will also be times where a sponsorship opportunity may conflict, so it is important to build a solid relationship with the sponsorship and marketing team. In addition, the sponsorship and marketing team will be interested in what you might need for the team and can help leverage a deal. Often the dealings will be for sports nutrition supplements or food products, where knowledge of the product and doping risks is crucial to signing a deal. A deal that adds no value to what you do or causes major conflicts needs to be addressed with care. When sponsorship deals are done, it is important to understand details such as the value of the deal (including contraindications or agreed spends), sponsor expectations (such as product placement during games) and club expectations (such as product batch-testing, product availability and ordering/purchasing arrangements).

Coaches will bring their own attitudes and philosophies to a team, and this includes beliefs about nutrition and nutrition services. Some coaches will have worked with sports dietitians before, while others may have had limited exposure to the role. Experiences may have been both positive and negative, so it is wise to establish rapport with coaching staff, learn their expectations and explain your role. Governance structures will vary. Some coaches like to have direct communication with the dietitian, while others may prefer to communicate through an intermediary such as a high-performance manager. A coach's personal philosophies around nutrition may not always align with current or optimal sports nutrition practices and can conflict with individual advice you give to a player—just another challenge for a sports dietitian in the team environment.

It is common for a sports dietitian to report to a manager of high performance or sports science and be included in the sports science team. Developing an open relationship with the high-performance manager is critical for the success of both roles but can be challenging if philosophies are not aligned. Be prepared to be challenged to find small performance gains through practice efficiencies, education and nutritional supplement strategies. Be prepared to defend nutrition strategies with evidence, but also to propose and trial new practices in a strategic way. The physical performance team will expect a level of innovation but be mindful if innovation becomes more important than getting basic practices right.

WORKING WITH NUTRITION SUPPORT STAFF

A sports dietitian is the best person to *oversee* team nutrition strategies, but the sports science team is critical to the *implementation* of team nutrition practices, with many roles not exclusive to sports dietitians. Sports science tasks may include taking anthropometric measurements such as skinfolds and organising DXA scans, monitoring hydration practices with urine specific gravity measurements, fluid balance and sweat studies, organising and monitoring recovery nutrition practices, helping with game-day nutrition practices, chasing player preferences and feedback, and providing feedback on team meals, particularly when teams travel without a dietitian. While sports dietitians in larger teams (such as AFL or rugby teams) will often assume these roles, in smaller teams with limited sports dietitian time these will often fall to sports science professionals (including students) instead. In most teams, the sports science staff will have far more frequent interactions with players and are well placed to observe practices, interpret training data, overhear conversations, monitor stock levels and usage, and liaise with coaches to provide valuable insights for the team sports dietitian.

Other support staff, such as team managers, trainers, volunteers, medical staff and other allied health professionals (physiotherapy, psychology, massage, player welfare), are important to engage in team-focused nutrition philosophies and strategies. An effective working relationship with all of these people will have a major impact on how successful team nutrition strategies are, as they will often be involved in the implementation. Involving support staff in decision-making and implementation of nutrition strategies is a great way to demonstrate your knowledge, skills and value within the team environment. Perhaps even more importantly, many of these staff are likely to be present in the team environment more often than the sports dietitian, so be mindful that the support staff will be crucial to maintaining nutrition strategies when the dietitian is not around.

Support staff are often able to provide significant observational feedback on individual practices and team nutrition strategies. Major sporting teams may take a sports dietitian when travelling for competition; however, this is a luxury for smaller teams, so a sports dietitian will rely on the game-day or competition-day observations of support staff.

Player welfare staff are often employed by sporting teams and can provide valuable insight into player living situations, personal relationships, mental health and coping strategies and other personal insights that can assist a sports dietitian to work effectively with individuals within a team environment. This insight can help the sports dietitian to be sensitive to personal issues that may impact on an athlete's ability to implement nutrition strategies and to identify issues that the athlete may disclose in a nutrition consultation.

A sports dietitian in a team environment will also spend a significant amount of time in contact with food service and catering suppliers, food companies, supplement companies and representatives. The range of activities can vary from arranging team meals during the training week and team meals for away trips, catering for club events, organising cooking sessions for players, sourcing new products for sampling and supply, and clarifying nutrition information. Good food product knowledge as well as knowledge of commercial cooking practices is essential for these roles. Cooking food in commercial quantities is very different from cooking at home, and products commonly used at home may not be available to commercial caterers. Catering for individual needs can be challenging with commercial catering but being prepared, having realistic expectations and investing time speaking with caterers can save unnecessary stress and negative feedback.

It is common for the sports dietitian in a team environment to be provided with samples of new products that need to be assessed for suitability. Endorsement by association is a common goal of product sales and marketing people, but remain objective and utilise other staff within the organisation to make decisions about new products.

It is common in elite sporting teams to have significant links with universities and academic researchers. Not only are these relationships valuable for keeping abreast of the latest research, they can also be useful for researching and validating nutritional interventions, and supporting students to complete projects and clinical placements within the team environment.

SUMMARY AND KEY MESSAGES

After reading this chapter, you should be familiar with the role of a sports dietitian in private practice and in team settings, and be able to describe a number of strategies for working with athletes and other members of sports organisations. You should also be familiar with the nutrition-related roles of other support staff in team environments. For more information about the differences in scope of practice for sport and nutrition professionals, refer to the Introduction.

Key messages

- Sports dietitians are highly trained and specialised nutrition professionals who work in a variety of settings.
- Communication and organisational skills are integral to successful practice in both one-on-one and team settings.
- It is important to invest time to observe and understand current practices when implementing change.
- Sports dietitians should understand the roles of other staff in the athlete support team and utilise their knowledge and skills to enhance their practice.
- There are a number of staff within sporting organisations who play a role in improving nutrition practices.

GLOSSARY

Absolute exercise intensity: The total amount of energy expended (expressed in kilojoules or kilocalories) to produce mechanical work.

Accredited Exercise Scientist: A specialist in the assessment, design and delivery of exercise and physical activity programs.

Acidosis: A process causing increased acidity in the blood and other body tissue.

Adenosine: A chemical that naturally occurs in humans and which causes a decrease in alertness and arousal when it binds to receptors on the surface of cells in the brain.

Aerobic: Exercise at an intensity that is low enough to allow the body's need for oxygen (to break down macronutrients) to be matched to the oxygen supply available.

Aerobic capacity: The ability of the body to take in and distribute oxygen to the working muscles during exercise.

Allometric scaling: Basing an individual's basal metabolic rate (BMR) and hence requirements on their body mass.

Amenorrhea: The absence or cessation of menstruation. Primary amenorrhea is defined as the delay of the first menstruation past 16 years of age. Secondary amenorrhea is defined as the absence of three to six consecutive cycles.

Amino acids: The building blocks of protein, composed of a central carbon to which is attached a hydrogen (H), an amino group (NH_2), a carboxylic acid group (COOH) and a side chain group.

Anabolic: An anabolic effect refers to the 'building up' and repair of tissues through increased protein synthesis and cell growth. It is the opposite of 'catabolism', which refers to the breakdown of molecules.

Anabolic reactions: Small molecules join to form a larger molecule in the presence of energy (ATP).

Anabolic steroids: Drugs which help the repair and build of muscle tissues, derived from the male hormone testosterone.

Anaerobic: Exercise at an intensity where the body's demand for oxygen is greater than the oxygen supply available, therefore relying on anaerobic metabolism and the production of lactate.

Anions: Negatively charged ions, which means they have lost electrons.

Anthropometry: The comparative study of measurement of sizes and proportions of the human body.

Antioxidants: Substances that decrease free radical damage by donating an electron to 'neutralise' free radicals.

Arginine: A conditionally essential amino acid that has been shown to have benefits in wound healing.

Beverage-hydration index: An index system that has been developed to describe the fluid retention capacity of different beverages by standardising values to the retention of still water.

Biomechanical: Pertaining to the mechanical nature of the body's biological processes, such as movements of the skeleton and muscles.

Body density: The compactness of a body, defined as the mass divide by its volume.

Body-image disorder: A mental disorder in which an individual continually focuses on one or more perceived flaws in appearance that are minor or not observable to others.

Bolus: A portion, with respect to food, that is swallowed at one time.

Bonking: An athletic term describing a sudden and overwhelming feeling of running out of energy, often also termed 'hitting the wall' during endurance events.

Brush border: The microvilli-covered surface of the epithelial cells in the surface of the small intestine.

Buffer: A chemical system within the body that aims to counteract a change in the blood pH, defined by the blood $[H^+]$.

Carbohydrate availability: Consideration of the timing and amount of carbohydrate (CHO) intake in the athlete's diet in comparison to the muscle fuel costs of the training or competition schedule. Scenarios of 'high carbohydrate availability' cover strategies in which body CHO supplies can meet the fuel costs of the exercise program, whereas 'low carbohydrate availability' considers scenarios in which endogenous and/or exogenous CHO supplies are less than muscle fuel needs.

Cardiac output: The product of an individual's heart rate (the amount of times the heart contracts per minute) and stroke volume (the volume of blood ejected from the heart per minute).

Cardiorespiratory exercise: Whole-body, dynamic exercise that taxes predominantly the cardiovascular and respiratory systems, such as running, cycling and swimming.

Cardiovascular system: A system of the body consisting of the heart, blood vessels and blood that delivers nutrients to the body and removes waste products.

Casein protein: Casein is a family of related phosphoproteins, which are found in mammalian milk. About 80 per cent of the protein in cow's milk is casein.

Catabolic reactions: Biochemical reactions that result in the breakdown of large molecules and give off energy in the form of ATP.

Cations: Positively charged ions, which means they have gained electrons.

Central nervous system: Composed of the brain and spinal cord, the central nervous system is responsible for control of our thoughts, movements and regulation.

Chyme: The mass of partially digested food that leaves the stomach and enters the duodenum.

Circadian process desynchronisation: Disruption of the sleep–wake cycle/circadian rhythm.

Cis form: In a molecule, the C atoms that have double bonds and the H atoms are on the same side.

Coeliac disease: Autoimmune disease in which the immune system reacts abnormally to gluten, causing damage to the small intestine.

Coenzyme: A substance that works with an enzyme to initiate or assist the function of the enzyme. It may be considered a helper molecule for a biochemical reaction.

Conduction: The transfer of heat from one object to another through contact. Heat is transferred from the warmer to the cooler object.

Convection: The transfer of heat through the movement of warmer liquids or gases towards areas that are cooler, usually due to air or water flow over the skin. The greater the flow of air or water, the greater the heat transfer.

Creatine supplementation: Supplementation with synthetic creatine can augment the level of creatine in the body and lead to enhanced performance of power activities.

Cytoplasm: The semifluid substance contained within a cell.

Denaturation: The change that occurs in a protein's shape and structure and resulting in loss of function. This denaturation may occur due to external stressors such as chemicals, temperature, digestion or other factors.

Direct calorimetry: A direct measure of heat transfer to determine energy expenditure.

Disordered eating: Eating behaviours that are not healthy or normal, including restrained eating, binge eating, fasting, heavy exercise, using excessive laxatives or purging.

Diuresis: Increased or excessive production of urine.

Diurnal: The 24-hour period or daily cycle, such as being active during the day and resting at night.

Docosahexaenoic acid: A long-chain n-3 fatty acid with 22– carbons and six double bonds, found in fatty fish and breast milk.

Ectopic fat depots: Excess adipose tissue in locations not usually associated with adipose tissue storage, such as in the liver or around the heart.

Electrolytes: Salts that dissolve in water and disassociate into charged particles called ions.

Electron: Negatively charged subatomic particles.

Electron transport chain: Electrons are passed through a series of proteins and molecules in the mitochondria to generate large amounts of ATP.

Emulsification of fat: Involves formation of smaller fat droplets suspended in the aqueous digestive juices. This process increases the surface area of fat for more efficient digestion.

Endocrine: Hormonal.

Endogenous: Substances that originate or derive from within the body, in this case from body stores.

Endogenous carbohydrate fuels: Carbohydrate fuel found inside the muscle cell (glycogen).

Enterocytes: Cells lining the intestine that are highly specialised for digestion and absorption.

Enzymes: Proteins that start or speed up a chemical reaction while undergoing no permanent change to their structure. Enzymes perform this function by lowering the minimum energy required (activation energy) to start a chemical reaction. Enzymes are involved in most biochemical reactions; without them, most organisms could not survive.

Epidemiological studies: Studies that analyse the distribution (who, when and where) and determinants of health and disease in a defined population by observation. Epidemiological studies include ecological, case-control, cross-sectional and retrospective or prospective longitudinal cohorts study designs.

Epithelial barrier: Surface cells lining the gastrointestinal tract.

Ergogenic: Enhancing physical performance.

Ergogenic aid: Any substance or aid that improves physical performance.

Euhydrated: Normal state of body water content.

Evaporation: Sweat from the surface of the skin accounts for the majority of heat transfer during exercise. The rate of sweating can increase significantly during exercise to increase the amount of evaporation and, therefore, the amount of heat transferred from the body.

Excess post-exercise oxygen consumption: An increased rate of oxygen consumption following high-intensity activity.

Exercise: Physical activity that is planned, structured, repetitive and purposeful with the aim to improve or maintain one or more components of physical fitness.

Exercise-associated hyponatraemia: Also called low blood sodium, and defined as 'hyponatraemia occurring during or up to 24 h after physical activity. It is defined by a serum, plasma or blood sodium concentration ([Na+]) below the normal reference range of the laboratory performing the test. For most laboratories, this is a [Na+] less than 135 mmol/L'.

Exercise-associated gastrointestinal syndrome: Describes the physiological responses that occur due to exercise, which may compromise gastrointestinal system function and gastrointestinal barrier integrity and trigger adverse symptoms.

Exercise-induced gastrointestinal syndrome: A term used to describe disruption to the structure and function of the gastrointestinal tract during exercise. This can result in gastrointestinal symptoms during exercise. Physical damage can also occur to the gut lining, allowing movement of bacteria and their by-products from the gut into the bloodstream. This causes a significant response from the immune system, which can further raise core body temperature, increasing the risk of exertional heat stroke.

Exertional heat stroke: An elevated core temperature associated with signs of organ system failure due to overheating.

Exogenous: Substances that come from outside of the body, in this case from food.

Exogenous carbohydrate fuels: Carbohydrate fuel taken up into the muscle from the circulation (blood glucose, which is greatly supplemented by the intake of carbohydrate during exercise).

Explosive: Requiring a maximum or near maximum power output from the athlete in a short amount of time.

Extracellular water: Water that is outside the cells, including the water between the cells and the plasma.

Fat soluble: Compounds that can be dissolved in lipids (fats or oils) and are found in the lipids of the body (or food). Fat-soluble vitamins are stored in the body.

Free radicals: Also referred to as reactive oxygen species, free radicals are highly reactive chemical species that can damage cellular components, resulting in cell injury or death. They are usually produced by oxidation and contain an unpaired electron.

Gastric pits: Specialised cells in the gastric glands that secrete gastric juices.

Gastrointestinal bleeding: Bleeding that occurs from any part of the gastrointestinal tract, but typically from the small intestine, large intestine, rectum or anus. Gastrointestinal bleeding is not a disease, but is a symptom of many diseases. For athletes, bleeding may occur due to sloughing of intestinal lining as a result of the continual jarring that occurs when running on hard surfaces.

Glycocalyx: A protective mucus on the epithelial cells that is weakly acidic and consists of mucopolysaccharides.

Glycolysis: The breakdown of glucose to form two molecules of ATP.

Gut microbiota: Microbe population living in the large intestine.

Haemoglobin: The protein unit in the red blood cell that carries oxygen.

Haemolysis: The rupture of red blood cells.

Heat acclimatisation: The process of adaptation by living and training in a naturally hot environment.

Heat acclimation: The process of adaptation from completing specific training sessions in artificially induced heat, such as a climate chamber or heated room.

Homeostasis: Processes used by living organisms to maintain steady conditions needed for survival.

Hydrochloric acid (HCl): An acid composed of hydrogen and chloride atoms that is produced by the gastric glands. HCl activates pepsinogen into the enzyme pepsin, which then aids digestion by breaking the bonds between amino acids.

Hydrolysis: The breakdown of a compound by chemical reaction with water.

Hydrolytic reaction: When the addition of water to another compound leads to the formation of two or more products; for example, the catalytic conversion of starch to sugar.

Hyperglycaemia: Elevated blood glucose levels.

Hypertonic: Having a higher concentration than a particular fluid—in this case, higher than body fluid or intracellular fluid.

Hypertrophy: An increase in skeletal muscle size through growth in size of its cells.

Hypoglycaemia: Low blood glucose levels.

Hypohydration: Dehydration of the body.

Hyponatraemia: Low blood sodium levels.

Hypoxia: Deficiency in the amount of oxygen reaching the tissues.

Ileocecal valve: The sphincter that separates the small and large intestine.

Indirect calorimetry: A method of estimating energy expenditure by measuring oxygen consumption and carbohydrate production.

Intrinsic factor: A glycoprotein produced in the gastric pits that binds with vitamin B12 to help in the absorption of vitamin B12.

Intermuscular adipose tissue: Adipose tissue located within the skeletal muscle.

Intervention studies: Studies in which researchers make changes to observe the effect on health outcomes; in nutrition, this will include changes to diet.

Iron deficiency anaemia: Depletion of iron levels in the blood that leads to low levels of haemoglobin and small pale red blood cells, which limits their capacity to carry oxygen.

Isoenergetic: Containing the same number of calories/kilojoules.

Isotope: Atoms that have the same number of protons and electrons but a different number of neutrons.

Jet lag: A physiological condition experienced when circadian processes do not correspond with the new external environment.

Joules: A unit of energy equal to the amount of work done by a force of 1 Newton to move an object 1 metre.

Kilocalories: A unit of energy equal to 1000 calories. A calorie is the energy required to increase the temperature of 1 gram of water by 1°C.

Kilojoules: A unit of energy equal to 1000 joules. A joule is a unit of energy equal to the amount of work done by a force of 1 Newton (the force required to accelerate 1 kilogram of mass at the rate of 1 metre per second squared in the direction of the applied force) to move an object 1 metre.

Kinetic energy: Energy due to motion.

Krebs cycle: A series of biochemical reactions that generate energy from the breakdown of pyruvate (the end-product of glycolysis).

Lactate shuttling: Lactate produced at sites of high glycolysis can be shuttled (moved) to other muscles where it can be used as an energy source.

Lactic acid: A by-product of anaerobic glycolysis that contributes to fatigue of the muscle.

Lactose intolerance: A condition that leads to the inability to digest lactose which results in bloating, abdominal discomfort, gas and diarrhoea.

Leucine: An essential amino acid, which is required for muscle protein synthesis.

Lingual lipase: An enzyme secreted by the tongue that breaks down triglycerides, a type of fat.

Lipoprotein: A cluster of lipids attached to proteins that act as transport vehicles for the lipids in the blood. They are divided according to their density.

Low-residue diet: Diet limiting higher-fibre foods.

Macrocycle: Refers to the overall training period, usually representing a year.

Macromolecules: Proteins (polypeptides), digestible carbohydrates and fats (triglycerides) digested by humans.

Maximal exercise: Exercise performed at an intensity equal to an individual's maximum capacity for the desired activity.

Maximally exhaustive: Exercise that requires the participant to work at their maximal capacity until exhaustion.

Maximum aerobic power ($\dot{V}O_{2max}$): The maximum amount of oxygen an individual can take up per minute during dynamic exercise using large muscle groups.

Metabolic acidosis: A decrease in blood pH below the body's normal pH of ~7.37–7.42.

Metabolic equivalents: Measures of energy expenditure typically used to describe the energy expended in physical activity. The standard resting metabolic rate is 1 MET, and is equivalent to 1.0 kcal/kg/hour, or 4.18 kJ/kg/hour.

Metabolism: Chemical processes that occur within a living organism to maintain life.

Morphological prediction: The prediction of the adult body shape from a growing child or adolescent.

Morphological prototype: The best body shape and distribution of soft tissue to maximise performance in a given sport.

Morphology: The body shape.

Motor unit: A motor neuron (nerve cell) and the skeletal muscle fibres that it innervates (services).

Neural: Relating to a nerve or the nervous system.

Neurological: Pertaining to the function of the nervous system in a healthy person.

Non-coeliac gluten/wheat sensitivity: A condition characterised by adverse gastrointestinal and/or extra-intestinal symptoms associated with the ingestion of gluten- or wheat-containing foods, in the absence of coeliac disease or wheat allergy.

Norepinephrine (or noradrenaline): A neurotransmitter that binds to α-adrenoreceptors of the sympathetic nervous system. It has effects such as constricting blood vessels, raising blood pressure and dilating bronchi, reducing blood flow to internal organs and increasing blood flow to the working muscles.

Nutrient-poor: A food or meal that has low content of nutrients relative to energy content.

Neuroendocrine: Relating to interactions between the neural and endocrine system, particularly relating to hormones.

Newton metres: A unit of torque.

Organoleptic: The aspect of substances, in this case food and drink, that an individual experiences via the senses of taste, texture, smell and touch.

Osmotic effect: The movement of water molecules from a higher water potential to a more negative water potential.

Osteoarthritis: A degenerative condition of the joints that occurs when the cartilage in the joint degenerates, which leads to loss of function.

Oxidation: Part of a chemical reaction that results in the loss of electrons. During fat oxidation, triglycerides are broken down into three fatty acid chains and glycerol.

Oxidative stress: Occurs when the body's production of free radicals occurs at a rate higher than the body's ability to neutralise them.

Oxygen reserve ($\%\dot{V}O_2R$): The difference between resting oxygen consumption and maximal oxygen consumption.

Pack mentality: For team sport athletes, a pack mentality occurs when individual athletes within the team act in a similar manner to others in the group.

Pathogenesis: The biological mechanism that leads to the development of diseases.

Pathology: A field in medicine which studies the causes of diseases.

Pepsinogen: Part of the zymogen enzyme family. These enzymes digest proteins and polypeptides (smaller proteins) in the body and are secreted in an inactive form to protect the digestive and accessory organ tissues themselves from being broken down. The enzymes can be activated by hydrochloric acid and other activated zymogens. The 'inactive' feature of these enzymes is very important to protect digestive and accessory organ tissues themselves from being broken down, as they are all made up of proteins.

Per cent heart rate reserve (%HRR): Heart rate reserve multiplied by the desired percentage of exercise intensity.

Periodisation: The timing of exercise bouts to ensure sufficient exercise stimulus and recovery is provided to elicit the greatest response and adaptation.

Peristalsis: The wave-like contractions of the longitudinal muscles of the digestive tract that propels food forward.

Personalised nutrition advice: Specific and individualised advice for each athlete based on their own personal situation including playing position, body composition, culture, taste preferences and past experiences.

Physical activity: Any bodily movement produced by skeletal muscles that results in energy expenditure.

Physiological: Pertaining to the functions of the body's systems in a healthy person.

Physiological conditions: The natural internal and/or external environmental conditions within which the body's physiological systems operate.

Placebo effect: When an individual experiences or perceives a benefit from a supplement due to the belief that it will be beneficial rather than any direct physiological effect.

Plyometric exercises: Exercises in which muscles exert maximum force in short intervals of time, with the goal of increasing power—for example, jump training.

Polyphenols: A group of over 500 compounds that are found in plants. They are important as they provide protection against disease.

Potential energy: Stored energy resulting from the relative position within a physical system.

Prebiotics: Food components that are not digested in the gastrointestinal system but are used by the bacteria in the colon to promote their growth.

Progressive overload: The continued incremental increase in training demand (duration or intensity) required to elicit an adaptive response.

Protocol: The official procedure or set of rules or methods that need to be followed.

Proton: A positively charged subatomic particle with a positive electric charge.

Pulmonary ventilation: The product of an individual's breathing frequency (the amount of breaths per minute) and tidal volume (the volume of gas inhaled per minute).

Pyruvate dehydrogenase (PDH): Mitochondrial enzyme complex that commits the breakdown products of glycolysis (the first step in glucose metabolism) into the citric acid (Krebs cycle) oxidation pathway. This step is irreversible and is the rate limiting step in carbohydrate oxidation.

Radiation: The transfer of heat through any medium, without contact, using thermal or infrared radiation.

RED-S: Relative energy deficiency in sport, a syndrome of impaired physiological function caused by relative energy deficiency.

Relative exercise intensity: Refers to exercise intensity that is expressed relative to an individual's maximal capacity for a given task or activity.

Resistance exercise: Exercise that predominantly involves the musculoskeletal system.

Respiratory exchange ratio: The ratio of carbon dioxide produced to oxygen consumed; used to indicate the relative contribution of substrates oxidised during submaximal exercise.

Rugae: The folds of the stomach that occur when the stomach is empty.

Salivary amylase (or α amylase): An enzyme in the saliva that breaks down amylose, a type of carbohydrate.

Satiety: The feeling of fullness and satisfaction after consuming food which inhibits the need to eat.

Segmentation: The contraction of the circular muscles of the digestive tract that leads to mixing and breaking up of food.

Sleep–wake cycle: Also known as circadian rhythm, a daily pattern that determines when it is time to sleep and when it is time to be awake.

Sliding filament theory: A theory explaining the mechanism of skeletal muscle actions whereby muscle proteins (myofilaments) slide past each other to produce movement.

Somatotype: Classification of the human physical shape according to the body build or shape.

Sphincters: Muscular rings that open or close to control passage of food along the digestive tract.

Splanchnic hypoperfusion: Splanchnic circulation refers to blood flow through the stomach, small intestine, colon, pancreas, liver and spleen. Hypoperfusion refers to *low* or *decreased* flow of fluid through the circulatory system. During exercise, blood flow to the splanchnic area (gastrointestinal organs) is decreased and instead shunted to working muscles.

Sports anaemia: Also referred to as dilutional anaemia or pseudo-anaemia, occurs when haemoglobin concentration is 'diluted' due to increased volume of the plasma (the liquid component of blood). Plasma volume generally increases in response to exercise; therefore, this 'anaemia' is transient and often fluctuates with training loads. Unlike the other anaemias described in this chapter, sports anaemia does not impair athletic performance or respond to nutritional changes.

Steady-state exercise: Exercise performed at an intensity whereby the body's physiological systems are maintained at a relatively constant value.

Stop-start sports: Sports in which the play is frequently stopped due to the ball going out of play or the referee stopping play because of violations of the rules. This includes sports like basketball and football.

Subconcussive: A hit to the head that does not meet the clinical criteria for concussion, but is hypothesised to have long-term adverse effects.

Subcutaneous adipose tissue: Adipose tissue directly under the skin.

Submaximal exercise: Exercise performed at an intensity below an individual's maximum capacity for the desired activity.

Substrate: The substance, in this case the components of food, on which enzymes work.

Sugar alcohols: Carbohydrates that have been chemically altered. They provide fewer kilojoules as they are not well absorbed and may have a laxative effect. They include sorbitol, mannitol and xylitol. While they have fewer kilojoules they can still lead to elevation in blood glucose levels and, hence, can have an impact on blood glucose control in people with diabetes; as such they need to be considered in the diet.

Sympathetic nervous system: Often termed the fight or flight response. It accelerates heart rate, dilates bronchial passages, decreases motility of the digestive tract, constricts blood vessels, increases sweating.

Synthesise: To form a substance by combining elements.

Tendinopathies: Diseases of the tendons, which may arise from a range of internal and external factors.

Thermoregulation: The maintenance of the body at a particular temperature regardless of the external temperature.

Total body water: The total sum of water in the body. It is the sum of water within the cells (intracellular) and outside the cells (extracellular).

Trachea: The tube leading to the lungs, more commonly known as the windpipe.

Training low: Training with low carbohydrate availability in the body.

Trans form: In a molecule, the C atoms that have double bonds and the H atoms are on opposite sides.

Transferrin: An iron transport protein in the blood.

Transit time: Duration of content movement through the colon. This can be affected by factors such as illness, infection and type and intensity of exercise. When transit time is accelerated there is not enough time for water and other macro- and micronutrients to be absorbed, resulting in their loss in stools.

Triglycerides: The main type of fat in our bodies and our diets. They are made up of a glycerol backbone with three fatty acids attached.

Villi: Cells that form finger-like projections from the intestinal lumen and have microvilli protruding from them. This greatly increases the absorption surface of the intestine.

Visceral adipose tissue: The adipose tissue within the abdominal cavity, which is wrapped around the organs.

Visceral hypersensitivity: Heightened sensation of pain in the internal organs.

Vitamin B12: An essential vitamin found in milk, eggs and meat. The active forms of this vitamin are methylcobalamin and deoxyadenosylcobalamin.

Water soluble: Compounds that can be dissolved in water and are found in the aqueous parts of the body (or food). Water-soluble vitamins are not stored in the body; they are excreted in the urine.

Weight-making: Any behaviour used to quickly lose weight regardless of what that 'weight' is (water, fat, muscle) before a competition weigh-in.

Whey protein isolate: A by-product of cheese production, which contains a high percentage of pure protein and is virtually lactose-free, carbohydrate-free, fat-free and cholesterol-free.

Window of opportunity: In sports nutrition and training this refers to the 1–2 hours after hard exercise in which the muscle is primed to absorb and store carbohydrate.

Wolff's Law: Bone in a healthy person will adapt to the loads under which it is placed. In this sense, an exercise stimulus results in bone remodelling that makes the bone stronger to resist that sort of loading.

Work capacity: The total amount of work a person can sustain over a defined period of time.

Zeitgebers: External or environmental cues which synchronises our biological rhythms to the Earth's 24-hour light–dark cycle.

INDEX